Practical Hemostasis and Thrombosis

Practical Hemostasis and Thrombosis

EDITED BY

Nigel Key, MB, ChB, FRCP

Harold R. Roberts Distinguished Professor of Medicine
Director, Hemophilia Treatment Center
The University of North Carolina at Chapel Hill
Division of Hematology & Oncology
Chapel Hill, North Carolina, USA

Michael Makris, MD

Director, Sheffield Haemophilia and Thrombosis Centre
Royal Hallamshire Hospital
Sheffield, UK

Denise O'Shaughnessy, DPhil, FRCP, FRCPath

Consultant Haematologist and Senior Medical Advisor (Blood Policy)
Department of Health
London, UK

David Lillicrap, MD, FRCPC

Professor, Department of Pathology and Molecular Medicine
Richardson Laboratory, Queen's University
Kingston, Ontario, Canada

SECOND EDITION

FOREWORD BY HAROLD R. ROBERTS, MD, FACP

Sarah Graham Kenan Distinguished Professor
Medicine and Pathology
University of North Carolina at Chapel Hill
Chapel Hill, North Carolina, USA

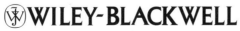

WILEY-BLACKWELL

A John Wiley & Sons, Ltd., Publication

Library of Congress Cataloging-in-Publication Data

Practical hemostasis and thrombosis. – 2nd ed. / edited by Nigel Key . . . [et al.] ; foreword by Harold R. Roberts.
p. ; cm.
Includes bibliographical references and index.
ISBN 978-1-4051-8460-1
1. Blood coagulation disorders.   2. Thrombosis.   3. Hemostasis.   I. Key, Nigel, 1956–
[DNLM: 1. Hemostasis–physiology.   2. Blood Coagulation Disorders.   3. Hemorrhagic Disorders.   4. Thromboembolism.   5. Thrombosis.   WH 310 P895 2009]
RC647.C55P734 2009
616.1′57–dc22

2008052785

ISBN: 978-1-4051-8460-1

A catalogue record for this book is available from the British Library.

Set in 8.75/12 pt Meridien by Aptara® Inc., New Delhi, India
Printed and bound in Singapore

1   2009

Contents

Contents

Contributors

Roopen Arya MA, PhD, FRCPath, FRCP
Consultant Hematologist
Department of Hematological Medicine
King's College Hospital
London, UK

Natalie Aucutt-Walter, MD
Vascular Neurology Fellow
Department of Neurology
University of North Carolina Hospitals
Chapel Hill, North Carolina, USA

Mary E. Bauman, RN, BA, MN, NP
Nurse Practitioner
Pediatric Thrombosis
Stollery Children's Hospital
University of Alberta
Edmonton, Alberta, Canada

Richard C. Becker, MD
Professor of Medicine
Divisions of Cardiology and Hematology
Duke University School of Medicine
Director, Cardiovascular Thrombosis Center
Duke Clinical Research Institute
Durham, North Carolina, USA

Jeffrey S. Berger, MD, MS
Cardiovascular Fellow
Duke Clinical Research Institute
Duke University Medical Center
Durham, North Carolina, USA

Victor S. Blanchette, MD, MA, MB, MRCS, LRCP, DCH,
MRCP, FRCPC, FRCP Chief
Division of Hematology/Oncology
Hospital for Sick Children
Professor of Pediatrics
University of Toronto
Toronto, Ontario, Canada

Paula Bolton-Maggs, DM, FRCP, FRCPath, FRCPCH
Consultant Haematologist
Manchester Royal Infirmary
Honorary Senior Lecturer
University of Manchester
Manchester, UK

Giancarlo Castaman
Department of Cell Therapy and Hematology
Hemophilia and Thrombosis Center
San Bortolo Hospital
Vicenza, Italy

Marco Cattaneo, MD
Professor
Unit of Hematology and Thrombosis
Ospedale San Paolo
Department of Medicine, Surgery and Dentistry
University of Milan
Milan, Italy

Adrian Copplestone, FRCP, FRCPath
Consultant Haematologist
Derriford Hospital, Plymouth
Honorary Reader in Haematology
Peninsula Medical School
Plymouth, UK

Benilde Cosmi, MD, PhD
Department of Angiology and Blood
Coagulation "Marino Golinelli"
University Hospital S. Orsola-Malpighi
Bologna, Italy

Anna Falanga, MD, PhD
Thrombosis and Hemostasis Center
Department of Hematology-Oncology
Ospedali Riuniti di Bergamo
Bergamo, Italy

Contributors

Ravi Gill
Consultant Anesthetist
Southampton University Hospitals Trust
Tremona Rd Southampton
London, UK

Paul Harrison, BSc, PhD, FRCPath
Clinical Scientist
Oxford Haemophilia & Thrombosis Centre
Churchill Hospital
Oxford, UK

John A. Heit, MD
Professor of Medicine
Mayo Clinic College of Medicine
Director, Mayo Clinic Special Coagulation
Laboratories and Clinic
Divisions of Cardiovascular Diseases, Hematology,
Hematopathology & Laboratory Genetics
Departments of Internal Medicine and Laboratory
Medicine and Pathology
Mayo Clinic
Rochester, Minnesota, USA

David Y. Huang, MD, PhD
Assistant Professor of Neurology
Department of Neurology
University of North Carolina Hospitals
Chapel Hill, North Carolina, USA

Beverley J. Hunt, FRCP, FRCPath, MD
Professor of Thrombosis & Haemostasis
King's College, London
Consultant in Departments of Haematology,
Pathology & Rheumatology
Guy's and St. Thomas' Trust
London, UK

Paula James, MD, FRCPC
Associate Professor
Department of Medicine
Queen's University
Kingston, Ontario, Canada

Valerie Jewells, DO
Assistant Professor of Radiology
Department of Radiology
University of North Carolina Hospitals
Chapel Hill, North Carolina, USA

Walter H.A. Kahr, MD, PhD, FRCPC
Assistant Professor of Pediatrics
University of Toronto
Division of Hematology/Oncology
The Hospital for Sick Children
Toronto, Ontario, Canada

Raj S. Kasthuri, MD
Fellow in Hematology and Oncology
Division of Hematology and Oncology and Transplantation
University of Minnesota Medical School
Minneapolis, Minnesota, USA

Clive Kearon, MB, MRCPI, FRCPC, PhD
Professor of Medicine
McMaster University
Hamilton, Ontario, Canada

Nigel S. Key, MB, ChB, FRCP
Harold R. Roberts Distinguished Professor of Mediciine
Director, Hemophilia Treatment Center
The University of North Carolina at Chapel Hill
Division of Hematology/Oncology
Chapel Hill, North Carolina, USA

Steven Kitchen, BSc, PhD
Clinical Scientist
Division of Coagulation
Royal Hallamshire Hospital
Sheffield, UK

David Lillicrap, MD, FRCPC
Professor
Department of Pathology and Molecular Medicine
Richardson Laboratory
Queen's University
Kingston, Ontario, Canada

Lori-Ann Linkins, MD, MSc(Epid), FRCPC
Assistant Professor
Department of Medicine
McMaster University
Hamilton, Ontario, Canada

Gordon D.O. Lowe, MD, FRCP, FFPH
Professor of Vascular Medicine
University of Glasgow
Royal Infirmary
Glasgow, UK

Alice D. Ma, MD
Associate Professor of Medicine
Department of Medicine
Division of Hematology/Oncology
University of North Carolina School of Medicine
Chapel Hill, North Carolina, USA

Rhona M. Maclean, MRCP, MRCPath
Consultant Hematologist
Sheffield Hemophilia and Thrombosis Centre
Royal Hallamshire Hospital
Sheffield, UK

Michael Makris, MD
Director
Sheffield Haemophilia and Thrombosis Centre
Royal Hallamshire Hospital
Sheffield, UK

Masina Marchetti, MSc
Thrombosis and Hemostasis Center
Department of Hematology-Oncology
Ospedali Riuniti di Bergamo
Bergamo, Italy

M. Patricia Massicotte, MSc, MD, FRCPC, MHSc
Peter Olley Chair
Pediatric Thrombosis Program
Stollery Children's Hospital
University of Alberta
Edmonton, Alberta, Canada

Dougald M. Monroe, PhD
Associate Professor of Medicine
University of North Carolina at Chapel Hill
School of Medicine
Division of Hematology/Oncology
Chapel Hill, North Carolina, USA

Thomas L. Ortel, MD, PhD
Professor of Medicine and Pathology
Director, Duke Hemostasis and Thrombosis Center
Director, Clinical Coagulation Laboratory
Division of Hematology
Department of Medicine
Duke University Medical Center
Durham, North Carolina, USA

Denise O'Shaughnessy, DPhil, FRCP, FRCPath
Consultant Haemotologist and
    Senior Medical Advisor (Blood Policy)
Department of Health
London, UK

Gualtiero Palareti
Department of Angiology and Blood
Coagulation "Marino Golinelli"
University Hospital S. Orsola-Malpighi
Bologna, Italy

Raj K. Patel, MD, MRCP, FRCPath
Consultant Hematologist
Department of Hematological Medicine
King's College Hospital
London, UK

Stephanie Perry, MD
Division of Hematology
Department of Medicine
Duke University Medical Center
Durham, North Carolina, USA

Rajiv K. Pruthi, MBBS
Assistant Professor of Medicine
Mayo Clinic College of Medicine
Director, Mayo Comprehensive Hemophilia Center
Co-Director, Special Coagulation Laboratories and Clinic
Divisions of Hematology, Hematopathology and
    Laboratory Genetics
Departments of Internal Medicine and Laboratory Medicine
    and Pathology
Mayo Clinic
Rochester, Minnesota, USA

Beverley J. Robertson, BSc, MB ChB, MRCP, FRCPath
Consultant Haematologist
Department of Haematology
Aberdeen Royal Infirmary
Aberdeen, UK

Jeremy D. Robertson, MBBS, FRCPA, FRACP
Consultant Hematologist
Department of Hematology
Royal Children's Hospital
Queensland, Australia

Francesco Rodeghiero
Director
Department of Cell Therapy and Hematology
Hemophilia and Thrombosis Center
San Bortolo Hospital
Vicenza, Italy

R. Campbell Tait, MB ChB, FRCP, FRCPath
Consultant Haematologist
Department of Haematology
Glasgow Royal Infirmary
Glasgow, UK

Ayalew Tefferi, MD
Division of Hematology
Mayo Clinic
Rochester, Minnesota, USA

Alberto Tosetto
Department of Cell Therapy and Hematology
Hemophilia and Thrombosis Center
San Bortolo Hospital
Vicenza, Italy

Isobel D. Walker, MD, MPhil, FRCP (Ed), FRCP (Glas),
FRCPath
Consultant Haematologist
Department of Haematology
Glasgow Royal Infirmary
Glasgow, UK

Contributors

Henry G. Watson, MD, FRCP, FRCPath
Consultant Haematologist
Department of Haematology
Aberdeen Royal Infirmary
Aberdeen, UK

Jonathan Wilde, MA, MD, FRCP, FRCPath
Consultant Hematologist
University Hospital Birmingham NHS Trust
Birmingham, UK

Foreword

There are many texts describing the blood clotting mechanism and the hemorrhagic and thrombotic problems related to it. Unfortunately, there are very few succinct, thorough, and practical textbooks on the subject. Many of the current texts are heavy, extremely detailed, and not readily available for quick and easy reference for questions related to thrombosis and hemorrhage. Thus, a more convenient yet complete textbook on this important topic is needed. Fortunately, the second edition of *Practical Hemostasis and Thrombosis* edited by Drs. Key, Makris, O'Shaughnessy, and Lillicrap is a welcome addition to the subject of blood coagulation and its disorders. This book is a handy, readable resource not only for hematologists but also for clinicians, medical interns, residents, and medical students. It is concise and succinct but covers all the information necessary to understand the clotting mechanism as well as how to prevent, diagnose, and treat bleeding and clotting disorders. The book covers the clinical aspects of both hemorrhage and thrombosis, including an in-depth description of platelet abnormalities and disseminated intravascular coagulation. In addition, there is an excellent section describing hemorrhagic and thrombotic problems in obstetrics, gynecology, surgery, hepatology, and transfusion medicine. There is also a helpful section devoted to laboratory and molecular biological tests needed for the diagnosis of bleeding and clotting disorders.

This is a practical, up-to-date, small textbook that contains all the important advances made since the first edition was published in 2005. I found this book to be very helpful, and I predict that it will be a handy and convenient reference book for all who need to look up information on patients who have suffered excessive hemorrhage or thromboembolic complications.

Harold R. Roberts, MD, FACP
Sarah Graham Kenan, Distinguished Professor
Medicine and Pathology
University of North Carolina at Chapel Hill

1 Basic principles underlying coagulation

Dougald M. Monroe

This chapter will discuss coagulation in the context of a hemostatic response to a break in the vasculature. *Coagulation* is the process that leads to fibrin formation; this process involves controlled interactions between protein coagulation factors. *Hemostasis* is coagulation that occurs in a physiological (as opposed to pathological) setting and results in sealing a break in the vasculature. This process has a number of components, including adhesion and activation of platelets coupled with ordered reactions of the protein coagulation factors. Hemostasis is essential to protect the integrity of the vasculature. *Thrombosis* is coagulation in a pathological (as opposed to physiological) setting that leads to localized intravascular clotting and potentially occlusion of a vessel. There is an overlap between the components involved in hemostasis and thrombosis, but there is also evidence to suggest that the processes of hemostasis and thrombosis have significant differences. There are also data to suggest that different vascular settings (arterial, venous, tumor microcirculation) may proceed to thrombosis by different mechanisms. Exploitation of these differences could lead to therapeutic agents that selectively target thrombosis without interfering significantly with hemostasis. Other chapters of this book will discuss some of the mechanisms behind thrombosis.

Healthy vasculature

Intact vasculature has a number of active mechanisms to maintain coagulation in a quiescent state. Healthy endothelium expresses ecto-ADPase (CD39) and produces prostacyclin (PGI$_2$) and nitric oxide (NO); all of these tend to block platelet adhesion to and activation by healthy endothelium [1]. Healthy endothelium also has active anticoagulant mechanisms, some of which

will be discussed below. There is evidence that the vasculature is not identical through all parts of the body [2]. Further, it appears that there can be alterations in the vasculature in response to changes in the extracellular environment. These changes can locally alter the ability of endothelium to maintain a quiescent state.

Even though healthy vasculature maintains a quiescent state, there is evidence to support the idea that there is ongoing, low-level activation of coagulation factors [3]. This ongoing activation of coagulation factors is sometimes termed "idling" and may play a role in preparing for a rapid coagulation response to injury. Part of the evidence for idling comes from the observation that the activation peptides of factors IX and X can be detected in the plasma of healthy individuals. Because levels of the factor X activation peptide are significantly reduced in factor VII deficiency but unchanged in hemophilia, the factor VIIa complex with tissue factor is implicated as the key player in this idling process.

Tissue factor is present in a number of tissues throughout the body [4]. Immunohistochemical studies show that tissue factor is present at high levels in the brain, lung, and heart. Only low levels of tissue factor are detected in skeletal muscle, joints, spleen, and liver. In addition to being distributed in tissues, tissue factor is expressed on vascular smooth muscle cells and on the pericytes that surround blood vessels. This concentration of tissue factor around the vasculature has been referred to as a hemostatic envelope. Endothelial cells in vivo do not express tissue factor, except possibly during invasion by cancer cells. Also, there is evidence to suggest that tissue factor may be present on microparticles in the circulation. The nature and function of this circulating tissue factor is being actively researched by a number of groups. The information to date suggests that this tissue factor accumulates in pathological thrombi. Further, there is general agreement in these studies that circulating tissue factor levels are extremely low in healthy individuals. Limited data suggest that tissue factor does not incorporate into hemostatic plugs [5], unlike the accumulation of tissue factor seen in thrombosis; and so, the model of hemostasis described in this chapter does not include a role for circulating tissue factor in hemostasis.

Given the location of tissue factor, it seems plausible that the processes associated with idling may not be intravascular but may rather occur in the extravascular space. At least two mechanisms are known that can concentrate plasma coagulation factors around the vasculature (Plate 1.1). Coagulation proteins enter the extravascular space in proportion to their size; small proteins readily get into the extravascular space, whereas large proteins do not seem to reach the extravasculature [6]. Because tissue factor binds factor VII so tightly, it can trap factor VII that moves into the extravascular space. This means that blood vessels already have factor VII(a) bound [7]. Also, factor IX binds tightly and specifically to the extracellular matrix protein collagen IV; this results in factor IX being concentrated around blood vessels [8]. A role for this collagen IV-bound factor IX in hemostasis is suggested by the observation that mice expressing a factor IX that cannot bind collagen IV have a mild bleeding tendency.

Initiation

A break in the vasculature exposes extracellular matrix to blood and initiates the coagulation process (Plate 1.2). Platelets adhere at the site of injury through a number of specific interactions [9]. The plasma protein von Willebrand factor (VWF) can bind to exposed collagen and, under flow, undergoes a conformational change such that it binds tightly to the abundant platelet receptor glycoprotein Ib. This localization of platelets to the extracellular matrix promotes collagen interaction with platelet glycoprotein VI. Binding of collagen to glycoprotein VI triggers a signaling cascade that results in activation of platelet integrins. Activated integrins mediate tight binding of platelets to extracellular matrix. This process adheres platelets to the site of injury.

In addition to platelet processes, plasma concentrations of factors IX and X are brought to the preformed factor VIIa/tissue factor complexes at the site of injury. Factor VIIa/tissue factor activates both factor IX and factor X; the activated proteins play distinct roles in the ensuing reactions. Factor IXa moves into association with platelets, where it plays a role in the later stages of hemostasis. Factor Xa forms a complex with factor Va to convert a small amount of prothrombin to thrombin. The source of factor Va for this reaction is likely protein released from the alpha granules of collagen adherent platelets [10]. Platelet factor V is released in a partially active form and does not require further activation to promote thrombin generation [10]. Thrombin formed on pericytes and in the extravascular space can promote local fibrin formation but is not sufficient to provide for hemostasis throughout the wound area.

The factor VIIa/tissue factor complexes are, over time, inhibited by tissue factor pathway inhibitor (TFPI). TFPI participates in a ternary complex with factor Xa and factor VIIa bound to tissue factor.

Deficiencies of tissue factor have not been seen in humans, and a knockout of the tissue factor gene in mouse models leads to embryonic lethality. Factor VII deficiency is associated with a bleeding phenotype, and many patients with <1% factor VII activity have spontaneous, severe bleeding.

Amplification

The thrombin formed in the initiation phase acts as an amplifier by acting on platelets and proteins to facilitate platelet-driven thrombin generation (Plate 1.3). Thrombin has a tight specific interaction with platelet glycoprotein Ib [11]. When bound to glycoprotein Ib, thrombin undergoes a conformational change that alters the activity of the protein and may protect it from inhibition. This conformational change enhances the ability of thrombin to cleave either of the two platelet protease-activated receptors (PARs). PARs are members of the seven transmembrane domain G-coupled family of proteins [12]. Cleavage of a PAR creates a new amino terminal, which can fold back on itself and bind to a receptor site in the transmembrane domain. This intramolecular binding initiates a signaling cascade. In platelets, cleavage of PAR1 leads to signaling that results in platelet activation. This process is initiated after exposure of platelets to very small amounts of thrombin.

Platelet activation leads to numerous significant changes. Platelets undergo cytoskeletal changes leading to a shape change. There are regulated changes in the platelet membrane such that expression of phosphatidylserine on the outer leaflet of the platelets is significantly enhanced [13]. Phosphatidylserine induces allosteric changes in the procoagulant complexes that significantly increase their activity. Platelets degranulate, releasing the contents of both alpha granules and dense granules. Dense granule contents, especially released-ADP, participate in a positive feedback loop either on the same platelet or on nearby platelets to further promote platelet activation. Among the alpha granule contents released when platelets are activated is partially activated factor V.

In addition to its action on platelet receptors, thrombin can also activate procoagulant cofactors. Platelet factor V or plasma factor V bound to platelets is activated by thrombin cleavage to release the B domain. VWF, in addition to participating in platelet adhesion, acts as a carrier of factor VIII. It seems reasonable that VWF bound to glycoprotein Ib might bring factor VIII into proximity of thrombin, also bound to glycoprotein Ib. Thrombin cleavage releases factor VIII from VWF as well as activating factor VIII. So the amplification phase results in activated platelets that have cofactors Va and VIIIa bound to the surface.

Some schemes of coagulation do not describe amplification as a separate step. But work from the Maastrich group, which was expanded on by Dale and colleagues, shows that platelets can be activated to different levels of procoagulant activity [13,14]. This suggests that in vivo the procoagulant activity of platelets may be modulated by local conditions. It also suggests that aspects of platelet activation could be targeted to reduce thrombin generation in pathological settings. So, amplification is included in this model as a discrete step.

Propagation

The activated platelet with activated cofactors is primed for a burst of thrombin generation (Plate 1.4).

Factor IXa formed during the initiation phase binds to activated platelets. One component of this binding is a saturable, specific, reversible site independent of factor VIIIa [15], and the other component of this binding is factor VIIIa. The factor IXa/VIIIa complex activates factor X on the platelet surface. This platelet surface-generated factor Xa can move directly into a complex with platelet surface factor Va. In the presence of prothrombin, this factor Xa is protected from inhibition by antithrombin or TFPI. Recent data suggest that these factor Xa/Va complexes are very stable for even extended times and, in the presence of a new supply of prothrombin, can immediately act to promote thrombin generation [16]. Platelet surface-generated factor Xa plays a different role than factor X activated by factor VIIa/tissue factor. Because of the rapid inhibition by TFPI of factor Xa that is not in a complex, it is likely that factor X generated by factor VIIa/tissue factor cannot reach the platelet surface. This conclusion is supported by the observation that, in hemophilia, when platelet factor Xa generation is absent or severely defective, the clot is very poor even though factor VIIa/tissue factor activity is normal and fibrin deposition can be observed at the margins of hemophilic wounds [17].

The burst of thrombin during the propagation phase leads to cleavage of fibrinopeptides from fibrinogen. Cleavage of these fibrinopeptides exposes new binding sites that fit with complementary sites on other fibrin molecules [18]. These interactions lead to fibrin molecules assembling in long, branched chains anchored at the platelet receptor glycoprotein IIb/IIIa. This process stabilizes the initial platelet plug into a consolidated fibrin plug. The nature and stability of the fibrin plug appear to depend on the rate of thrombin generation during the propagation phase [19].

In addition to its role in cleaving fibrinopeptides, thrombin generation participates in a positive feedback loop by activating factor XI on the platelet surface [20]; this factor XIa can activate factor IXa to enhance factor Xa generation. And the high levels of thrombin generated during the burst phase can cleave PAR4. Signaling downstream from PAR4 contributes to platelet shape changes that might be important in stabilization of the hemostatic plug. Finally, high levels of thrombin generated during the propagation phase bind to fibrin and, when bound, are protected from inhibition by antithrombin. This fibrin-bound thrombin provides an important role in maintaining hemostasis. Disruption of a plug brings fibrinogen into contact with the bound thrombin, where fibrin formation can be initiated immediately without the need for thrombin generation. One aspect of the bleeding associated with hemophilia may be both the initial poor structure of the fibrin plug and the lack of bound thrombin to stabilize the plug.

Deficiencies of proteins in the propagation phase are associated with bleeding. X chromosome-linked hemophilia in males is associated with deficiencies in factors VIII and IX (hemophilia A and B, respectively). Because both genes are located on the X chromosome, the hemophilic phenotype results from a single-gene defect in males. Bleeding risk in hemophilia A and B is linked to factor level. Factor XI deficiency is also associated with bleeding risk. However, bleeding in factor XI deficiency shows a somewhat weak association with factor level [21]. The proposed model is consistent with this observation in that factor XI is not primary to the pathway leading to thrombin generation, but rather contributes through the positive feedback loop to boost thrombin generation.

Localization

A hemostatic plug should, by definition, seal the break in the vasculature but not continue platelet accumulation and thrombin generation to the point that the entire vessel is occluded. Thrombin released from a platelet plug into flowing blood is swept downstream. At plasma concentrations of antithrombin, the expected half-life of thrombin in blood is well under a minute. Also, factor Xa, either released into the blood or generated on healthy endothelium, is rapidly inhibited by TFPI in solution or TFPIβ, which is associated with the endothelial cell surface through a glycosylphosphatidylinositol linkage [22].

Healthy endothelial cells, in addition to the mechanisms described above for blocking platelet activation, have active mechanisms to downregulate thrombin generation [23]. Thrombin on the platelet surface participates in a positive feedback loop that promotes additional thrombin generation. By contrast, thrombin on healthy endothelium participates in a negative feedback loop that blocks additional thrombin generation (Plate 1.5).

Thrombin that reaches an endothelial cell binds to thrombomodulin. This binding causes a conformational change in thrombin such that it can no longer cleave fibrinogen. Thrombin bound to thrombomodulin is rapidly inhibited by protein C inhibitor [24]. This thrombin/inhibitor complex rapidly dissociates so that thrombomodulin can again bind thrombin, and thrombin bound to thrombomodulin can rapidly activate protein C. The endothelial cell protein C receptor enhances protein C activation by thrombin/thrombomodulin. Activated protein C, in coordination with protein S, inactivates factors Va and VIIIa. The net result is that thrombin generation is confined by healthy endothelium to a site of injury. Deficiencies of protein C or S, or defects that prevent cleavage and inactivation of factor V (factor V Leiden), allow for the spread of thrombi into the vasculature and are associated with venous thrombosis.

Coagulation assays

The two most common assays in the clinical coagulation laboratory are the Prothrombin Time (PT) and Activated Partial Thromboplastin Time (APTT). In the PT assay, a large excess of thromboplastin (tissue factor) is added to plasma. There is rapid activation of factor X, leading to thrombin generation and clot formation. The assay is sensitive to deficiencies of factors VII, X, V, and prothrombin, but not factors XI, IX, or VIII. Thus, the PT evaluates the factors involved in the initiation phase (Plate 1.2).

Because the PT does not assess factors VIII or IX (the factors that are deficient in hemophilia A and B, respectively), the APTT assay was developed to diagnose hemophilia and monitor therapy. The original APTT used a dilution of thromboplastin, but kaolin was substituted in 1961 [25], resulting in a simple, reproducible, reliable assay (that no longer has a thromboplastin component). The current APTT takes advantage of the ability of factor XII and high molecular weight kininogen, even though they are not involved in physiological hemostasis, to be activated by a negatively charged surface. With this initiator, the clotting reaction proceeds through, and is sensitive to deficiencies of, factors XI, IX, VIII, X, V, and prothrombin. Thus, the APTT assays the factors involved in the platelet surface propagation phase (Plate 1.4).

Summary

This model of hemostasis views the process as having three overlapping phases: initiation, amplification, and propagation. The hemostatic plug is localized to the area of injury by healthy endothelium, which has active processes to downregulate thrombin generation. It is important to focus on the cellular location of the steps rather than the proteins involved. The protein factors overlap between the steps, but, for example, thrombin bound to platelet surface glycoprotein Ib plays a different role than thrombin bound to endothelial cell thrombomodulin. So, each of the cellular steps must contribute for the overall process to result in a coordinated hemostatic plug. A defect in initiation means that the coagulation reactions will not be started. Tissue factor deficiency is lethal in animals models, and factor VII deficiency is associated with bleeding. Platelet adhesion or activation defects, such as Scott Syndrome, are associated with bleeding. Hemophilia is a defect of factor X activation on the platelet surface during the propagation phase. Factor X activation by factor VIIa/tissue factor during initiation cannot substitute for the platelet surface reactions. Factor Xa is confined to the tissue factor bearing surface, where it is formed because, when released from the surface, it is rapidly inhibited by TFPI and antithrombin. So, for normal hemostasis, a factor X-activating complex must be formed on activated platelets. The localization process confines platelet deposition and fibrin formation to keep the clot from expanding over healthy endothelium. This is consistent with the observation that defects in antithrombin, TFPI, and proteins C and S are associated with thrombosis. The tie between this model and the standard coagulation assays is that the PT and APTT assess the initiation and propagation phases, respectively.

References

1 Jin RC, Voetsch B, Loscalzo J. Endogenous mechanisms of inhibition of platelet function. *Microcirculation* 2005;12:247–58.

2 Aird WC. Vascular bed-specific thrombosis. *J Thromb Haemost* 2007;5(Suppl 1):283–91.

3 Bauer KA, Mannucci PM, Gringeri A, et al. Factor IXa-factor VIIIa-cell surface complex does not contribute to the basal activation of the coagulation mechanism in vivo. *Blood* 1992;79:2039–47.

4 Drake TA, Morrissey JH, Edgington TS. Selective cellular expression of tissue factor in human tissues. Implications for disorders of hemostasis and thrombosis. *Am J Pathol* 1989;134:1087–97.

5 Hoffman M, Whinna HC, Monroe DM. Circulating tissue factor accumulates in thrombi, but not in hemostatic plugs. *J Thromb Haemost* 2006;4:2092–3.

6 Miller GJ, Howarth DJ, Attfield JC, et al. Haemostatic factors in human peripheral afferent lymph. *Thromb Haemost* 2000;83:427–32.

7 Hoffman M, Colina CM, McDonald AG, et al. Tissue factor around dermal vessels has bound factor VII in the absence of injury. *J Thromb Haemost* 2007;5: 1403–8.

8 Gui T, Lin H, Jin D, et al. Circulating and binding characteristics of wild-type factor IX and certain Gla domain mutants in vivo. *Blood* 2002;100:153–8.

9 Varga-Szabo D, Pleines I, Nieswandt B. Cell adhesion mechanisms in platelets. *Arterioscler Thromb Vasc Biol* 2008;28:403–12.

10 Monković DD, Tracy PB. Functional characterization of human platelet-released factor V and its activation by factor Xa and thrombin. *J Biol Chem* 1990;265: 17132–40.

11 De Marco L, Mazzucato M, Masotti A, et al. Localization and characterization of an alpha-thrombin-binding site on platelet glycoprotein Ib alpha. *J Biol Chem* 1994;269:6478–84.

12 Coughlin SR. Protease-activated receptors in hemostasis, thrombosis and vascular biology. *J Thromb Haemost* 2005;3:1800–14.

13 Bevers EM, Comfurius P, Zwaal RF. Changes in membrane phospholipid distribution during platelet activation. *Biochim Biophys Acta* 1983;736:57–66.

14 Dale GL. Coated-platelets: an emerging component of the procoagulant response. *J Thromb Haemost* 2005;3: 2185–92.

15 Ahmad SS, Rawala-Sheikh R, Walsh PN. Comparative interactions of factor IX and factor IXa with human platelets. *J Biol Chem* 1989;264:3244–51.

16 Orfeo T, Brummel-Ziedins KE, Gissel M, et al. The nature of the stable blood clot procoagulant activities. *J Biol Chem* 2008;283:9776–86.

17 Sixma JJ, van den Berg A. The haemostatic plug in haemophilia A: a morphological study of haemostatic plug formation in bleeding time skin wounds of patients with severe haemophilia A. *Br J Haematol* 1984;58:741–53.

18 Lord ST. Fibrinogen and fibrin: scaffold proteins in hemostasis. *Curr Opin Hematol* 2007;14:236–41.

19 Wolberg AS. Thrombin generation and fibrin clot structure. *Blood Rev* 2007;21:131–42.

20 Oliver JA, Monroe DM, Roberts HR, et al. Thrombin activates factor XI on activated platelets in the absence of factor XII. *Arterioscler Thromb Vasc Biol* 1999;19: 170–7.

21 Seligsohn U. Factor XI in haemostasis and thrombosis: past, present and future. *Thromb Haemost* 2007;98:84–9.

22 Piro O, Broze GJ. Comparison of cell-surface TFPIalpha and beta. *J Thromb Haemost* 2005;3:2677–83.

23 Esmon CT. The protein C pathway. Chest 2003;124: 26S–32S.

24 Rezaie AR, Cooper ST, Church FC, et al. Protein C inhibitor is a potent inhibitor of the thrombin-thrombomodulin complex. *J Biol Chem* 1995;270: 25336–9.

25 Proctor RR, Rapaport SI. The partial thromboplastin time with kaolin. A simple screening test for first stage plasma clotting factor deficiencies. *Am J Clin Pathol* 1961;36:212–19.

2 Laboratory tests of hemostasis

Steven Kitchen and Michael Makris

Introduction

In the laboratory investigation of hemostasis, the results of clotting tests can be affected by the collection and processing of blood samples and by the selection, design, quality control, and interpretation of screening tests and specific assays. Such effects can have important diagnostic and therapeutic implications.

Sample collection and processing

Collection

For normal screening tests, venous blood should be collected gently but rapidly using a syringe or an evacuated collection system, when possible, from veins in the elbow. Application of a tourniquet to facilitate collection does not normally affect the results of most tests for bleeding disorders, although prolonged application must be avoided and the tourniquet should be applied just before sample collection.

Tests of fibrinolysis

Minimal stasis should be used because venous stasis causes local release of fibrinolytic components into the vein. The needle should not be more than 21 gauge (for infants, a 22- or 23-gauge needle may be necessary).

Venous catheters

Collection through peripheral venous catheters or nonheparinized central venous catheters can be successful for prothrombin time (PT) and activated partial thromboplastin time (APTT) testing, but is best avoided; if used, sufficient blood must be discarded to prevent contamination or dilution by fluids from the line (typically 5–10 mL of blood from adults).

Mixing with anticoagulant

If there is any delay between collection and mixing with anticoagulant, or delay in filling of the collection system, the blood must be discarded because of possible activation of coagulation. Once blood and anticoagulant are mixed, the container should be sealed and mixed by gentle inversion five times, even for evacuated collection systems. Vigorous shaking should be avoided.

Any difficulty in venepuncture can affect the results obtained, particularly for tests of platelet function. Prior to analysis, the sample should be visually inspected and discarded if there is evidence of clotting or hemolysis. Partially clotted blood is typically associated with a dramatic false shortening of the APTT together with the loss of fibrinogen.

Anticoagulant and sample filling

The recommended anticoagulant for collection of blood for investigations of blood clotting is normally trisodium citrate. Different strengths of trisodium citrate have been employed but:
- A strength of 0.105–0.109 mol/L has been recommended for blood used for coagulation testing in general, including factor assays. One volume of anticoagulant is mixed with nine volumes of blood, and the fill volume must be at least 90% of the target volume for some test systems to give accurate results.
- Although 0.129 mol/L trisodium citrate has been considered acceptable in the past, this is not currently recommended. Samples collected into 0.129 mol/L may be more affected by underfilling than samples collected into the 0.109 mol/L strength.

Table 2.1 The volume of anticoagulant required for a 5-mL sample.

Hematocrit (%)	Volume of anticoagulant (mL)	Volume of blood (mL)
25–55	0.5	4.5
20	0.7	4.3
60	0.4	4.6
70	0.25	4.75
80	0.2	4.8

• If the patient has a hematocrit greater than 55%, results of PT and APTT can be affected, and the volume of anticoagulant should be adjusted to account for the altered plasma volume. Table 2.1 is a guide to the volume of anticoagulant required for a 5-mL sample.

Alternatively, the anticoagulant volume of 0.5 mL can be kept constant and the volume of added blood varied accordingly to the hematocrit. The volume of blood to be added (to 0.5 mL of 0.109 mol/L citrate) is calculated from the formula:

$$\frac{60}{100 - \text{hematocrit}} \times 4.5$$

Container

The inner surface of the sample container employed for blood sample collection can influence the results obtained (particularly for screening tests) and should not induce contact activation (non-siliconized glass is inappropriate). For factor assays, there is evidence that results on samples collected in a number of different sample types are essentially interchangeable.

Processing and storage of samples prior to analysis

Centrifugation

For preparation of platelet-rich plasma to investigate platelet function, samples should be centrifuged at room temperature (18–25°C) at 150–200 g for 15 minutes, and analyzed within 2 hours of sample collection.

For most other tests related to bleeding disorders, samples should be centrifuged at a speed and time that produces samples with residual platelet counts below 10×10^9/L; for example, using 2000 g for at least 10 minutes.

Centrifugation at a temperature of 18–25°C is acceptable for most clotting tests. Exceptions include labile parameters, such as many tests of fibrinolytic activity. After centrifugation, prolonged storage at 4–8°C should be avoided, as this can cause cold activation, increasing factor VII (FVII) activity and shortening of the PT or APTT.

Stability

Samples for APTT should be analyzed within 4 hours of collection. The results of some other clotting tests, such as the D-dimer and the PT of samples from warfarinized subjects are stable for 24 hours or longer. Unless a laboratory has data on the stability of testing plasmas at room temperature for a specific test, the plasmas should be deep frozen within 4 hours of collection for future analysis.

Some clotting factor test results are stable for samples stored at −24°C or lower for up to 3 months and for samples stored at −74°C for up to 18 months (results within 10% of baseline defined as stable). Storage in domestic grade −20°C freezers is normally unacceptable.

If frozen samples are shipped to another laboratory for testing on dry ice, care must be taken to avoid exposure of the plasma to carbon dioxide, which may affect the pH and the results of screening tests.

Prior to analysis, frozen samples must be thawed rapidly at 37°C for 3–5 minutes. Thawing at lower temperatures is not acceptable because some cryoprecipitation is possible.

Recommendations and summary: sample collection and processing

- Avoid prolonged venous stasis.
- Use a 21-gauge or lower gauge needle for adults.
- Avoid indwelling catheters or lines.
- Mix immediately with 0.105–0.109 mol/L trisodium citrate.
- Discard sample if any delay or difficulty in collection.
- Discard if marked hemolysis or evidence of clotting.
- Underfilling (<80–90% of target volume) prolongs some screening tests.
- If hematocrit is >55%, adjust anticoagulant: blood ratio.

Table 2.2 Interpretation of abnormalities of coagulation screening tests.

PT*	APTT	Thrombin time	Fibrinogen	Possible conditions
Prolonged	Normal	Normal	Normal	Factor VII (FVII) deficiency
Normal	Prolonged	Normal	Normal	Deficiency of FVIII, FIX, FXI, FXII, contact factor, or lupus anticoagulant
Prolonged	Prolonged	Normal	Normal	Deficiency of FII, FV, or FX
				Oral anticoagulant therapy
				Vitamin K deficiency
				Combined deficiency of FV and FVIII
				Combined deficiency of FII, FVII, FIX, and FX
				Liver disease
Prolonged	Prolonged	Prolonged	Normal or low	Hypo- or dysfibrinogenemia
				Liver disease
				Massive transfusion
				DIC

Abbreviations: PT, prothrombin time; APTT, activated partial prothrombin time; DIC, disseminated intravascular coagulopathy.

- Sample collection system can affect results by up to 10%.
- For plasma tests, centrifuge at 2000 g for at least 10 minutes at room temperature.
- Store at room temperature.
- Only centrifuge and store at 4°C if necessary.
- Test within 4 hours (unless evidence for longer stability).
- Freezing may affect results depending on temperature and time of storage.
- Any deep-frozen plasma should be thawed rapidly at 37°C.

Use of coagulation screening tests

Laboratories usually offer a set of tests (the coagulation screen) that aims to identify most clinically important hemostatic defects. Invariably this includes the PT, APTT, fibrinogen, and usually thrombin time. It is important to perform a full blood count to quantify the platelet count, but assessment of platelet function is not usually offered or performed in the initial tests. The pattern of abnormalities of the coagulation screen, as shown in Table 2.2, suggests possible diagnoses and allows further tests to be performed to define the abnormality.

Prothrombin time

Tissue factor (in the form of thromboplastin) and calcium are added to plasma that has been anticoagulated with citrate during collection. Tissue factor reacts with FVIIa to activate the "extrinsic" pathway and thus form a clot.

Use of the PT test

The PT is sensitive to and thus prolonged in patients with deficiencies of factors VII, X, V, and II and fibrinogen. It is particularly useful in monitoring anticoagulation in patients on warfarin.

Figure 2.1 suggests a pathway for investigation of a patient with a prolonged PT.

Activated partial thromboplastin time

Phospholipid (lacking tissue factor, hence the term "partial" thromboplastin) and particulate matter (such as kaolin) are added to plasma to generate a clot. Abnormalities in the "intrinsic" and "common" pathway will result in prolongation of the APTT [1].

Use of the APTT

This test is abnormal in patients:
- with deficiencies of factors XII, XI, X, IX, VIII, V, II, and fibrinogen;
- on heparin therapy; or
- who have the lupus anticoagulant.

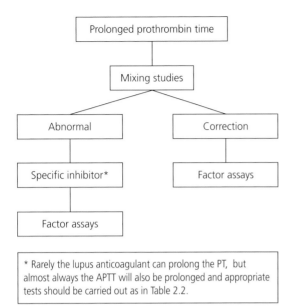

* Rarely the lupus anticoagulant can prolong the PT, but almost always the APTT will also be prolonged and appropriate tests should be carried out as in Table 2.2.

Figure 2.1 Investigation of a prolonged PT.

Figure 2.2 suggests a pathway for investigation of patients with prolonged APTT. Prolongation of the APTT, sometimes to a dramatic degree, can be seen in patients without a bleeding diathesis (Table 2.3).

Mixing studies

These are central in the investigation of a prolonged APTT. The principle is that the test is repeated, with 50% of the test plasma being replaced by normal plasma (which assumes that this contains normal amounts of all the clotting factors). The result of the mixing study is that the test will have all the clotting factors to a minimum of 50%, and thus should result in:

• a normal APTT if the cause of the abnormality was a deficiency of a clotting factor; or
• a prolonged APTT if an inhibitor (either to a specific factor or a lupus anticoagulant) is present.

Thrombin time

The thrombin time measures the rate of conversion of fibrinogen to polymerized fibrin after the addition of thrombin to plasma. It is sensitive to and thus prolonged in:

• hypo- and dysfibrinogenemia;
• heparin therapy (or heparin contamination of the sample); and

• the presence of fibrin(ogen) degradation products and factors that influence the fibrin polymerization (e.g. the presence of a paraprotein in myeloma).

Figure 2.3 suggests a pathway for investigation of a prolonged thrombin time. Heparin contamination in a sample can also be confirmed by correction of a prolonged thrombin time after treatment of a sample with heparinase, hepzyme, reptilase, or mixing with protamine, an agent that antagonizes heparin.

Fibrinogen

A number of methods are available for measurement of fibrinogen concentration. Most automated coagulation analyzers now provide a measure of fibrinogen concentration, calculated from the degree of change of light scatter or optical density during measurement of the PT (PT-derived fibrinogen). Although this is simple and cheap, it is inaccurate in some patients, such as those with disseminated intravascular coagulopathy, liver disease, renal disease, dysfibrino-genemia, following thrombolytic therapy, and in those with markedly raised or reduced fibrinogen concentrations. The recommended method for measuring fibrinogen concentration as originally described by Clauss is based on the thrombin time and uses a high concentration of thrombin solution.

Screening tests: Assay issues

The sensitivity of the PT and APTT to the presence of clotting factor deficiencies is dependent on the test system employed. The degree of prolongation in the presence of a clotting factor deficiency can vary dramatically between reagents [2]. There is no clear consensus on what level of clotting factor deficiency is clinically relevant, and therefore the level that should be detected as an abnormal screening test result has not been defined. In relation to the APTT, one important application is the detection of deficiencies associated with bleeding, in particular factors VIII, IX, and XI.

A number of APTT methods are available for which abnormal results are normally present when the level of clotting factor is below 30 U/dL, and only methods for which this is the case should be used to screen for possible bleeding disorders. In the case of FVIII, it has been recommended in the past that the APTT technique selected should have a normal reference range

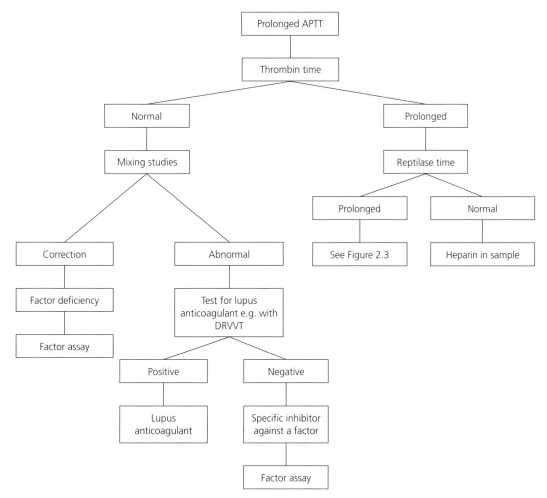

Figure 2.2 Investigation of a prolonged APTT.

that closely corresponds to a FVIII reference range of 50–200 U/dL. However, it should be noted that, for most methods, normal APTT results will be obtained in at least some patients with FVIII in the range

Table 2.3 Conditions associated with a prolonged APTT but without a bleeding diathesis.

Deficiency of:
   factor XII
   high molecular weight kininogen
   Prekallekrein
Lupus anticoagulant
Excess citrate anticoagulant

30–50 U/dL, and few, if any, reagents will be associated with prolonged results in every patient of this type.

For most techniques, the APTT is less sensitive to the reduction of FIX levels than for FVIII, and most, if not all, currently available techniques will be associated with normal APTT results in at least some cases with FIX in the range 25–50 U/dL.

Data from published studies and from external quality-assessment programs suggest that most widely used current APTT reagents will have:
• prolonged APTT results in samples from patients with FIX or FXI below 20–25 U/dL; and
• a more mixed pattern of normal and abnormal results when FIX or FXI is in the range of 25–60 U/dL.

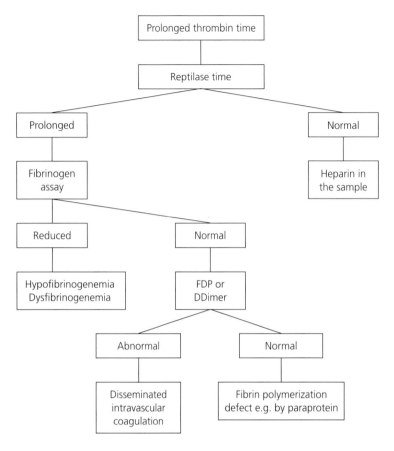

Figure 2.3 Investigation of a prolonged thrombin time.

Lower limit of normal range

The lower limit for FXI activity is probably between 60 and 70 U/dL. The lower limit of normal for FVIII or FIX is approximately 50 U/dL. A normal APTT does not always exclude the presence of a mild deficiency. In plasma from subjects with FIX or FXI deficiency, marked elevation of FVIII, if present, may normalize the APTT.

Variation with reagents

There is marked variation between results:
• with different APTT reagents, partly because of the use of different *activators* in the APTT as well as the *phospholipid profile*. For these reasons, locally determined reference ranges are essential.
• with different PT *thromboplastins* used in the assays of FVII or FX. Sensitive PT techniques will show prolongation of the PT above the upper limit of normal

when there is an isolated deficiency of FVII, FX, or FV with a level below 30–40 U/dL. In general, the level of FII (prothrombin) associated with prolongation of the PT is lower than for the other factors.

In the case of both the PT and APTT, it is useful to repeat borderline results on a fresh sample. It should be noted that the within subject variation of the PT and APTT over time may be 6–12%.

For both the PT and APTT, the degree of prolongation may be small in the presence of mild deficiency, and therefore there is a need for adequate quality-control procedures and for carefully established accurate normal or reference ranges. In view of the limitations of screening tests, it is important that results are interpreted in conjunction with all relevant personal and family history details when screening for bleeding disorders. *Normal screening tests do not always exclude the presence of mild deficiency states.*

Recommendations and summary: Screening tests

- PT and APTT methods vary in sensitivity to factor deficiency.
- Mild deficiency may be associated with normal PT or APTT.
- For bleeding disorders, select a method for which APTT is normally prolonged when FVIII, FIX, or FXI is 30 IU/dL or less.
- Elevated FVIII may normalize APTT in mild FIX or FXI deficiency.
- Assessments of APTT sensitivity should employ samples from patients.

Clotting factor assay design

One-stage assays

For many years, the most commonly performed assays for clotting factors have been one-stage clotting assays based on:

- the APTT in the case of factors VIII, IX, or XI; or
- the PT in the case of factors II, V, VII, or X.

There are a number of general features of the design of one-stage clotting assays that are necessary to ensure accurate, reliable, and valid results. In factor assays, the principle depends on the ability of a sample containing the factor under investigation to correct or shorten the delayed clotting of a plasma completely deficient in that factor. Such deficient plasmas must contain less than 1 U/dL of the clotting factor under investigation and normal levels of all other relevant clotting factors.

It is important that the clotting time measured by the APTT or PT depends directly on the amount of factor present in the mixture of deficient and reference or test plasma. For example, in a FVIII assay, the level of FVIII must be rate-limiting in relation to the clotting time obtained. This requires dilution of a reference or standard plasma of known concentration. Preparation of several different dilutions of the reference plasma allows construction of a calibration curve in which the clotting time response depends on the dose (concentration) of factor present. At lower plasma dilutions or higher factor concentrations, the factor under investigation may not be rate-limiting, and the assay is no longer specific and therefore invalid. It may

be necessary to extend the calibration curve by testing additional dilutions when analyzing test plasmas with concentrations below 10 U/dL. At very low concentrations of an individual factor (<1–2 U/dL), the clotting time of the deficient plasma may not be even partially corrected by addition of the test plasma dilution. Dilutions are selected so that there is a linear relationship between concentration (logarithmic scale) and the response in clotting time (logarithmic or linear scale). The reference curve should be prepared using at least three different dilutions, and a calibration curve should be included each time the assay is performed unless there is clear evidence that the responses are so reproducible that a calibration curve can be stored for use on other occasions. The reference plasma should be calibrated by a route traceable back to WHO international standards where these are available. Test plasmas should be analyzed by using three dilutions so that it is possible to confirm that the dose–response curve of the test plasma is linear and parallel to the dose–response curve of the reference plasma. It is not acceptable to test a single test dilution because this reduces the accuracy substantially and may lead to major underestimation of the true concentration when inhibitors are present. If a dose–response curve of a test plasma is not parallel to the reference curve, and the presence of an inhibitor (such as an antiphospholipid antibody) is confirmed or suspected, then the estimate of activity obtained from the highest test plasma dilution is likely to be closest to the real concentration; but, it should be noted that the criteria for a valid assay cannot be met and results must be interpreted with caution. In the case of one-stage, APTT-based assays, the interference by antiphospholipid antibodies is frequently dependent on the APTT reagent used and its phospholipid content. Some APTT reagents, such as Actin FS, contain a high phospholipid concentration, and this type of reagent is much less affected by these antibodies and is particularly suitable for use in factor assays in such cases.

Recommendations and summary: Factor assays

- Assays should be calibrated with reference plasmas traceable back to WHO standards where available.

- Deficient plasmas must have <1 U/dL of the clotting factor being assayed and normal levels of other relevant factors.
- No less than three dilutions of test plasmas should be tested.
- A valid assay requires test and calibration lines to be parallel.
- Interference by antiphospholipid antibodies can be minimized by use of an APTT reagent with a high phospholipid content.

Thrombophilia testing

This section addresses some laboratory aspects of testing for heritable thrombophilia: protein C (PC), protein S (PS), antithrombin (AT), activated protein C resistance (APC-R), FV Leiden (FVL), and the prothrombin 20210A allele [3,4].

Sample collection, processing, and assay

For thrombophilia testing, as for other coagulation tests:
- A citrate concentration of 0.105–0.109 mol/L should be used for sample collection, because citrate strength may affect results, at least for APC-R testing.
- Centrifugation should be as for other coagulation tests described above.
- Residual platelets in plasma following centrifugation can also affect results of APC-R tests, and plasmas should be centrifuged as described above, separated, and recentrifuged a second time to ensure maximum removal of platelets. (Such a procedure is not necessary for AT, PC, or PS testing but can be used for convenience without adverse effects if the same plasma is to be used for these investigations in addition to APC-R.)
- Such double-centrifuged plasma can then be stored deep frozen prior to analysis for at least 6 months for clotting PS activity and at least 18 months for PC and AT.
- In general, activity assays are preferable to antigen assays because antigen assays will be normal in some patients with type 2 defects where a normal concentration of a defective protein is present.

In the case of PS, this is complicated by the problems associated with interference by FVL in many different activity assays and can lead to important underestimation of the true level, with misdiagnosis a possibility.

At present, the standardization of PS activity assays is poor in that results of different assays may differ substantially even in normal subjects. For these reasons, PS activity assays must be used with caution.

FVL can also cause underestimation of the true PC level in clotting assays. A chromogenic PC assay may be used to avoid this problem, or alternatively the PC clotting assay can be modified to include predilution of test sample 1 in 4 in PC-deficient plasma to restore specificity. A similar procedure can be employed to improve performance of clotting PS assays in the presence of FVL.

Clotting assays of PC and PS may also be influenced adversely by elevated FVIII, causing underestimation. The presence of the lupus anticoagulant may be associated with falsely high results, with the possibility of a false normal result in the presence of deficiency.

When assaying PC, PS, and AT, calibration curves should include a minimum of three dilutions, and, in general, the most precise test results will be obtained if a calibration curve is prepared with each group of patient samples. As for other tests of hemostasis, it is important to use a reference plasma traceable back to WHO standards, which are available for AT, PC, and PS.

Testing for APC-R is largely based on the APTT in the presence and absence of APC, and therefore many of the variables that affect the APTT will in turn influence APC-R test results. These include the presence of heparin or lupus anticoagulant by prolonging clotting times, or elevated FVIII, which shortens clotting times and manifest as acquired APC-R. The original APC-R test also requires normal levels of clotting factors, including FII and FX, which are reduced by warfarin therapy. Valid APC-R testing as originally used requires a normal PT and APTT.

There is evidence that standardization of results obtained by the original assay can be improved by calculation of the normalized APC-R ratio (test APC ratio divided by APC ratio of a pooled normal plasma tested in the same batch of tests). The test can be significantly improved by predilution of test plasma in FV-deficient plasma, making the test 100% sensitive to the presence of FVL. This modification also makes the test specific for FVL, and will be associated with normal results where APC resistance in the classic assay is not a consequence of FVL. This must be borne in mind when interpreting results. In some versions of the test, there is clear separation between results obtained in heterozygotes and homozygotes; but, even for such assays, confirmation by genetic testing may be necessary because it is important to identify homozygotes with certainty.

When genetic testing for the FVL or prothrombin alleles is undertaken, there are fewer relevant preanalytical variables than for phenotypic tests on plasma. Whole blood samples are stable for several weeks, at least for some of the genotyping methods.

Because of the many differences between results of apparently similar assays in thrombophilia testing, it is particularly important to establish locally a reference or normal range (as discussed in Appendix 1).

Recommendations and summary: thrombophilia tests

- Double centrifugation is required for APC-R testing.
- Presence of FVL may cause significant underestimation of clotting PC or PS activity.
- Results of PS activity assays are highly dependent on reagents used.
- Elevated FVIII or lupus anticoagulant can interfere with PC or PS clotting assays.
- Results of AT assays may depend on the enzyme used in the assay.
- APC-R with FV-deficient plasma dilution is the most sensitive and specific for FVL.
- Genetic testing for FVL or prothrombin allele may not be error free.

Quality assurance

All laboratory tests of blood coagulation require careful application of quality-assurance procedures to ensure reliability of results. Quality assurance is used to describe all the measures that are taken to ensure the reliability of laboratory testing and reporting. This includes the choice of test, the collection of a valid sample from the patient, analysis of the specimen, and the recording of results in a timely and accurate manner, through to interpretation of the results, where appropriate, and communication of these results to the referring clinicians.

Internal quality control (IQC) and external quality assessment (EQA) are complementary components of a laboratory quality-assurance program. Quality assurance is required to check that the results of laboratory investigations are reliable enough to be released to assist clinical decision-making, monitoring of therapy, and diagnosis of hemostatic abnormalities.

Internal quality control

IQC is used to establish whether a series of techniques and procedures are performing consistently over a period of time (precision). It is therefore deployed to ensure day-to-day laboratory consistency. It is important to recognize that a precise technique is not necessarily accurate; accuracy being a measure of the closeness of an estimated value to the true value.

IQC procedures should be applied in a way that ensures immediate and constant control of result generation. Within a laboratory setting, the quality of results obtained is influenced by maintenance of an upto-date manual of standard operational procedures; use of reliable reagents and reference materials; selection of automation and adequate maintenance; adequate records and reporting system for results; and an appropriate complement of suitably trained personnel.

For screening tests, it is important to include regular and frequent testing of quality-control material, which should include a normal material and at least one level of abnormal sample. For batch analysis, a quality-control sample can be included with each batch. For continuous processing systems, the frequency of quality-control testing must be tailored to the work pattern and should be adjusted until the frequency of repeat patient testing resulting from the limits of the quality control studies is at a minimum. For many random access coagulometers, performing screening tests, this could typically be every 2 hours of continuous work or every 30–40 samples. For factor assays and parameters typically tested in batches, a quality-control sample should be included with each group of tests. Patient results should only be released if quality-control results remain within acceptable target limits. It is frequently useful to include IQC material at different critical levels of abnormality.

External quality assessment

EQA is used to identify the degree of agreement between one laboratory's results and those obtained by other centers, which can be used as a measure of accuracy. The main function of EQA is proficiency testing of individual laboratory testing, but larger programs provide information concerning the relative performance of analytical procedures, including the method principle, reagents, and instruments. As a general principle, all centers undertaking investigations of hemostasis should participate in an accredited EQA program for all tests where available.

Recommendations and summary: quality control

• Quality-control samples should be analyzed regularly and frequently for screening tests and with each group of factor assays.

• Centers should participate in accredited EQA programs for all tests where available.

References

1 Koepke JA. Partial thromboplastin time test: proposed performance guidelines. ICSH Panel on the PTT. *Thromb Haemost* 1986;55:143–4.

2 Lawrie AS, Kitchen S, Purdy G, Mackie IJ, Preston FE, Machin SJ. Assessment of actin FS and actin FSL sensitivity to specific clotting factor deficiencies. *Clin Lab Haematol* 1998;20:179–86.

3 Jennings I, Cooper P. Screening for thrombophilia: a laboratory perspective. *Br J Biomed Sci* 2003;60: 39–51.

4 Walker ID, Greaves M, Preston FE. Investigation and management of heritable thrombophilia. *Br J Haematol* 2001;114:512–18.

Laboratory evaluation and thrombophilia

Rajiv K. Pruthi and John A. Heit

Overview

Venous thromboembolism (VTE) is a prototype of a multifactorial disease model in which interaction of genetic and environmental risk factors (termed thrombophilia) predispose to VTE. Patients who develop a VTE are considered to have thrombophilia; however, this term should not be considered to be a disease, but a risk factor for (venous or arterial) thrombosis, thus it is important to note that presence of thrombophilia in an individual is not absolutely predictive of thrombosis. The most common clinical presentation of thrombophilia is VTE; other presentations are listed in Table 3.1. The currently recognized inherited and acquired thrombophilias (Tables 3.2 and 3.3) predispose to VTE; however, selected conditions (lupus anticoagulants and hyperhomocysteinemia) may also predispose to arterial thrombosis. The presence of thrombophilia determines a patient's risk for initial and subsequent (recurrent) VTE, which influences (primary and secondary) VTE prevention strategies.

Assessment for presence of thrombophilia

Clinical assessment
Assessment of presence of thrombophilia is not solely confined to laboratory testing but begins with a detailed history and physical examination. Detailed inquiry into symptoms and signs of acquired risk factors (coexisting diseases, medication exposure, and clinical circumstances) that are associated with thrombosis (Tables 3.2–3.4) are an important part of the initial evaluation as is a complete physical examination.

In addition to judicious laboratory testing appropriate for the patient's age and symptoms, objective confirmation of venous thromboembolism is critical prior to embarking on extensive laboratory testing for thrombophilia. Because indiscriminate, extensive testing for occult cancer in patients presenting with idiopathic VTE has not clearly been shown to improve cancer-related survival, such an evaluation should be confined to age-appropriate cancer screening and further evaluation of patient symptoms and signs.

Laboratory testing
Currently, there is no single laboratory global assay that will 'screen' for the presence of thrombophilia. Thus, laboratory testing can be broadly categorized into (1) general diagnostic testing, (2) specialized coagulation testing, and (3) ancillary testing for disorders known to predispose to thrombotic disorders.

General diagnostic testing
All patients with objectively confirmed VTE should have the following tests prior to initiation of anticoagulant therapy: complete blood count (CBC), tests of kidney and liver function (these tests are primarily to assess for safety of anticoagulation with heparin and warfarin); obtaining baseline prothrombin time (PT) and activated partial thromboplastin time (APTT) tests aid in optimal monitoring of anticoagulation (Table 3.5).

Specialized coagulation testing
Special Coagulation testing consists of a battery of complex (protein and DNA-based) thrombophilia assays to detect presence of an inherited or acquired thrombophilia. As discussed below, multiple preanalytical conditions affect results of these assays (e.g. anticoagulants, acute thrombosis, liver disease, etc.),

Table 3.1 Thrombophilia: clinical manifestations.

Strongly supportive data:
1) VTE: Superficial or DVT, PE
2) Thrombosis of "unusual" venous circulations (e.g. cerebral, hepatic, mesenteric, and renal veins; possibly arm, portal, and ovarian veins; not retinal vein or artery)
3) Warfarin-induced skin necrosis
4) Purpura fulminans (neonatalis or adult)
5) Recurrent fetal loss

Weakly supportive data:
6) Possibly arterial thrombosis (e.g. stroke, acute myocardial infarction)
7) Possibly complications of pregnancy (e.g. intrauterine growth restriction, stillbirth, severe pre-eclampsia, abruptio placentae)

Table 3.3 Acquired thrombophilia.

Strongly supportive data:
A. Hematologic malignancies:
   1) Myeloproliferative disorders
   2) Paroxysmal nocturnal hemoglobinuria
B. Solid organ malignancies:
C. Chemotherapy
   1) L-asparaginase, thalidomide, anti-angiogenesis therapy
D. Drugs:
   1) Heparin-induced thrombocytopenia
E. Nephrotic syndrome
F. Acquired coagulopathies:
   1) Disseminated intravascular coagulation and fibrinolysis
   2) Antiphospholipid antibody syndromes (lupus anticoagulant, anticardiolipin antibody, anti-beta2 glycoprotein-1 antibody)
G. Estrogens and progestational agents
   1) Oral contraceptives
   2) Hormone replacement therapy
   3) Pregnancy/postpartum state
H. Others
   1) Thrombotic thrombocytopenic purpura
   2) Sickle cell disease
   3) Selective estrogen receptor modulator (SERM) therapy (tamoxifen and raloxifene)
   4) Wegener granulomatosis

Supportive data:
1) Inflammatory bowel disease
2) Thromboangiitis obliterans (Buerger disease) Bechet syndrome
3) Varicose veins
4) Systemic lupus erythematosus
5) Venous vascular anomalies (e.g. Klippel Trenaunay syndrome)
6) Progesterone therapy
7) Infertility "therapy"
8) Hyperhomocysteinemia
9) HIV infection
10) Dehydration

so interpretation of results needs to be done within the context of the circumstances surrounding testing. An additional factor affecting the yield of testing is the ethnicity of the patient population being studied. Prevalence of factor V Leiden (FVL) varies from

Table 3.2 Hereditary thrombophilia: laboratory associations.

Strongly supportive data:
A. Procoagulant protein abnormalities
   1) APC-R (FVL)
   2) Prothrombin G20210A
   3) Selected dysfibrinogenemia variants
B. Anticoagulant protein abnormalities
   1) Antithrombin deficiency
   2) Protein C deficiency
   3) Protein S deficiency
C. Others
   1) Homocysteinuria

Supportive data:
1) Increased procoagulant proteins: FII, FVIII, FIX, FXI, and fibrinogen
2) Factor XIII polymorphisms
3) Hyperhomocysteinemia
4) Reduced tissue factor pathway inhibitor

Weakly supportive data:
1) Deficiency of protein Z
2) Elevated levels: tissue plasminogen activator inhibitor (PAI-1), thrombin activatable fibrinolysis inhibitor (TAFI)

3% to 7% in Caucasians of European ancestry, but has a very low prevalence in individuals of other ethnic groups: 0% among Native Americans/Australians and Africans, 0.16% among the Chinese, and 0.6% among individuals from Asia Minor (India, Pakistan, Sri Lanka) (Table 3.5) [1]. No such data are available for other known thrombophilias for non-Caucasian European populations.

Table 3.4 Independent risk factors for venous thromboembolism [5].

Baseline characteristics	Odds ratio	95% CI
Hospitalization: Acute medical illness	7.98	4.49–14.18
Hospitalization: Major surgery	21.72	9.44–49.93
Trauma	12.69	4.06–39.66
Active cancer without chemotherapy	4.05	1.93–8.52
Active cancer with chemotherapy	6.53	2.11–20.23
Central venous catheter or transvenous pacemaker	5.55	1.57–19.58
Prior superficial venous thrombosis	4.32	1.76–10.61
Neurologic disease with extremity paresis	3.04	1.25–7.38
Serious liver disease	0.1	0.01–0.71

In general, specialized coagulation thrombophilia assays can be broadly divided into assays that detect a clot-based endpoint (e.g. lupus anticoagulant, protein S activity), chromogenic assays (e.g. protein C and antithrombin activities), or variants of enzyme-linked immunosorbent assays (ELISAs). An ideal approach to testing consists of performing activity assays with reflexive antigenic assays if indicated (e.g. a low antithrombin activity is typically followed up by performing an antithrombin antigen, primarily to classify the type of deficiency).

Factors affecting results of coagulation testing

Effect of acute thrombosis

During the acute thrombotic episode, levels of antithrombin, protein C, and protein S may be transiently reduced [2]; thus, if testing is not repeated, remote from the thrombotic event and from anticoagulant therapy, the patient may be misdiagnosed as having a congenital deficiency.

Effect of anticoagulants

Heparin. Heparin therapy can falsely reduce antithrombin levels. Although most lupus anticoagulant (LAC) reagents [e.g. dilute russel viper venom time (DRVVT) and Staclot APTT] contain heparin neutraliz-

ers that can neutralize up to 1 U/mL of heparin, presence of excess heparin may result in a false-positive test result, which impacts the duration of secondary prophylaxis. Thus, positive results of LAC testing performed while on heparin should be reconfirmed when the patient is off heparin.

Vitamin K antagonist (VKA) therapy. Protein C and S levels are lowered by VKA therapy (e.g.warfarin since they are vitamin K-dependent proteins). In addition, VKA therapy may result in a false-positive LAC with certain assays (e.g. DRVVT).

Direct thrombin inhibitors (DTIs; e.g. argatroban, lepirudin, bivalirudin). Because the majority of anticoagulant activity assays rely on generation of thrombin to achieve an endpoint of clot detection, presence of DTIs interfere with this endpoint and delay clot formation. This can lead to a false-positive LAC or falsely reduced protein C and S levels. Results of chromogenic assays are likely reliable.

Effect of liver disease

The majority of anticoagulant and procoagulant proteins are produced in the liver. In advanced liver disease, levels of both the anticoagulant and procoagulant proteins are reduced.

Sample collection and processing issues

Practically speaking, ordering physicians have limited impact on specimen collection and processing; however, knowledge of such effects may lead one to consider repeat testing, if the data are unexpected or do not fit the expected pattern [e.g. reduced activated protein C resistance (APC-R) ratio suggesting presence of APC-R, yet the FVL test is negative].

Effect of type of anticoagulant in specimen collection tube

Standard specimen collection tubes contain 0.105–0.109 mol/L citrate for optimal results. Specimens may inadvertently be collected in ethylenediaminetetraacetic acid (EDTA), which will result in falsely reduced protein levels and a reduced APC-R ratio.

Effect of specimen processing

Specimens should be double centrifuged as soon as possible after collection in order to reduce the amount of residual platelets to a minimum. The presence of residual platelets can result in a false-negative test for LAC.

Table 3.5 Laboratory evaluation for suspected familial or acquired thrombophilia (tests are suggested and should be performed selectively based on clinical judgment; see text).

General diagnostic testing:
1) CBC with peripheral blood smear.
2) Prothrombin time as a baseline prior to initiation of warfarin.
3) APTT (using a thromboplastin that is relatively sensitive to the presence of a lupus anticoagulant)
4) Serum creatinine
5) Liver enzymes

Specialized coagulation and DNA-based testing:
Protein-based testing:
1) APC-R ratio with reflexive molecular (DNA-based) testing for factor V R506Q (Leiden) mutation
2) Anticoagulant proteins (protein C, protein S, and antithrombin)
3) LAC panel
4) Anticardiolipin and anti-beta2 glycoprotein 1 antibodies (IgG and IgM isotypes)
5) Disseminated intravascular coagulation and fibrinolysis screen (fibrinogen, soluble fibrin monomer complex and quantitative plasma fibrin D-dimer)
6) Thrombin time with reflexive reptilase time (to detect a heparin or DTI effect, and to screen for dysfibrinogenemia)

Molecular (DNA-based) testing
1) Prothrombin G20210GA mutation genotyping (direct genomic DNA mutation testing)
Additional specialized testing.
1) Homocysteine (basal)

Ancillary testing based on clinical suspicion and/or results of history and examination findings:
1) Flow cytometry (CD55 and CD59) for PNH
2) Plasma ADAMTS13 activity (for acquired or familial thrombotic thrombocytopenic purpura)
3) Heparin-induced thrombocytopenia testing [plasma anti-PF4/glycosaminoglycan antibodies (ELISA); platelet 14C-serotonin release assay; heparin-dependent platelet aggregation]
4) Quantitative PCR assay for JAK2 V617F mutation (for suspicion of myeloproliferative disease).
5) Age-appropriate cancer screening or testing based on results of history and examination findings:
   Tumor markers (e.g. prostate-specific antigen)
   Urinalysis
   Radiography: Posteroanterior/lateral chest x-ray; mammogram; abdominal imaging (CT); colon imaging
   Speciality consultations: otolaryngology consultation, especially for smokers
   Specialized procedures as indicated: UGI/upper endoscopy; endometrial biopsy if endometrial cancer suspected

Factors affecting molecular (DNA-based) testing

The main patient-related factors affecting currently available DNA-based testing include liver and hematopoeitic stem cell transplantation, the type of anticoagulant in the collection tube, and the white blood cell count.

Effect of liver transplantation

Anticoagulant proteins are produced in the liver. A patient with thrombophilia (e.g. APC-R) who receives a liver transplant from an unaffected donor may be "cured" of APC-R, yet will still carry the FVL muta-

tion in their peripheral blood genomic DNA, resulting in discordant results. In contrast, patients previously unaffected with APC-R, who receive a liver from an individual with APC-R, will test negative for the FVL mutation, yet have APC-R on protein-based testing.

Effect of hematopoeitic stem cell transplantation (HSCT)

A carrier of FVL mutation who receives HSCT from an unaffected donor will still have APC-R, but peripheral blood genomic DNA testing will be negative for FVL mutation.

Effect of patient white blood cell count

Because the large majority of testing is performed on sample from peripheral blood leukocytes, leucopenia caused by intrinsic hematologic disorders, or as a result of chemotherapy, may make it technically difficult to perform the assays.

Type of anticoagulant in the collection tube

In general, peripheral blood for DNA-based testing is collected in acid-citrate-dextrose (ACD) or EDTA. Heparin interferes with the polymerase chain reaction (PCR)-based testing.

Ancillary testing

Additional testing to detect disorders known to predispose to VTE should be pursued if clinically indicated. Flow cytometry for CD55 and CD59 is indicated in patients with evidence of intravascular hemolysis with or without pancytopenia for detection of paroxysmal nocturnal hemoglobinuria (PNH). Assays for ADAMTS-13 in patients with microangiopathic hemolytic anemia, thrombocytopenia, with or without neurological symptoms, fever, and renal insufficiency detect thrombotic thrombocytopenic purpura. In patients exposed to heparin, testing should be done for the heparin-induced thrombocytopenia (HIT) antibody using either a functional assay (serotonin release assay, heparin-dependent platelet aggregation) or ELISA. Patients with evidence of erythrocytosis, thrombocytosis, or mesenteric or portal venous thrombosis should be evaluated for myeloproliferative disease; testing consists of assessment for the JAK-2 V617F mutation, which can be performed on peripheral blood or bone marrow aspiration/biopsy specimens. At this time, routine in-depth testing for a malignancy is discouraged; however, age-appropriate cancer screening and symptom/signs-directed testing for case detection should be pursued (see Table 3.5).

Management of patients with thrombophilia

Primary prevention

There are at least 300,000 first-lifetime cases of VTE per year in the United States (US), and, given the aging population, the incidence is expected to rise. Because 25% of patients experience sudden death as the initial presentation of pulmonary embolism (PE), mortality is also expected to rise.Thus, primary prevention of VTE in the hospitalized patient is imperative. Currently, VTE prophylaxis recommendations for patients hospitalized for surgery or medical illness are based solely on the presence or absence of clinical predictors of thrombosis (Tables 3.2 and 3.3) [3]. Although VTE is a multifactorial disease in which inherited thrombophilias interact with clinical risk factors to compound the risk of incident VTE, routine thrombophilia testing with the intent of tailoring a prophylaxis regimen for an inherited thrombophilia is not recommended. However, given the increased risk of symptomatic VTE after high-risk surgery, patients with known thrombophilia should be considered for a longer duration (e.g. out-of-hospital) of prophylaxis.

Acute therapy

The aims of anticoagulation for acute VTE include prevention of extension or embolism of an acute thrombosis. Except for selected circumstances described below, acute management of VTE in patients with familial or acquired thrombophilia should be no different than in those with no identifiable thrombophilia. This involves initial intravenous unfractionated heparin (UFH), low-molecular-weight heparin (LMWH) or fondaparinux, and the simultaneous initiation of warfarin with an overlap until a therapeutic international normalized ration (INR) is achieved [4].

Antithrombin deficiency

Some patients with antithrombin (AT) deficiency may be relatively heparin-resistant as defined by an apparently subtherapeutic APTT despite high doses of UFH (>35,000 U of UFH per 24 hours). Supplemental AT concentrate could be considered in these patients.

Hereditary protein C deficiency

Protein C has a short half-life of approximately 6 hours and thus rapidly declines upon initiation of warfarin, whereas the decline in factor II levels is slower (4 to 5 days). Without therapeutic heparin (UFH or LMWH) overlap, this transitional period results in a "hypercoagulable" state and puts patients at risk for warfarin-induced skin necrosis or progression of the thrombosis. To reduce this risk, warfarin should be started only after therapeutic heparinization, at a low initial dose (e.g. 2 mg) that is slowly increased.

Lupus anticoagulant

Therapeutic monitoring of UFH is based on the APTT; however, presence of an LAC typically prolongs the baseline APTT, precluding accurate UFH monitoring, hence the importance of measuring a baseline APTT prior to initiation of UFH. In this situation, UFH can be monitored with an anti-Xa assay (heparin assay); alternatively, administration of weight-based LMWH may be considered.

Secondary prophylaxis

In general, a first-lifetime VTE occurring in association with a transient clinical risk factor does not warrant secondary prophylaxis. However, in patients with idiopathic VTE, those with identifiable thrombophilia, or a clinical risk factor known to predict recurrence, consideration of secondary prophlaxis is reasonable [4]. Currently, VTE is viewed as a chronic disease with episodic recurrence, with up to 30% of patients experiencing a recurrence over 10 years [5] and with the majority of recurrences occurring within 6 to 12 months after discontinuation of anticoagulation. Thus, the aim of secondary prophylaxis is to prevent recurrent VTE. The decision regarding duration of secondary prophylaxis is complex, and the risks (based on clinical predictors and thrombophilia) and consequences of VTE recurrence need to be balanced with the risk of anticoagulant-related bleeding and patient preference. The hazards of incident and recurrent VTE based on the presence of clinical predictors and thrombophilia are shown in Tables 3.4 and 3.6.

Secondary prophylaxis based on clinical predictors

Secondary prophylaxis may be considered for idiopathic, recurrent, or life-threatening VTE (e.g. hemodynamically significant PE phlegmasia with threatened venous gangrene, or purpura fulminans). Other factors predictive of high risk of recurrence include active cancer, chronic neurologic disease with extremity paresis, and persistent residual deep vein thrombosis (DVT). Additional factors influencing the decision on secondary prophylaxis include the site of incident event and patient comorbidities. Although the site of incident event (e.g. DVT alone vs. PE) is not a predictor of recurrence, those that experience a recurrence are more likely do so in the same vascular territory as the incident event. Given that the 7-day patient

fatality rate is significantly higher for recurrent PE (34%) compared with recurrent DVT alone (4%), secondary prophylaxis should be considered for incident PE, especially for patients with reduced cardiopulmonary functional reserve (e.g. congestive heart failure, chronic obstructive pulmonary disease, etc.).

Note that a family history of VTE is not predictive of an increased risk for VTE recurrence and should not influence the decision regarding secondary prophylaxis.

Secondary prophylaxis based on the presence of thrombophilia

Secondary prophylaxis is reasonable in selected thrombophilias that are predictive of a high-recurrence risk, including a persistent LAC, high-titer IgG or IgM antiphospholipid antibody (anti-cardiolipin and/or anti-beta2 glycoprotein I antibodies), congenital anticoagulant deficiencies (antithrombin, protein C, or protein S), heterozygous carriers for more than one familial thrombophilia (e.g. heterozygous for the FVL and prothrombin G20210A mutations), or homozygous carriers of FVL.

Other predictors of increased risk of recurrence include significant hyperhomocysteinemia, increased factor VIII and factor IX activities, decreased tissue-factor pathway inhibitor activity, and a persistently increased D-dimer measured at least 1 month after stopping warfarin therapy independent of residual venous obstruction.

The risk of recurrence among isolated heterozygous carriers for either the FVL or Prothrombin G20201A mutations is relatively low and insufficient to warrant secondary prophylaxis after a first-lifetime thrombotic event in the absence of other independent predictors of recurrence [6].

The risks of recurrent VTE must be weighed against the risks of anticoagulant-related bleeding. Predictors of hemorrhagic complications include age (1.5-fold for every 10-year increase in age), associated malignancy (2-fold increased risk) [7], patient's functional status (increased risk associated with falls), prior anticoagulation experience (prior hemorrhage and history of widely fluctuating INR), poor compliance, prior gastrointestinal bleeding or stroke, recent myocardial infarction, anemia (hematocrit <30%), impaired renal function (serum creatinine >1.5 mg/dL), impaired liver function, and thrombocytopenia. Risks of hemorrhage can be reduced with optimal management of warfarin by anticoagulation management services or patient self-testing or self-management. With appropriate patient selection and management, the risk of major bleeding can be reduced to about 1% per year.

Given that risk of recurrent VTE decreases over time and risk of anticoagulant-related hemorrhage varies, the need for secondary prophylaxis should be continually reevaluated at appropriate intervals (e.g. annually). It is inappropriate to recommend "lifelong" or "indefinite" anticoagulation therapy.

Controversial aspects of thrombophilia testing

Who should be tested?
At the present time, population screening for thrombophilia is not indicated. Populations typically considered for testing include symptomatic patients with a first apparently idiopathic VTE, those with recurrent VTE, venous thrombosis in an unusual vascular territory (e.g. cerebral, hepatic, mesenteric, or renal vein thrombosis), neonatal purpura fulminans, and warfarin-induced skin necrosis. The presence of two or more of these characteristics may increase the yield of finding one or more coexisting thrombophilic traits, thus a complete thrombophilia profile is recommended.

Currently, populations in whom testing is controversial include patients with a first VTE associated with a known temporary risk factor, asymptomatic family members of symptomatic patients with known thrombophilia, or individuals at increased risk for VTE (e.g. prior to pregnancy, oral contraception or estrogen therapy, high-risk surgery, or chemotherapy with angiogenesis inhibitors). A selective approach (e.g. APC-R/FVL, prothrombin G20210A mutation) is reasonable for first-degree relatives with known thrombophilia.

Timing of thrombophilia testing
Given the effects of acute thrombosis, heparin and warfarin on the results of thrombophilia testing, and a lack of significant impact on the acute management of VTE, it is reasonable to delay thrombophilia testing until completion of the appropriate duration of anticoagulation. For situations in which interruption of warfarin therapy is felt to be unsafe (e.g. possible LAC based on a prolonged baseline APTT), LMWH can be substituted for warfarin with the test sample being obtained prior to administration of the morning LMWH dose. However, the effect of warfarin on protein S levels may not resolve for 4 to 6 weeks. Any abnormal result should be confirmed with repeat testing and/or by testing symptomatic relatives.

Counseling issues related to thrombophilia testing

Because thrombophilia testing involves assessment of genetic risk factors, it is imperative that patients receive appropriate pre- and posttest counseling, with a detailed balanced discussion on the pros and cons of testing. Points to cover include the impact of finding of a genetic thrombophilic trait in the patient (including potential impact on the personal health, life insurability and employment, stigmatization, and mental anguish) and the impact on family members, especially the possibility of uncovering nonpaternity. A discussion on the impact of results of testing on the overall management of increased risk of thrombosis and the risk of adverse pregnancy outcomes (in women of reproductive age) should be undertaken.

Providing estimates of the absolute risk of VTE is generally more useful than providing relative risk estimates. As an example, the relative risk of VTE among women on estrogenic oral contraceptives who are heterozygous FVL carriers is increased about 30-fold; however, the VTE incidence is only about 300 per 100,000 woman-years, or about 0.3% per woman-year (Table 3.6). These absolute risk estimates will vary with age; for example, the incidence of VTE is 123 per 100,000 woman-years among peri-menopausal women (50 to 54 years), which increases exponentially with age. Among FVL carriers of perimenopausal age, the relative risk of VTE associated with hormone replacement therapy (HRT) may be increased 7- to 15-fold; although the relative risk for VTE is less for HRT than estrogenic oral contraceptives, the absolute risk is substantially higher (approximately 900–1800 per 100,000 woman-years, or approximately l–2% per woman-year).

Table 3.6 Estimated prevalence of thrombophilia by population, incidence, and relative risk of incident and recurrent VTE.

Thrombophilia	Prevalence (%)			Incident VTE		Recurrent VTE	
	Normal	Incident VTE	Recurrent VTE	Incidence* (95% CI)	Relative risk (95% CI)	Incidence (95% CI)	Relative risk (95% CI)
FVL[†]	3-7	12-20	40-50	150 (80-260)	4.3[‡] (1.9-9.7)	3500 (1900-6100)	1.3 (1.0-3.3)
Prothrombin G20210A[†]	1-3	3-8	15-20	350	1.9 (0.9-4.1)		1.4 (0.9-2.0)
Antithrombin deficiency	0.02-0.04	1-2	2-5	500 (320-730)	17.5 (9.1-33.8)	10,500 (3800-23,000)	2.5
Protein C deficiency	0.02-0.05	2-5	5-10	310 (200-470)	11.3 (5.7-22.3)	5100 (2500-9400)	2.5
Protein S deficiency	0.01-1	1-3	5-10	710 (530-930)	32.4 (16.7-62.9)	6500 (2800-11,800)	2.5
Hyper homocysteinemia							2.5
Antiphospholipid antibody							2.5
Factor VIII (>200%)							1.8 (1.0-3.3)
Combined thrombophilia[§]				840 (560-1220)	46.7 (22.5-97.1)	5000 (2000-10,300)	

*Per 100,000 person-years.
[†]Heterozygous carriers.
[‡]Homozygous carriers, relative risk 80.
[§]FVL or prothrombin G20210A with either antithrombin, protein C, or protein S deficiency.

Conclusion

The characterization of clinical and laboratory thrombophilic influences is playing an increasingly important role in the long-term management of VTE. Although the currently recognized risk factors provide estimates of risk for groups of patients, the discovery of novel laboratory risk factors and their integration with clinical risk factors may provide better models to risk stratify individual patients. This will provide optimal prophylactic and therapeutic regimens for individual patients rather than groups of individuals.

References

1 Rees DC, Cox M, Clegg JB. World distribution of factor V Leiden. *Lancet* 1995;346(8983):1133–4.
2 Kovacs MJ, Kovacs J, Anderson J, Rodger MA, Mackinnon K, Wells PS. Protein C and protein S levels can be accurately determined within 24 hours of diagnosis of acute venous thromboembolism. *Clin Lab Haematol* 2006;28(1):9–13.
3 Geerts WH, Bergqvist D, Pineo GF, et al. Prevention of venous thromboembolism: American College of Chest Physicians Evidence-Based Clinical Practice Guidelines (8th Edition). *Chest* 2008;133(6 Suppl):381S–453S.
4 Kearon C, Kahn SR, Agnelli G, et al. Antithrombotic therapy for venous thromboembolic disease: American College of Chest Physicians Evidence-Based Clinical Practice Guidelines (8th Edition). *Chest* 2008;133(6 Suppl):454S–545S.
5 Heit JA, Mohr DN, Silverstein MD, Petterson TM, O'Fallon WM, Melton LJ 3rd. Predictors of recurrence after deep vein thrombosis and pulmonary embolism: a population-based cohort study. *Arch Intern Med* 2000;160(6):761–8.
6 Ho WK, Hankey GJ, Quinlan DJ, Eikelboom JW. Risk of recurrent venous thromboembolism in patients with common thrombophilia: a systematic review. *Arch Intern Med* 2006;166(7):729–36.
7 Vink R, Kraaijenhagen RA, Levi M, Büller HR. Individualized duration of oral anticoagulant therapy for deep vein thrombosis based on a decision model. *J Thromb Haemost* 2003;1(12):2523–30.

4 Molecular diagnostic approaches to hemostasis

Paula James and David Lillicrap

Introduction

The first coagulation factor gene, factor IX, was cloned and characterized in 1982, and since that time, progressive advances have been made in the use of molecular genetic strategies to assist in the diagnosis of coagulation disorders. This chapter summarizes the current state of molecular diagnostics for the more common hemostatic conditions, with a discussion of both hemorrhagic and thrombotic problems for which genetic tests are now available.

It is important to emphasize that, for most hemostatic conditions encountered in clinical practice, the initial diagnostic test of choice will still be one that is performed in a routine hemostasis laboratory. For example, the diagnosis of hemophilia A will still, in the vast majority of cases, be made using a factor VIII clotting assay. The role of molecular genetic testing for this condition will be to assist in genetic counseling and to provide predictive information relating to certain aspects of clinical management. To date, the number of conditions for which the initial diagnostic strategy demands a genetic test is small. One such example is the test for the prothrombin 20210 thrombophilic variant.

A second, general issue that merits brief discussion concerns the appropriate venue for molecular genetic testing for hemostatic disorders. The successful implementation of a molecular diagnostic service for hemostatic conditions requires access to appropriate expertise and technology, and these tests cannot readily be added to the repertoire of a routine clinical coagulation laboratory. Increasingly, optimal molecular genetic testing approaches incorporate methodologies that require access to expensive

equipment that will not be found in a hemostasis laboratory. However, genetic testing for hemostatic problems can easily be incorporated into a general molecular diagnostic facility, although the involvement of personnel with an additional interest in the phenotypic aspects of clotting is undoubtedly beneficial for optimizing testing strategies and test interpretation.

Molecular diagnostics of bleeding disorders

Molecular genetic testing for the hemophilias have been available since the cloning of the factor VIII and IX genes in 1984 and 1982, respectively [1,2]. Since then, with the cloning of all the known coagulation factor genes, molecular characterization of the rare inherited bleeding disorders has also been possible.

Hemophilia A

To date, all inherited cases of isolated factor VIII deficiency have been linked to mutations of the factor VIII locus, which is located at the telomeric end of the long arm of the X chromosome (Xq28) and encompasses 186 kilobases (kb) of genomic DNA (Fig. 4.1). The large size of the gene, which contains 26 exons, was originally a challenge for the development of molecular diagnostic testing. Two diagnostic strategies can be used to investigate this condition: an indirect test of transmission of the hemophilic FVIII gene (polymorphism linkage) and direct detection of the disease-causing mutation.

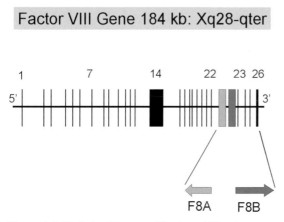

Factor VIII Gene 184 kb: Xq28-qter

1   7   14   22   23 26

5'   3'

F8A   F8B

Figure 4.1 The factor VIII gene and the two additional transcripts originating from the factor VIII genetic locus (F8A and F8B).

Polymorphism linkage analysis in hemophilia A

Although linkage analysis is used far less frequently than in the past, where there is a family history of hemophilia and informative intragenic polymorphisms are identified, polymorphism linkage testing can still be a useful and inexpensive strategy for performing carrier diagnosis and prenatal testing. However, linkage analysis is limited in its utility by a number of factors, the most frequently encountered of which are:

• an isolated case of hemophilia (lack of prior family history);
• the absence of informative polymorphic markers; and
• the problem of non-participating family members.

In an isolated case of hemophilia, linkage data can still be used to exclude further transmission of the mutant allele by the propositus. However, because the time at which the mutation arose within the pedigree is unclear, predictions about previous transmission of the mutant allele to others within the family are not possible. There are highly informative simple sequence repeat polymorphisms in introns 13 and 22 of the gene and a *Bcl*I dimorphism in intron 18. Together, these polymorphic markers are informative in approximately 90% of families tested, regardless of ethnic background. These studies can produce results for reporting within a few days from the receipt of the test

material, an interval that is acceptable for most prenatal testing situations.

If the assays for these markers are uninformative, further analysis of less frequent polymorphisms in introns 22 (*Xbal*) and 7 (G/A dimorphism) may also be helpful. The number of instances in which a linked extragenic polymorphism has to be used, with the accompanying risk of recombination, is fortunately very low.

Direct mutation testing for hemophilia A

With the rapid advancement of molecular genetic technology over the past decade, even genes as large and complex as factor VIII are now readily accessible to direct analysis of the disease-causing mutations. Extensive investigations since the cloning of the factor VIII gene have documented mutations at this locus in approximately 98% of patients with hemophilia A. To date, the only other genetic locus that has been associated with isolated factor VIII deficiency is the von Willebrand factor gene in type 2N von Willebrand disease (see below), although two different genes have been implicated in combined inherited factor V and VIII deficiency (LMAN1 and MCFD2). The current Internet-accessible Hemophilia A Mutation Database, HAMSTeRS (http://europium. csc.mrc.ac.uk/WebPages/Main/main.htm) lists more than 1000 different factor VIII mutations [3]. The majority of these changes represent single-nucleotide substitutions that have now been reported in all 26 exons of the gene. The database also lists many small [<200 nucleotides (nt)] and large deletions and a number of factor VIII gene insertions. A single factor VIII transcriptional mutation has been reported.

Rationale for direct mutation testing in hemophilia A

Genetic testing for hemophilia is still performed most frequently to determine the carrier status of potential heterozygous females and for prenatal diagnostic purposes. One of the most frequent groups of subjects for whom direct mutation testing is beneficial are those in whom an isolated report of severe hemophilia precludes the use of linkage analysis to track the mutant factor VIII gene. These individuals require direct mutation analysis to identify the carrier state and for accurate prenatal identification of affected offspring. Direct detection of the hemophilic mutation will also eliminate the uncertainties posed by potential germline mosaicism in the setting of a newly acquired mutation.

The second reason for pursuing the causative mutation in hemophilia A is the evidence that specific factor VIII genotypes are more predictive for the risk of acquiring a factor VIII inhibitor [4]. Patients with null genotypes (large deletions, nonsense mutations, and the factor VIII inversion mutations) have significantly higher risks for developing an inhibitor [between 20% (inversion mutations) and 70% (large, multidomain deletions)] than those whose hemophilia is caused by missense mutations, small deletions, and gene insertions for whom the risk of inhibitor development is less than 10%. Although the pathogenesis of inhibitor development is complex and multifactorial, given the clinical consequences of inhibitor development and the potential benefit of various forms of immune tolerance protocols, one can reasonably make the case for early mutation testing in all new severe cases of hemophilia A. Furthermore, there is also preliminary evidence that the outcome of immune tolerance protocols is also influenced significantly by the factor VIII genotype.

Strategies for direct mutation detection in hemophilia A

Two basic approaches can be taken to identifying the causative mutation in hemophilia A (Fig. 4.2) [5]:

1 A mutation screening strategy followed by sequencing of the abnormal region of the gene.
2 Direct sequencing of the factor VIII coding region.

A variety of screening techniques have now been developed for the detection of subtle mutations, including:

- single-strand conformation polymorphism analysis;
- denaturing gradient gel electrophoresis;
- chemical mismatch cleavage;
- conformation-sensitive gel electrophoresis;
- denaturing high-performance liquid chromatography; and
- DNA microarray analysis

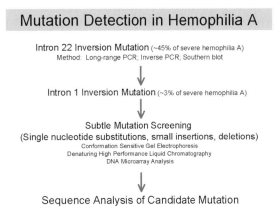

Figure 4.2 Molecular genetic testing algorithm for severe hemophilia A.

In laboratories using any one of these methods on a regular basis, the sensitivity for detecting point mutations is likely to be between 85% and 95%.

Following the identification of an abnormality in one region of the gene, the abnormal fragment can be sequenced (Fig. 4.3 and Plate 4.1). With the rapid development of automated sequencing technology, the cost and efficiency of direct sequence analysis has now improved to the point where this strategy is now being used routinely for factor VIII mutation detection by many molecular diagnostic laboratories.

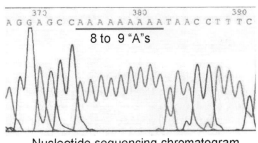

Nucleotide sequencing chromatogram

Exon 14 Factor VIII

"A" Insertion into a Run of Adenines—Frameshift

Figure 4.3 Sequencing chromatogram from a severe hemophilia A patient. In this woman, The factor VIII mutation is a single adenine insertion into a run of 8 adenine residues in exon 14. The "A" insertion results in a reading frameshift.

Factor VIII inversion mutations

There are two significant exceptions to the mutational heterogeneity of hemophilia A:

1 The intron 22 factor VIII inversion mutation, found in approximately 45% of patients with a severe hemophilia A phenotype [6]. This inversion involves exons 1–22 of the factor VIII gene and is caused by an intrachromosomal recombination event between a copy of the F8A gene within intron 22 of factor VIII and additional F8A copies approximately 400 kb 5′ (telomeric) of factor VIII. The inversion is only found in patients with a severe phenotype. In the molecular diagnostic laboratory, testing for the inversion mutation should be the first step in the analysis of any kindred affected by severe hemophilia A. The inversion can be detected with either a Southern blot (Fig. 4.4) or a long-range (>10 kb) inverse polymerase chain reaction (PCR)-based approach. The choice of methodology will depend on a combination of the amount and quality of the sample DNA and the laboratory expertise. In approximately 83% of cases, the recombination event will have been with the distal extragenic copy of F8A (type 1 inversions), in approximately 16% with the proximal F8A copy (type 2), and in approximately 1% of inversions rare rearrangement patterns are seen.

2 A second recurring factor VIII mutation is seen in ~3% of severe hemophilia A cases and involves an inversion event with sequences in intron 1 [7]. This mutation can readily be detected with a PCR-based approach.

Hemophilia B

All reported cases of hemophilia B have been linked to defects in the factor IX gene, which is centromeric to the factor VIII gene on the X chromosome (Xq27). As with hemophilia A, the inherited deficiency of factor IX demonstrates both phenotypic and mutational heterogeneity. The molecular diagnostic strategies employed for hemophilia B testing are similar to those discussed for hemophilia A, with the exception that, in hemophilia B, there is no single predominant mutation equivalent to the factor VIII inversions in hemophilia A.

Polymorphism linkage analysis in hemophilia B

The factor IX gene contains a number of polymorphisms that can be used for linkage analysis in kindreds in which hemophilia B is known to be segregating. There are no multiallelic repeat elements in the factor IX gene, and the ethnic variability of several of the factor IX polymorphisms is extreme. For instance, in Oriental populations, analysis of the intragenic markers is invariably uninformative.

Direct mutation testing for hemophilia B

In contrast to hemophilia A, where the large size of the gene has limited direct mutational analysis, most laboratories will now proceed to direct mutation analysis for the smaller and less complex factor IX gene (186 kb/26 exons for factor VIII vs. 34 kb/8 exons for factor IX). A worldwide Hemophilia B Mutation Database has been in existence since 1990, and the current Internet-accessible registry [8] lists information on more than 1000 different mutations in over 2500 patients, making hemophilia B one of the most extensively investigated monogenic diseases at the molecular genetic level. As with hemophilia A, most of the mutations resulting in this phenotype are single-nucleotide variations located throughout the gene from the promoter to the end of the coding region. In comparison with hemophilia A, missense mutations are a far more frequent cause of the clotting factor deficit in hemophilia B.

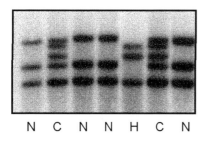

N C N N H C N

Factor VIII Intron 22 Inversion Mutation Southern Blot

Alternative Methodologies: Long-range PCR or inverse PCR

Figure 4.4 A Southern blot autoradiograph of the intron 22 inversion mutation in factor VIII, the cause of ~45% of the cases of severe hemophilia A. N, normal; H, hemophilia A due to the inversion mutation; and C, carrier female for the intron 22 inversion.

Hemophilia B mutations of particular clinical significance

Many of the factor IX missense mutations have provided knowledge of the basic structure and function correlates of the factor IX protein. However, several clinically important mutation types are worth highlighting from a molecular diagnostic standpoint.

The first group of mutations of note are a variety of gross factor IX gene deletions and rearrangements that result in severe hemophilia B. These can be complicated by the development of inhibitors and anaphylactic reactions to factor IX replacement therapy [9]. This constellation of findings has now been reported in small numbers of patients worldwide, and has further emphasized the proposal that all new cases of severe hemophilia B should be screened as soon as possible for gross factor IX deletions or rearrangements by both PCR and Southern blotting with a cDNA probe.

The second, recently described type of factor IX mutation with important clinical consequences involves missense mutations in the propeptide-encoding sequence, resulting in a markedly reduced affinity of the mutant protein for the vitamin K-dependent carboxylase [10]. Two different missense mutations have been described at amino acid residue −10 in the propeptide, and these patients have normal baseline factor IX levels but show marked sensitivity to treatment with vitamin K antagonists, leading to a significantly increased risk of bleeding on oral anticoagulant therapy.

The final group of factor IX mutations that merit recognition are those in the factor IX promoter (18 different point mutations have now been described in the approximately 40 nucleotides adjacent to the transcription start site). These mutations are associated with the hemophilia B Leyden phenotype, where factor IX deficiency undergoes at least a partial spontaneous phenotypic resolution following puberty, as a result of androgen-dependent factor IX gene expression [11]. For some of these mutations (e.g. nt ~6 G to A), the phenotype is less severe and patients appear to recover factor levels of approximately 30% by age 4 or 5 years. In contrast to the normal hemophilia B Leyden phenotype, four patients have been reported with a mutation at nt ~26, in whom no recovery of factor IX levels has been documented. Finally, at least one patient with a mutation at nt +13 in the Leyden-specific region of the promoter and with apparently normal sexual growth and development has failed to recover normal factor IX levels by middle age [12]. This case suggests that caution should be exercised in predicting phenotypic recovery in all instances of Leyden mutations.

von Willebrand disease (VWD)

VWD is the most common inherited bleeding disorder known in humans, and there has been much interest in the genetic pathology over the past decade. This is a complex hemostatic disorder and, despite significant advances in our understanding of molecular genetic mechanisms responsible for VWD, the role of molecular diagnostics for disease diagnosis is still somewhat limited. Furthermore, with 52 exons encompassing 178 kb of genomic DNA, molecular genetic analysis of the von Willebrand factor (VWF) gene has proved to be a significant challenge (Fig. 4.5). This testing is further complicated by the presence on chromosome 22 of a partial pseudogene sequence that replicates exons 23–34 of the chromosome 12 gene with 3% sequence variation [13,14]. Thus, any analysis of this region of the gene must ensure that PCR primers and probes are designed for the chromosome 12 gene. The final challenge in testing for and interpreting VWF genetic data is the extreme polymorphic nature of this gene. Indeed, in many instances, a clear distinction between neutral polymorphic changes and disease-causing variants is still unresolved.

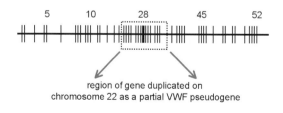

Figure 4.5 The VWF gene with an indication of the region of the gene (exons 23–34) that is duplicated on chromosome 22 in a partial pseudogene.

Type 3 VWD

Although this disorder is rare (prevalence of ~1 per million population), molecular studies of families with type 3 VWD represent one instance in which molecular diagnostics can be beneficial, as parents with children diagnosed with type 3 VWD may choose prenatal testing in future pregnancies. Given the recessive nature of this condition, the disease incidence is significantly higher in countries in which consanguinous marriages are more frequent.

Highly informative repeat sequence polymorphisms are available for linkage analysis, both within the VWF gene (intron 40) and in the 5′ flanking region of the gene. As with the hemophilias, an Internet-accessible mutation database is also maintained for VWD [15].

A review of this database and the current literature indicates that type 3 VWD can result from a variety of VWF gene mutations, all of which have the consequence of an absence of VWF protein in the plasma. The first group of type 3 mutations to be characterized were complete or partial deletions of the VWF gene. Type 3 patients with deletion mutation may develop anti-VWF antibodies on exposure to VWF replacement therapy, with the development of anaphylaxis in some patients. Thus, the screening of type 3 VWD patients for complete or partial VWF gene deletions with a strategy such as multiplex ligation-dependent probe amplification and/or cDNA Southern blotting might be helpful, both for direct mutation detection and also to evaluate the risk of anti-VWF antibody development. More extensive analysis of type 3 VWD patients has shown that some of these patients synthesize a mutant VWF protein that is presumably grossly misfolded and never leaves the cell of synthesis. Most of these missense mutants involve either the loss or gain of cysteine codons, and thus, disruption of dimer and/or multimer assembly is likely.

Type 2 VWD

Type 2 variants of VWD comprise approximately 15% of these patients in most surveys. Although initial investigation of these cases should rely on the use of standard coagulation tests to evaluate the VWF–factor VIII complex, molecular genetic analysis can be used to confirm or refute first diagnostic impressions (Fig. 4.6). Type 2A, 2B, and 2M VWD are transmitted as dominant traits with high penetrance, whereas type 2N disease is recessive in nature.

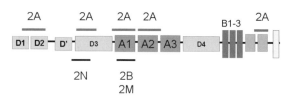

Figure 4.6 Diagram of the VWF protein (pro-polypeptide and mature subunit) with localization of the molecular defects responsible for type 2 VWD.

Type 2A VWD

Type 2A VWD involves loss of high-molecular-weight (HMW) VWF multimers and a resultant decrease in platelet-mediated VWF function.

Two molecular mechanisms have been described for type 2A disease:

1 In group 1, HMW multimers are synthesized ineffectively by the cell.

2 In group 2, HMW multimers secreted into the plasma are more susceptible to proteolysis by ADAMTS13.

Both forms of the disorder are the result of heterozygous missense mutations affecting regions of the VWF protein involved in dimer and multimer formation. Thus, to date, type 2A VWD mutations have been documented in the VWF propeptide, the D3, A1, A2, and C-terminal domains of the protein. Examination of VWF multimer patterns can, in some instances, predict where the mutations will be found.

In general, molecular diagnostic testing for type 2A VWD should be reserved for those cases in which phenotypic analysis, and particularly VWF:RCo, VWF multimer profiles and ristocin-induced platelet agglutination results are equivocal. No therapeutic benefit is derived from acquiring a molecular genetic diagnosis of type 2A disease.

Type 2B VWD

Type 2B VWD involves dominant gain-of-function changes, enhancing the affinity of mutant VWF for its platelet receptor, glycoprotein (Gp) Ib. These missense mutations are consistently clustered in the region of the gene encoding the A1 protein domain (rarely A2).

Direct sequencing of exon 28 sequences can provide molecular genetic confirmation of the type 2B phenotype. This region of the VWF gene is duplicated, with sequence variation, in the partial pseudogene on chromosome 22, and thus choice of amplification primers should take this fact into consideration. Ninety percent of type 2B VWD cases are caused by the missense mutations R1308C, R1306C, V1316M, and R1341Q.

Given the localized nature of type 2B mutations, molecular genetic confirmation of the phenotypic diagnosis is easily achieved through examination of exon 28 PCR products.

Type 2B VWD demonstrates hemostatic test results that are very similar to those seen in the dominantly inherited platelet disorder, platelet-type VWD. Molecular genetic analysis offers a definitive approach to differentiating between these two conditions (see below).

Type 2M VWD

The type 2M VWD variant has reduced platelet-mediated VWF function with normal VWF multimers. Here again, as with type 2B disease, the molecular pathology represents a variety of missense mutations localized to exon 28, the A1 domain-coding region of the gene. Type 2M disease is essentially the loss-of-function equivalent of type 2B VWD, with the A1 substitutions resulting in disruption of the interaction with platelet GpIb. As with type 2B disease, genetic confirmation of the type 2M phenotype can be achieved through exon 28 sequencing.

Type 2N VWD

Type 2N VWD is a recessively inherited trait. This condition should be considered in the differential diagnosis of mild–moderate isolated factor VIII deficiency and can easily be confused with mild hemophilia A. Phenotypic testing involves a direct assessment of the FVIII binding potential of VWF using a microtiter plate-based assay. The most efficient molecular genetic approach to confirm a diagnosis of type 2N disease is to sequence the PCR products amplified from exons 18–25 of the VWF gene, the region encoding the N-terminal D'/D3 factor VIII binding domains of VWF. In patients with type 2N VWD, this analysis will show either homozygous or compound heterozygous missense mutations affecting the factor VIII binding domain of the protein. In addition, coinheritance of a type 2N allele with a severe type 1 or type 3 null allele

will also result in this phenotype. The R854Q missense mutation is the most frequent type 2N variant, resulting in factor VIII levels around 20%. Levels of factor VIII of approximately 10% are seen with some of the other mutations, such as R816W and T791M.

Type 1 VWD

Despite being the most prevalent form of the disorder, representing approximately 75% of all VWD cases, the molecular pathogenesis of type 1 VWD remains the least well understood. Diagnosis can often be difficult and is influenced by a variety of factors, including the temporal variability of VWF levels and the ABO blood group of patients, accounting for approximately 30% of the variability in VWF levels, with blood group O subjects having the lowest levels. Another significant complicating factor in attempting to address the genetic basis for type 1 VWD is the marked variability in penetrance and expression of the phenotype within families, which makes the use of classic linkage analysis problematic. Therefore, much of the knowledge gained in this area has relied on labor-intensive strategies, such as direct sequencing of genomic DNA.

The recent completion of 3 population-based studies of the molecular genetic pathology of type 1 VWD has provided information from 300 patients with this diagnosis [16–18]. The findings from these studies have been similar and demonstrate the following:
• The type 1 VWD phenotype is linked to the VWF gene in approximately 60% of families.
• Candidate VWF gene mutations can be found in approximately 65% of type 1 VWD patients.
• More than 100 different candidate VWF gene mutations have been identified.
• Approximately 65% of the candidate VWF mutations are missense substitutions.
• Candidate VWF gene mutations are found throughout the VWF locus from the 5' flanking region to the C-terminal domain of the protein.
• In approximately 15% of patients, more than a single candidate VWF mutation is present.

An analysis of the mutations found in the three population studies has also shown that certain candidate mutations are recurrent. This group of mutations includes Y1584C (found in between 8% and 25% of the type 1 VWD population), R924Q, R1205H, R1315C, R1374H, and R854Q. Suffice it to say that, even with these common variants, the understanding of pathogenic mechanisms is incomplete.

The information derived from these initial molecular surveys of type 1 VWD indicate that, in addition to incomplete penetrance and variable expressivity, the genetics of this complex trait is further complicated by mutational and locus heterogeneity. Whereas most type 1 cases with plasma VWF levels <30% will demonstrate candidate VWF mutations, patients with mild VWF deficiency (30–50%) are more likely to have a phenotype in which contributions from several loci (including the ABO blood group locus) are playing an important pathogenic role. To date, the identity of these additional genetic modifiers is unknown.

Given the size and complexity of the VWF gene and the problems of mutational and locus heterogeneity, the application of molecular genetic analysis to the diagnosis of type 1 VWD is not currently warranted. This situation may change with further advances in technology and the potential identification of key genetic modifiers.

Less common inherited coagulation factor deficiencies

As the genes for all of the procoagulant proteins have been cloned and characterized, molecular genetic testing is feasible for the inherited deficiency of any of these factors. However, the diagnosis of these disorders (factor XI and X deficiencies and others) remains firmly based in the clinical hemostasis laboratory through the performance of biological clotting assays.

Although specific research laboratories may be interested in determining the disease-causing mutations in these families, primarily as a means to assist in structure and function analysis, the performance of these tests for diagnostic purposes is not usual. An exception is the documentation of mutations in the LMAN1 and MCFD2 genes in patients with inherited combined factor V and VIII deficiencies. Most cases of this rare disorder are caused by one of several recurring point mutations in these intermediate compartment processing proteins; thus, documentation of one of these mutations would definitively establish an otherwise unusual diagnosis.

Inherited platelet disorders

As with the less common coagulation factor deficiencies, the diagnosis of inherited platelet disorders is predominantly by phenotypic analysis. Standard morphology, platelet aggregation studies, and an evaluation of platelet receptor density will usually establish or exclude a diagnosis of Bernard–Soulier syndrome or Glanzmann's thrombasthenia, the two most frequently encountered, but nevertheless rare, recessive inherited platelet disorders [19].

In unusual instances, knowledge of the causative mutation in these patients could be useful, perhaps for prenatal testing. In the Bernard–Soulier syndrome, a heterogeneous mutational pattern has been documented, with both homozygous and compound heterozygous mutations identified in the genes encoding Gp Ibα, Ibβ, and IX [19]. A variety of different mutations has been found at these loci, including deletions, frameshifts, and nonsense and missense changes. To date, no Bernard–Soulier mutations have been identified in the GpV gene.

In Glanzmann's thrombasthenia, a similarly varied pattern of mutations has been documented in the genes for Gp IIb and IIIa.

As alluded to above, the standard coagulation studies in platelet-type (pseudo) VWD (PT-VWD) are very similar to those encountered in patients with type 2B VWD. Here, clarification of the diagnosis most effectively involves molecular genetic analysis of exon 28 of the VWF gene (for type 2B VWD missense mutations) and the GpIbα gene (for PT-VWD) [20]. In PT-VWD, heterozygous dominant missense mutations can be found in the GpIbα gene, which have been shown through the analysis of recombinant mutant protein to possess an increased binding affinity for the A1 domain of VWF. One partial deletion mutation in GpIbα has also been identified as being causative for PT-VWD.

Molecular diagnostics for thrombotic disease

Although an inherited tendency for excessive bleeding can often be ascribed to single gene abnormalities, there is ample evidence to suggest that, in contrast, the clinical manifestations of hypercoagulability are usually the result of adverse interactions between multiple genes and the environment [21]. Thus, the use of molecular diagnostics to document markers of thrombotic risk (thrombophilia) will prove to be far more challenging than with the inherited hemorrhagic disorders. To further complicate matters, despite the fact that with appropriate testing, thrombophilic mutations can be identified in approximately 50% of patients following a first clinical episode of venous thromboembolism, interpretation of these results remains problematic in some cases.

Over the past decade, after an initial enthusiasm to use molecular testing for the identification of thrombophilic traits, more recent analysis has tended to be far more conservative with the application of this diagnostic approach. In particular, the presence of a strong family history of thrombotic disease is probably, on its own, a significant predictor of risk, and likely represents the combined influences of known and currently unresolved genetic factors responsible for this phenotype.

Inherited resistance to activated protein C: Factor V Leiden

Until 1994, the investigation of patients with clinical evidence of hypercoagulability was usually unproductive. However, with the discovery by Dahlback and Hildebrand of an inherited form of resistance to the proteolytic effects of activated protein C [22], and the subsequent finding of a common missense mutation in the factor V gene by Bertina and colleagues in Leiden [23], a major advance was made in the laboratory assessment of thrombotic risk.

The Leiden mutation substitutes a glutamine for an arginine at amino acid residue 506 in factor V, the initial cleavage site for activated protein C. The mutation is readily detected by a number of PCR-based approaches. Between 2% and 5% of individuals in Western populations have been documented to be heterozygous for factor V Leiden. In contrast, the mutation is extremely rare in subjects of Asian and African descent.

In some laboratories, initial screening for resistance to activated protein C is performed using the prolongation of an activated partial thromboplastin time-based

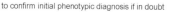

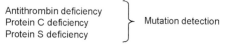

Figure 4.7 Molecular genetic testing approaches for thrombophilic traits.

assay as an indicator; patients testing positive (prolongation in the presence of factor V-deficient plasma) are subsequently evaluated by a PCR assay (Fig. 4.7).

Increasingly, where access to PCR-based molecular analysis is routine, laboratories will more often choose to proceed directly to the genetic test, as the result is definitive and more than 95% of activated protein C resistance is a result of this single mutation. Rare, alternative factor V mutations have been documented at arginine 306 (Arg to Thr and Arg to Gly), but it seems unlikely that these variants are significant markers of a thrombotic risk.

Persons heterozygous for the factor V Leiden mutation have an approximately five-fold increased relative risk of venous thrombosis. It is found in 15–20% of patients experiencing their first episode of venous thrombosis and in 50–60% of thrombosis patients with a family history of thrombotic disease. The hypercoagulable phenotype associated with factor V Leiden shows incomplete penetrance, and some individuals may never manifest a clinical thrombotic event. In contrast to the increased relative risk for an initial venous thrombotic event associated with factor V Leiden, this genetic variant is not associated with increased risks for either arterial thrombosis or a recurrence of venous thrombosis. Coinheritance of other inherited thrombotic risk factors or exposure to environmental risk factors (i.e. oral contraceptives) can dramatically enhance the thrombotic risk in carriers of factor V Leiden. Many clinicians test for this disorder in patients with a family history of thrombosis who are about to be exposed to an acquired thrombotic risk factor. Individuals homozygous for the mutation have a 70-fold enhanced relative risk of venous thrombosis, indicating that this phenotype is transmitted as a codominant trait.

Prothrombin 20210 3′ non-coding sequence variant

In 1996, Poort and colleagues described an association between a G to A nucleotide polymorphism at position 20210 in the 3′ untranslated region (UTR) of the prothrombin gene, increased plasma levels of prothrombin, and an enhanced risk for venous thrombosis [24]. This polymorphic nucleotide substitution is at the very end of the 3′ UTR and exerts its effect on prothrombin levels in the heterozygous state. Although the plasma levels of prothrombin in subjects heterozygous for this polymorphism are higher on average than those in individuals with a normal prothrombin genotype, levels are usually still within the normal range. As a consequence, this polymorphism can only be evaluated by genetic testing, which is achieved by a PCR-based assay, most often now involving a form of real-time quantitative assay.

As with the factor V Leiden genotype, the prevalence of the prothrombin 20210 G to A variant in the general population is relatively high at 1–5%. This variant is also rare in persons of Asian and African descent. The heterozygous state is associated with a two- to four-fold increase in the relative risk for venous thrombosis. There is no influence on venous thrombotic recurrence or arterial thrombosis.

Thermolabile C677T 5,10-methylene-tetrahydrofolate reductase variant

The third, high-prevalence genetic variant that was initially thought to be associated with an increased thrombotic risk is the C to T variant at nucleotide 677 (an alanine to valine substitution) in the 5,10-methylene-tetrahydrofolate reductase (MTHFR) gene. This genotype results in expression of an enzyme with increased thermolability. Homozygosity for the variant is associated with hyperhomocysteinemia, particularly in the presence of folate deficiency. In many populations (southern Europeans and Hispanic Americans),

approximately 10% of subjects are homozygous for the C677T variant, a sequence change that can easily be detected by a PCR-based strategy. After further extended analysis, in contrast to the factor V Leiden and prothrombin 20210 variants, the role of the MTHFR C677T polymorphism as an independent risk factor for venous thromboembolism appears minor.

Deficiencies of antithrombin, protein C, and protein S

Deficiencies of the major anticoagulant proteins antithrombin, protein C, and protein S have long been known to represent individual risk factors for the development of venous thromboembolism. The protein deficiencies manifest thrombotic phenotypes in the heterozygous state, but penetrance and expression of the phenotype are extremely variable and relate to both the individual protein deficiency (antithrombin deficiency being the most severe condition) and the specific molecular defect. Homozygosity for antithrombin and protein C deficiencies results in the severe neonatal thrombotic condition, pupura fulminans.

Diagnosis of these three disorders relies on standard functional tests or immunoassays that should be performed in the diagnostic hemostasis laboratory. All three of the deficiency states are associated with significant mutational heterogeneity, and routine molecular diagnostic investigation of these mutations is not warranted. However, these are lifelong diagnoses, and if any doubt exists about the phenotypic test results, confirmation of the diagnosis by genetic testing should be considered (Fig. 4.7).

The role of genetic testing in the clinical management of oral anticoagulation

Studies in the past couple of years have now indicated that individual anticoagulant responses to the vitamin K antagonist, Coumadin (Warfarin), can be predicted to some extent through the analysis of genotypes for two proteins involved in the metabolism of this drug: cytochrome P-450 2C9 (CYP2C9) and vitamin K epoxide-reductase complex 1 (VKORC1). Analysis of polymorphic haplotypes of the CYP2C9 and VKORC1 genes by PCR testing has been shown to be helpful in identifying patients who may be especially sensitive to oral anticoagulant administration [25]. This appears to be particularly the case for VKORC1 analysis during the initiation phase of oral anticoagulation. Thus, rapidly reported VKORC1 genotyping may prove to be a useful adjunctive testing strategy to international normalized ratio testing in this clinical situation; and, indeed, in the United States, the Food and Drug Administration have recommended that this laboratory-monitoring approach be added to the drug insert information.

The future for diagnostic molecular hemostasis

With the completion of the Human Genome Project and the ongoing analysis of complex genetic traits through the performance of genome-wide association studies, additional information pertaining to genetic influences on hemostasis is likely to be derived in the next few years. This fact, along with further advances in genetic methodologies, including more accessible microarray-based testing approaches may well provide further opportunities for the application of molecular diagnostic testing in the area of clinical hemostasis. However, as has already been witnessed with thrombophilic testing, initial enthusiasm for test adoption will need to be tempered by formal evidence of clinical benefit deriving from the tests. Indeed there is a significant possibility that the major genetic influences on most hemostatic phenotypes have already been identified and that any new associations are unlikely to play a clinically important role. An area where this possibility may well be tested in the next decade is that of genetic risk factors for arterial thrombosis. To date, very little benefit can be derived from genetic testing for this phenotype, and it may well be that the combined genetic and environmental background of this condition will be too complex for the useful application of a genetic testing strategy.

References

1 Gitschier J, Wood WI, Goralka TM, et al. Characterization of the human factor VIII gene. *Nature* 1984;312:326–30.

2 Kurachi K, Davie EW. Isolation and characterization of a cDNA coding for human factor IX. *Proc Natl Acad Sci USA* 1982;79:6461–4.

3 HAMSTeRS: The Haemophilia A Mutation, Structure, Test and Resource Site. 2008. http://europium. csc.mrc.ac.uk/WebPages/Main/main.htm.

4 Goodeve AC, Peake IR. The molecular basis of hemophilia A: genotype-phenotype relationships and inhibitor development. *Semin Thromb Hemost* 2003;29:23–30.

5 Keeney S, Mitchell M, Goodeve A. The molecular analysis of haemophilia A: a guideline from the UK haemophilia centre doctors' organization haemophilia genetics laboratory network. *Haemophilia* 2005;11: 387–97.

6 Lakich D, Kazazian HH Jr, Antonarakis SE, Gitschier J. Inversions disrupting the factor VIII gene are a common cause of severe haemophilia A. *Nat Genet* 1993;5:236–41.

7 Bagnall RD, Waseem N, Green PM, Giannelli F. Recurrent inversion breaking intron 1 of the factor VIII gene is a frequent cause of severe hemophilia A. *Blood* 2002;99:168–74.

8 Haemophilia B Mutation Database: Version 13. 2008. http://www.kcl.ac.uk/ip/petergreen/haemBdatabase. html.

9 Thorland EC, Drost JB, Lusher JM, et al. Anaphylactic response to factor IX replacement therapy in haemophilia B patients: complete gene deletions confer the highest risk. *Haemophilia* 1999;5: 101–5.

10 Oldenburg J, Quenzel EM, Harbrecht U, et al. Missense mutations at ALA-10 in the factor IX propeptide: an insignificant variant in normal life but a decisive cause of bleeding during oral anticoagulant therapy. *Br J Haematol* 1997;98:240–4.

11 Picketts DJ, Mueller CR, Lillicrap D. Transcriptional control of the factor IX gene: analysis of five cis-acting elements and the deleterious effects of naturally occurring hemophilia B Leyden mutations. *Blood* 1994;84:2992–3000.

12 James PD, Stakiw J, Leggo J, Walker I, Lillicrap D. A case of non-resolving hemophilia B Leyden in a 42-year-old male (F9 promoter + 13 A>G). *J Thromb Haemost* 2008;6:885–6.

13 Mancuso DJ, Tuley EA, Westfield LA, et al. Structure of the gene for human von Willebrand factor. *J Biol Chem* 1989;264:19514–27.

14 Mancuso DJ, Tuley EA, Westfield LA, et al. Human von Willebrand factor gene and pseudogene: structural analysis and differentiation by polymerase chain reaction. *Biochemistry* 1991;30:253–69.

15 ISTH SSC VWF Database. 2008. http://www.vwf.group.shef.ac.uk/.

16 Goodeve A, Eikenboom J, Castaman G, et al. Phenotype and genotype of a cohort of families historically diagnosed with type 1 von Willebrand disease in the European study, Molecular and Clinical Markers for the Diagnosis and Management of Type 1 von Willebrand Disease (MCMDM-1VWD). *Blood* 2007;109:112–21.

17 James PD, Notley C, Hegadorn C, et al. The mutational spectrum of type 1 von Willebrand disease: Results from a Canadian cohort study. *Blood* 2007;109:145–54.

18 Cumming A, Grundy P, Keeney S, et al. An investigation of the von Willebrand factor genotype in UK patients diagnosed to have type 1 von Willebrand disease. *Thromb Haemost* 2006;96:630–41.

19 Nurden P, Nurden AT. Congenital disorders associated with platelet dysfunctions. *Thromb Haemost* 2008;99:253–63.

20 Othman M, Lillicrap D. Distinguishing between non-identical twins: platelet type andtype 2B von Willebrand disease. *Br J Haematol* 2007;138:665–6.

21 Reitsma PH, Rosendaal FR. Past and future of genetic research in thrombosis. *J Thromb Haemost* 2007;5(Suppl 1):264–9.

22 Dahlback B, Hildebrand B. Inherited resistance to activated protein C is corrected by anticoagulant cofactor activity found to be a property of factor V. *Proc Natl Acad Sci USA* 1994;91:1396–400.

23 Bertina RM, Koeleman BP, Koster T, et al. Mutation in blood coagulation factor V associated with resistance to activated protein C. *Nature* 1994;369:64–7.

24 Poort SR, Rosendaal FR, Reitsma PH, Bertina RM. A common genetic variation in the 3'-untranslated region of the prothrombin gene is associated with elevated plasma prothrombin levels and an increase in venous thrombosis. *Blood* 1996;88:3698–703.

25 Schwarz UI, Ritchie MD, Bradford Y, et al. Genetic determinants of response to warfarin during initial anticoagulation. *N Engl J Med* 2008;358:999–1008.

5 Tests of platelet function

Paul Harrison

Structure of platelets

Human blood platelets are small, anucleated cells that play a critical role in hemostasis and thrombosis. Human platelets normally circulate for approximately 10 days, constantly surveying the integrity of the vessel wall. Normal human platelets are small and discoid in shape (0.5×3.0 μm), have a mean volume of 7–11 fL, and normally circulate in relatively high numbers between 150 and 400×10^9/L.

A cross-section of a typical discoid platelet is shown in Fig. 5.1.

Function

Their small disc shape enables the platelets to be marginated toward the edge of vessels so that the majority circulate adjacent to the vascular endothelial cells that line all blood vessels. Upon detection of vessel wall damage, they undergo rapid but controlled adhesion, activation, and aggregation to form a hemostatic plug and thus rapidly prevent blood loss.

Endothelial cells produce a number of potent antiplatelet substances (e.g. nitric oxide, prostacyclin, and CD39) that normally inhibit vessel wall–platelet interactions. Vessel wall damage exposes highly adhesive substrates [e.g. P selectin, Von Willebrand factor (VWF), collagen, and many other extracellular matrix components], which result in a sequence of stepwise events resulting in the formation of a hemostatic plug (Plate 5.1):

- Initial adhesion, transient rolling of platelets along the vessel wall, and slowing of the cells. Consequently, platelets are more likely to undergo stable adhesion.
- Stable adhesion through additional receptor–ligand interactions.
- Platelet activation (if there is more extensive damage or stimuli-promoting platelet activation).
- Platelet aggregation (Plate 5.1).
- Generation of platelet procoagulant activity and stabilization of the hemostatic plug.
- Clot retraction.

The platelets interact with and sense the environment through many types of surface receptors (major receptors and their ligands are summarized in Table 5.1). The net balance between activating or inhibitory stimuli thus controls whether platelets continue to circulate, begin to reversibly interact with the vessel wall, or become irreversibly adherent to either the vessel wall or each other.

During adhesion, platelets become activated through signal transduction pathways, which mediate shape change, degranulation, and spreading upon areas of exposed subendothelium. Activated platelets recruit additional platelets into the growing platelet aggregate or thrombus via a number of positive feedback pathways, including release of dense granular adenosine diphosphate (ADP) and generation of thromboxane. Activated platelets also express negatively charged phospholipids on their surface, facilitating the local generation of high amounts of thrombin, which not only further activates other platelets, but also stabilizes the platelet plug through fibrin formation. In this manner, platelets rapidly seal any areas of vessel wall damage and provide a catalytic surface for coagulation to occur, resulting in the formation of a stable hemostatic plug.

Thrombosis is usually the consequence of inappropriate activation of platelets, especially in regions of abnormal vessel wall lesions or damage (e.g. atherosclerotic plaques). The high shear stress that

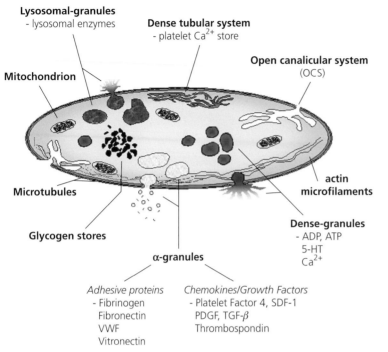

Figure 5.1 Platelet structure and organelles. This diagram summarizes the key structural elements of a platelet, including the open canalicular system (OCS), the dense tubular system (DTS), action microfilaments and microtubules, mitochondria, glycogen stores, dense granules, lysosomes, and alpha granules. (Reproduced with permission from Watson S, Harrison P. The vascular function of platelets. In: Hoffbrand V, Tuddenham E, Catovsky D, eds. *Postgraduate Haematology* (5th Edition). Oxford: Blackwell, 2005:813.)

often occurs in these regions also significantly contributes to thrombus formation (via promotion of VWF-dependent platelet adhesion and aggregation) along with the events described above.

Anti-platelet drug therapy thus provides an important means to prevent thrombosis in high-risk patients with arterial disease. In contrast, there are also many defects in platelet function that can occur in patients, often resulting in an increased risk of bleeding.

Classification of platelet defects

Platelet abnormalities can be broadly classified into quantitative (abnormal in number) and qualitative defects (abnormal in function). Defects in number include many types of thrombocytopenia (e.g. caused by immune or nonimmune destruction or decreased production) and thrombocytosis (increased platelet number). Functional defects can either be inherited or more commonly acquired (secondary to disease, surgical procedures or drugs, and anti-platelet therapy).

Inherited platelet-related disorders include many abnormalities, such as the following:

- defects in various platelet receptors for both adhesive proteins and soluble agonists;
- defects in adhesive proteins that mediate platelet adhesion and aggregation;
- defects in the storage or release of platelet granules;
- defects in signal transduction pathways;
- defects in exposure of negatively charged phospholipid; or
- inherited thrombocytopenias.

Table 5.2 summarizes the classification of inherited platelet function defects.

Platelet function testing

Before platelet function tests are performed, the full clinical history (including family and recent drug-taking history) is obtained and a physical examination of the patient is performed. Platelet disorders are usually associated with excessive bleeding (especially after trauma), and other classic symptoms including petechiae, epistaxis, and menorrhagia. Coagulation protein defects, in contrast, are usually associated with a delayed pattern of bleeding and the presence of hemarthroses and hematomas.

Table 5.1 Major platelet agonists and their surface receptors.*

Agonist	Receptor	Effect and physiological role
Adhesion molecules		
Collagen	Gp VI	Major signaling receptor for collagen
	$\alpha_2\beta_1$	Supports adhesion by collagen
Fibrinogen	$\alpha_{IIb}\beta_3$	Aggregation, spreading and clot retraction
Fibronectin	$\alpha_5\beta_1$, $\alpha_{IIb}\beta_3$	$\alpha_5\beta_1$ mediates adhesion
Laminin	$\alpha_6\beta_1$	Adhesion
von Willebrand factor	Gp Ib-IX-V, $\alpha_{IIb}\beta_3$	Platelet tethering (also fibrinogen)
Amines		
Adrenaline	α_2	
5-HT	5-HT_{2A}	Mediates vasoconstriction
Cytokines		
TPO	c-Mpl	Maturation of megakaryocytes
Immune complexes		
Fc portion of antibodies	$Fc\gamma RIIA$	Immune-based platelet activation
Lipids		
Lysophospholipids		
PAF	PAF	
Prostacyclin	IP	Endothelial-mediated inhibition
Sphingosine 1-phosphate		
Thromboxanes	TP	Major positive feedback agonist
Nucleotides		
Adenosine	A_{2A}	
ADP	$P2Y_1$	Early role in platelet activation
	$P2Y_{12}$	Major positive feedback receptor
ATP	$P2X_1$	Possible early role in platelet activation
Proteases		
Thrombin	PAR_1, PAR_4	Coagulation-dependent platelet activation
Surface molecules		
CD40 ligand	CD40 and $\alpha_{IIb}\beta_3$	
Tyrosine kinase receptors		
Angiopoietin 1 and 2	Tie-1	
EphrinB1	EphA4 and EphB1	Late events in platelet activation?
Vitamin K-dependent		
Gas6	Sky, Axl and Mer	Supports platelet activation?

*Platelets express a remarkable number and variety of receptors for a wide range of ligands. For many of these receptor–ligand combinations, however, the effect on platelet activation is weak and of uncertain significance. [Reproduced with permission from Watson S, Harrison P. The Vascular function of platelets. In: Hoffbrand V, Tuddenham E, Catovsky D, eds. *Postgraduate Haematology* (5th Edition). Oxford: Blackwell, 2004:819.]

As many patients present with a transiently acquired defect of platelet function (e.g. often caused by aspirin or diet), repeat testing is often necessary to ensure correct results and diagnosis. If a hemostatic defect is suspected, then laboratories will use a range of initial screening tests. These tests include:

• full blood count and blood film;
• coagulation tests [prothrombin time (PT), activated partial thromboplastin time (APTT), and thrombin time (TT)];
• bleeding time or platelet function analysis with the PFA-100® (as the in vivo bleeding time is considered

Table 5.2 Classification of inherited platelet defects.

Defect	Disorder
Platelet adhesion	Bernard–Soulier syndrome
	Von Willebrand disease
Platelet aggregation	Glanzmann thrombasthenia
	Congenital afibrinogenemia
Platelet activation (receptor defects)	Collagen receptor defects: $\alpha_2\beta_1$ or Gp VI deficiency
	ADP receptor defects: $P2Y_{12}$ deficiency
	Thromboxane receptor defects
Secretion defects	Storage pool disease
	Hermansky–Pudlak syndrome
	Chédiak–Higashi syndrome
	Grey platelet syndrome
	Quebec platelet disorder
	Wiskott–Aldrich syndrome
Signaling pathways	$G\alpha q$ deficiency
	Cyclooxygenase deficiency
	Phospholipase C deficiency
	Thromboxane synthase deficiency
	Lipoxygenase deficiency
	Calcium mobilization defects
Platelet size	Inherited macrothrombocytopenia
Membrane phospholipids	Scott syndrome

unreliable, some laboratories are now beginning to use in vitro alternatives, such as the PFA-100® or Impact® device, see below);

• light transmission platelet aggregation (still considered the gold standard although time-consuming; some laboratories use whole blood impedance aggregometry as an alternative); and

• factor VIII/VWF levels.

The biggest problems still faced by platelet function testing are a number of quality-control issues, including anticoagulation, sample quality, sample handling (collection and processing and lack of standardization of methodologies used).

Platelets are not only prone to artefactual in vitro activation but also to desensitization. Most functional tests have to be performed relatively quickly (e.g. less than 2 hours from sampling). It is also impossible to use standard quality-control material apart from freshly drawn blood from healthy normal volunteers.

Global tests of platelet function

Bleeding time

The skin bleeding time has been clinically used for almost a century and has been modified several times in attempts to improve reliability. Briefly, a constant blood pressure of 40 mm Hg is applied to the upper arm, and a disposable, sterile, automated template device is applied to inflict standardized cuts into the forearm. Excess blood is then removed with filter paper at regular intervals, and the time for the cessation of bleeding recorded. Normal bleeding times are less than 10 minutes. Prolonged bleeding times are encountered in patients with severe platelet defects, and so the test has been widely used as a screening tool.

The clear advantages of the bleeding time are that it is a simple test of natural hemostasis including the important contribution of the vessel wall and it also avoids potential anticoagulation artefacts. The disadvantages are that bleeding time results can be both poorly reproducible and insensitive to milder forms of platelet dysfunction.

The consensus is that the test does not necessarily correlate well with the bleeding risk and that an accurate clinical history is more valuable. A number of different in vitro methods have therefore been devised to try to measure global platelet function within whole blood exposed to conditions that attempt to simulate in vivo hemostasis, such as the PFA-100®.

Platelet function analyzer: PFA-100®

This analyzer, developed by Dade–Behring, is based on the original principle and prototype instrument described by Kratzer and Born. Widespread experience with the instrument is increasing, but how the test should be used within normal laboratory practice remains to be fully defined.

All test components are within disposable cartridges that are loaded into the instrument at the start of the test. Citrated whole blood (800 μL) is pipetted into the cartridge and, after a short incubation period, exposed to high shear (5000–6000/s) through a capillary tube before encountering a membrane with a central aperture of 150 μm diameter. The membrane is coated with collagen and either ADP or epinephrine. The instrument monitors the drop in flow rate as platelets form a hemostatic plug that seals the aperture and stops blood flow. This parameter is recorded as the closure time (CT). The maximal value obtainable is 300 s.

To ensure optimal PFA-100® performance and data interpretation, there are a number of quality-control procedures and good practice guidelines that need to be kept in mind:

• Mandatory daily instrument checks; PFA-100® self-test should always be performed.
• Ensuring the quality of blood sampling.
• Ensuring consistency in anticoagulation, 3.8% (0.129 mol/L) or 3.2% (0.105 mol/L) buffered trisodium citrate.
• Checking for cartridge batch variation.
• Testing within 4 hours of sampling.
• Always perform a full blood count to help interpret the results.
• A control group within each laboratory setting should be established. These individuals should ideally exhibit CTs within the middle of the established laboratory reference range.
• Each laboratory should also ideally establish their own reference ranges on both cartridges using normal volunteers from their institution.

Typical normal ranges obtained with 3.8% trisodium citrate are 58–151 s for collagen/ADP and 94–202 s for collagen/epinephrine. With 3.2% trisodium citrate, typical ranges are 55–112 s for collagen/ADP and 79–164 s for collagen/epinephrine (Oxford Hemophilia and Thrombosis Centre, unpublished results).

Within-sample coefficients of variation (CVs) have been reported as approximately 10%, which, although acceptable for a platelet function test, may obviously cause problems with values obtained close to upper normal range cut-off values.

The advantages of the test are that it is simple, rapid, and does not require specialist training (apart from training in the manipulation of blood samples). It is a potential screening tool for assessing patients with many types of platelet abnormality. Within a typical population of patients tested, the overall negative predictive value of the test can be high (more than 90%), although the test is clearly not 100% sensitive to all platelet defects. The test is particularly useful in pediatric settings where the availability of blood is often a limiting factor, particularly for potentially assessing platelet function in nonaccidental injury cases. Given the high shear conditions to which platelets are ex-

posed during the test, it is not surprising that the test is highly VWF-dependent and is useful not only for detecting VWD, but also for monitoring therapy, particularly with DDAVP. The instrument thus provides laboratories with a limited but optional screening tool that gives rapid and reliable data with a high negative predictive value.

A number of studies suggest that the PFA-100® is a potential in vitro replacement of the bleeding time. The disadvantages are that, like the in vivo bleeding time, the test is sensitive to both the platelet count and hematocrit, and it is therefore crucial that a full blood count is performed to help interpret abnormal results. The test is usually insensitive to coagulation protein defects, including afibrinogenemia, hemophilia A and B, and other clotting factors. False-negative results are sometimes obtained; for example, in patients with storage pool disease, primary secretion defects, Hermansky–Pudlak syndrome, type 1 VWD, and the Quebec platelet disorder. Diagnosis of these disorders could therefore be missed if relying on the PFA-100® as a screening test alone. In patients with apparently normal platelet function, the instrument has also been shown to occasionally give false-positive results, which then require further detailed testing.

Many studies are also in progress to assess whether the PFA-100® can reliably predict either thrombotic or bleeding complications in different patient groups. As more interlaboratory experience is gathered, eventually it should be feasible to define the exact role(s) for this instrument in routine laboratory testing. A recent ISTH SSC document by Hayward and colleagues (2006) provides a useful up-to-date consensus review of the utility of the test.

Impact® Cone and Plate(let) Analyzer

The cone and plate(let) analyzer originally developed by Varon and colleagues monitors platelet adhesion and aggregation to a plate coated with collagen or extracellular matrix under high shear conditions of $1800\ s^{-1}$. In the commercial version of the device, the Impact®, a plastic plate is used instead. The test is now fully automated, simple to operate, uses a small quantity of citrated whole blood (0.12 mL), and displays results within 6 minutes. The instrument contains a microscope and performs staining and image analysis of platelets that have adhered and aggregated on the plate. The software permits storage of the images from each analysis and records a number of parameters, including surface coverage, average size, and distribution histogram of the adhered platelets. There is also a research version of the instrument, called the Impact-R®, that requires some of the steps to be manually performed and facilitates adjustment of the shear rate. To ensure optimal Impact® performance and data interpretation, many of the quality-control procedures and good practice guidelines used for the PFA-100® also apply. Typical normal ranges are 7.8–19% for Surface Coverage and 35–70 μm^2 for aggregate size within 3.2% citrated blood, and typical CVs are <15% (Oxford Hamophilia and Thrombosis Centre, unpublished results).

Preliminary data suggest that the test can also potentially be used for the screening of platelet defects and VWD and monitoring anti-platelet therapy. The test is dependent on the platelet count and hematocrit, and a full blood count should always be performed. As the test also measures platelet adhesion to polystyrene, it also important to be aware that fibrinogen is also an important variable within the test. Because the commercial test has only been available for a relatively short time, widespread experience is still limited at present. The overall sensitivity and specificity of the Impact® as a screening test remains to be fully evaluated.

Diagnostic tests

Light transmission platelet aggregometry

In the 1960s, the invention of platelet aggregometry revolutionized the analysis of platelet function within routine laboratory testing. Still regarded as the "gold standard," it is the most widely used platelet function test. Citrated platelet-rich plasma (PRP) is normally stirred under conditions of low shear within an incubated cuvette (37°C between a light source and a photocell. Anticoagulated whole blood may also be used in some commercial multichannel impedance-based aggregometers, such as the Chronolog or Multiplate aggregometers. These have the significant advantage that the blood does not require further processing for analysis.

The addition of different dosages of a panel of agonists triggers platelet activation, shape change, and primary and secondary aggregation events that increase light transmission over time, and this is recorded on the aggregation trace (Fig. 5.2). By using a panel of agonists at differing concentrations, it is possible to detect a number of classic platelet defects. Modern instruments usually offer multichannel capability and computer analysis and storage of data, although samples and reagents still have to be prepared manually.

A fully automated and near patient testing aggregation system called the VerifyNow® device (Accumetrics) is now available solely for the monitoring of the three major classes of anti-platelet drugs (e.g. Gp IIb/IIIa inhibitors, aspirin, and P_2Y_{12} inhibitors/antagonists) using specific cartridges.

The light transmission method is as follows:
• Citrated PRP (prepared by centrifugation at 150–200 g for 10 minutes; non-adjusted count as this introduces an artefact) is added to cuvette at 37°C and preincubated for 5 minutes.
• The PRP is stirred at a recommended speed (e.g. 1000 rpm using a magnetic stir bar) to allow platelets to come in contact with each other.
• 100% transmission is set with autologous platelet-poor plasma (PPP) (prepared by centrifugation at 1500 g for 20 minutes).
• 0% transmission is set with PRP and a stable baseline established before addition of agonist.
• Agonist is added (up to 10% total volume).
• Aggregation is recorded (10–15 minutes).
• Calculate percentage aggregation (maximum or final) and slope (rate of aggregation).
• Hemolyzed or very lipemic samples may interfere with light transmission.
• Thrombocytopenic samples are also unsuitable for analysis.

A typical panel of agonists (stored in frozen aliquots) are:
• ADP (0.1–20 $\mu mol/L$).
• Epinephrine (1.0–10 $\mu mol/L$).
• Collagen (1–5 $\mu g/mL$), usually mediates a steep aggregation curve but after a characteristic lag phase of more than 1 minute.
• Arachidonic acid (1.0–2.0 $mmol/L$).
• Ristocetin (0.5–1.5 mg/mL) is not strictly an agonist but stimulates platelet agglutination through binding of plasma VWF to Gp Ib and therefore will also give abnormal results in VWD; usually used at a single low and high dose.
• Thrombin (0.1–0.5 IU/mL).

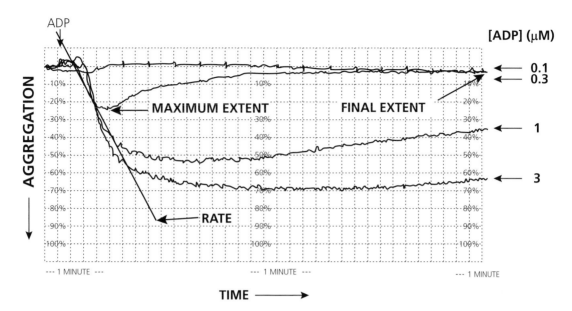

Figure 5.2 Typical example of a trace recording of ADP-induced aggregation generated by a PAP-4 aggregometer, illustrating the indices of aggregation used to characterize the response. The concentration-dependency of the response is clearly evident. At the lower concentrations of ADP, the response is transient and reversible, resulting in different values for the maximum and final extents of aggregation. (Reproduced with permission from Jarvis et al. *Br J Pharmacol* 2000;129:282, published by Macmillan.)

A typical aggregation curve can often be divided into primary and secondary aggregation responses (see Fig. 5.2), the latter being characterized by degranulation and thromboxane generation, which mediate irreversible aggregation. Thus, any defects in either thromboxane generation or storage granules will result in a reduced secondary aggregation response to certain agonists. Some laboratories also use an extended panel of agonists, which can include thrombin receptor-activating peptide (TRAP; to activate PAR-1), collagen-related peptide; to activate GPVI), U46619 (to activate the thromboxane receptor), and A23187 (calcium ionophore).

There are no commercially available quality-control kits for platelet function testing. Aggregometers can be checked by using the PRP and PPP to check percentage aggregation settings, and dilutions (mixes of PRP and PPP) can be performed to check linearity. Normal ranges for each concentration of agonists should ideally be established; normal controls can be run in parallel and new batches of reagents always checked for the same performance as the previous batch. Platelet aggregometry is remarkably poorly standardized (e.g.

in the choice and range of concentrations of agonists) as highlighted in many recent surveys, and there are few up-to-date guidelines available (although this is likely to change in the near future). Typical expected aggregation responses to the more commonly encountered platelet defects are detailed below

Glanzmann thrombasthenia
There is complete absence of aggregation to agonists such as ADP, but a normal agglutination response to ristocetin.

Bernard–Soulier syndrome
Platelets aggregate to all of the physiologic agonists but do not agglutinate to ristocetin.

VWD
Patients with VWD will have defective ristocetin-induced agglutination. This can be corrected by addition of normal plasma or cryoprecipitate. A low dose of ristocetin (<0.6 mg/mL) will also only mediate platelet agglutination in type 2B VWD or platelet-type VWD.

Storage pool or release defects

Patients with storage pool or release defects typically show an impaired secondary aggregation response. In order to confirm the diagnosis, platelet nucleotide content should also be additionally measured using either lumiaggregometry or within lysed platelet preparations that can be stored and batched for analysis. Defects in thromboxane generation (e.g. COX-1 deficiency caused by aspirin) will also be characterized by defective arachidonic acid-induced aggregation coupled with impaired secondary aggregation to other agonists.

Flow cytometry

Whole blood flow cytometry offers a very attractive and reliable test for the diagnosis of various platelet receptor, granular, and other defects. Flow cytometry can rapidly measure the properties and characteristics of a large number of individual platelets.

The method is as follows:

• Diluted whole blood (preferred, minimizing activation) or PRP preparations are labeled with fluorescently conjugated monoclonal antibodies.

• The diluted suspension of platelets is then analyzed at a rate of 1000–100,000 cells/minute through a focused laser beam within the instrument flow cell.

• The cytometer then detects both scattered and fluorescent light emitted by each platelet. The intensity of each signal is directly proportional to antigen density or the size/granularity of the platelet, and usually 5000–20,000 platelet events are collected in total for each sample.

• Only platelets should be analyzed or gated on by the flow cytometer. This is normally achieved by studying

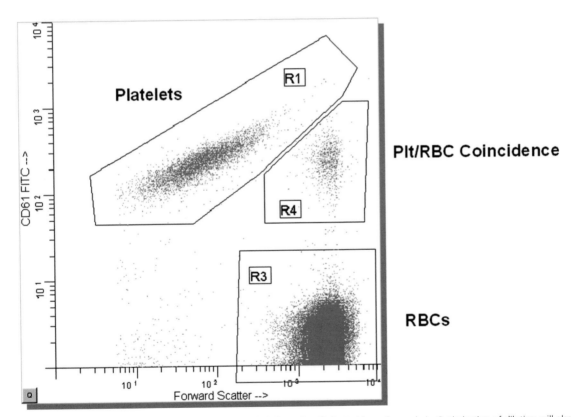

Figure 5.3 A flow cytometry plot using a fluorescent-labeled platelet-identifying antibody (anti-CD61) when triggering on a low value of forward scatter (FS). If the instrument is triggered on this fluorescence, all other nonplatelet events shown (RBCs) will be eliminated from the analysis. Optimization of dilution will also eliminate the coincident events. (Reproduced with permission from Harrison et al. *Am J Clin Pathol* 2001;115:448–59, published by Lippincott-Raven.)

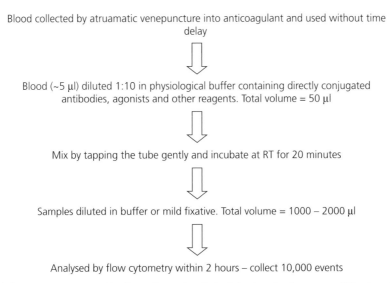

Blood collected by atruamatic venepuncture into anticoagulant and used without time delay

Blood (~5 µl) diluted 1:10 in physiological buffer containing directly conjugated antibodies, agonists and other reagents. Total volume = 50 µl

Mix by tapping the tube gently and incubate at RT for 20 minutes

Samples diluted in buffer or mild fixative. Total volume = 1000 – 2000 µl

Analysed by flow cytometry within 2 hours – collect 10,000 events

Figure 5.4 A typical flow cytometry protocol for the testing and analysis of platelets. Small amounts of blood are incubated with test reagents, diluted, and analyzed. New reagents are easily incorporated into this standard procedure.

the characteristic light scatter pattern that is obtained with platelets, which normally allows their resolution from RBCs, WBCs, and background "noise" in most samples. However, in some situations where there is an abnormal platelet distribution which overlaps with the RBCs (e.g. macrothrombocytopenia and Bernard–Soulier disease), it is often useful to use a specific identifying antibody (e.g. Gp Ib or IIb/IIIa) to resolve the fluorescent population of platelets from non-fluorescent RBCs/WBCs and debris/ noise (Fig. 5.3).

• Double labeling using another antibody with a different fluorophore is also possible.

Care needs to be taken that:

• the subject is rested (20–30 minutes);

• the venepuncture is clean (discarding the first few milliliters of blood); and

• there are no time delays between sampling and analysis.

It is recommended that daily quality-control procedures be performed with stable, fluorescently labeled bead preparations to ensure optimal instrument and laser performance.

The increasing availability of commercial platelet reagents (e.g. antibodies, ligands, and probes) has facilitated the development of many types of platelet assay, which can be incorporated into a standard protocol (Fig. 5.4).

Table 5.3 summarizes the various types of platelet function that can be tested using a flow cytometer. The most commonly used assay is for the diagnosis of the two major platelet glycoprotein abnormalities: Bernard–Soulier syndrome (Gp Ib deficiency) and Glanzmann thrombasthenia (Gp IIb/IIIa deficiency). Diagnostic assays are also available for quantifying copy number of any major glycoprotein, studying granular defects (e.g. storage pool disease), heparin-induced thrombocytopenia, and defects in platelet aggregation, secretion, or procoagulant activity.

The use of whole blood has several advantages over purified platelet preparations and PRP:

• Platelets are analyzed in the presence of erythrocytes and leucocytes;

• Only small quantities of blood are required per tube (2–5 µL);

• There is no loss of subpopulations of cells during separation procedures;

• Providing the venepuncture is well standardized, minimal manipulation of fresh samples results in little artefactual in vitro platelet activation;

• It is possible to study platelets from patients with thrombocytopenia and in a pediatric setting; and

• Both the in vivo resting activation state and dose–response to classical agonists can be measured with high sensitivity.

Table 5.3 Flow cytometric platelet function tests.

Diagnosis of platelet defects	Bernard–Soulier syndrome
	Glanzmann thrombasthenia
	Storage pool disease
	HIT
Platelet activation markers	Degranulation markers: CD62p, CD63, and CD40L
	Gp IIb/IIIa conformation
	Platelet–leukocyte conjugates
	Platelet-derived microparticles
Monitoring anti-platelet therapy	Gp IIb/IIIa antagonists
	Clopidogrel and ticlopidine
	Aspirin and COX-1 inhibitors
Measuring platelet production	Reticulated platelets
Accurate platelet counting	Platelet: RBC ratio – new reference method
Platelet-associated IgG	ITP
	Alloantibodies
Blood bank tests	Quality control of concentrates
	Leukocyte contamination
	Platelet HPA-1a
	Cross-matching

Abbreviations: HIT, heparin-induced thrombocytopenia; ITP, idiopathic thrombocytopenic purpura.

When diagnosing any platelet function or receptor defect, it is good practice to analyze a normal control sample in parallel to ensure that normal results can be obtained with the test in question. This will also facilitate the eventual calibration of a normal range. Results are normally expressed as mean fluorescent intensity (MFI) or as a percentage of the gated platelet population (Table 5.4). Absolute quantification of receptor density is now possible by using calibrated fluorescent standards, some of which are available in kit form (e.g. Dako, Sigma, Biocytex). The lowest limit of detection by these techniques is quoted as approximately 500 molecules/platelet.

A panel of activation-dependent antibodies (e.g. CD62p, CD63, PAC-1) can be used to assess a patient's platelet response to dose–response curves of agonists that are also used for aggregation (e.g. TRAP, ADP, collagen).

Table 5.4 MFI and percentage of positive cells showing antibody staining in normal platelets and in platelets from a patient with Glanzmann thrombasthenia (Gp IIb/IIIa deficiency).

Receptor (Mab)	Normal		Patient (LK)	
	Positive cells (%)	MFI	Positive cells (%)	MFI
Mouse IgG (PE)	0.5	–	0.5	–
Gp Ib (anti-CD42b PE)	97.5	557	98.24	851
Mouse IgG (FITC)	0.5	–	0.5	–
Gp IIb (anti-CD41 FITC)	95.99	13.97	1.55	
Gp IIIa (anti-CD61 FITC)	98.42	598	0.8	1.63

Further reading

BCSH Haemostasis and Thrombosis Task Force. Guidelines on platelet function testing. *J Clin Pathol* 1988;41:1322–30.

Bolton-Maggs PH, Chalmers EA, Collins PW, et al. A review of inherited platelet disorders with guidelines for their management on behalf of the UKHCDO. *Br J Haematol* 2006;135(5):603–33.

Fressinaud E, Veyradier A, Truchaud F, et al. Screening for von Willebrand disease with a new analyzer using high shear stress: a study of 60 cases. *Blood* 1998;91:1325–31.

Gresele P, Fuster V, Lopez H, Page C, Vermylen J, eds. *Platelets in Hematologic and Cardiovascular Disorders.* Cambridge: Cambridge University Press, 2008.

Harrison P. Platelet function analysis. *Blood Rev* 2005; 19:111–23.

Hayward CP, Harrison P, Cattaneo M, Ortel TL, Rao AK. The Platelet Physiology Subcommittee of the Scientific and Standardization Committee of the International Society of Thrombosis and Haemostasis. *J Thromb Haemost* 2006;4(2):212–9.

Hayward CP, Rao AK, Catteneo M. Congenital platelet disorders: an overview of their mechanisms, diagnostic evaluation and treatment. *Haemophilia* 2006;12(Suppl 3):128–36.

Hayward CP. Diagnostic approach to platelet function disorders. *Transfus Apher Sci* 2008;38:65–76.

Hayward CP, Eikelboom J. Platelet function testing: quality assurance. *Semin Thromb Hemost* 2007;33:273–82.

Jilma B. Platelet function analyzer (PFA-100): a tool to quantify congenital or acquired platelet dysfunction. *J Lab Clin Med* 2001;138:152–63.

Linnemann B, Schwonberg J, Mani H, Prochnow S, Lindhoff-Last E. Standardization of light transmittance aggregometry for monitoring antiplatelet therapy: an adjustment for platelet count is not necessary. *J Thromb Haemost* 2008;6(4):677–83.

Michelson AD. Flow cytometry: a clinical test of platelet function. *Blood* 1996;87:4925–36.

Michelson AD. *Platelets* (2nd edition). New York: Academic Press, 2007.

Ruggeri ZM. Platelets in atherothrombosis. *Nat Med* 2002;8:1227–34.

Schmitz G, Rothe G, Ruf A, et al. European Working Group on Clinical Cell Analysis: Consensus protocol for the flow cytometric characterization of platelet function. *Thromb Haemost* 1998;79:885–96.

Zhou L, Schmaier AH. Platelet aggregation testing in platelet-rich plasma: description of procedures with the aim to develop standards in the field. *Am J Clin Pathol* 2005;123(2):172–83.

6 Evaluation of the bleeding patient

Alice Ma

Introduction

Few evaluations in hematology provoke as much diagnostic uncertainty as that of the patient with a suspected bleeding diathesis. The evaluation, including history, physical examination, and laboratory testing, is aimed at determining the likelihood that the patient has an underlying hemorrhagic disorder, as well as the treatment of future bleeding episodes. The evaluation is fraught with diagnostic uncertainty, because many historical features are shared by individuals without bleeding diatheses, laboratory studies may have a significant false-positive rate, and external pressures (such as insurance coverage) may limit the diagnostic testing available to the patient and physician. This chapter will attempt to present a systematic approach to the individual with a suspected bleeding disorder.

The bleeding history

A detailed history of bleeding episodes, including a family history, is critical in elucidating whether a bleeding diathesis is present. To that end, questions are aimed at determining the likelihood of a bleeding disorder being present as well the type of the putative bleeding diathesis (is this a disorder of primary or secondary hemostasis?) and inheritance pattern.

The history should include an orderly description of bleeding during infancy and childhood, including umbilical stump bleeding (characteristic of FXIII deficiency), bleeding with circumcision (characteristically seen in boys with severe hemophilia A or B), bleeding with loss of deciduous teeth, and bleeding with childhood trauma and surgeries. Bleeding with dental pro-

cedures, including wisdom tooth removal, should be explored. Questions such as "Did you have to go back for stitches? Did you awaken with a pillow covered with blood?" are more specific than "Did you bleed with tooth removal?" Patients with milder bleeding disorders may only bleed with procedures involving mucosal surfaces, due to the high levels of fibrinolytic activity at these sites. Epistaxis may be a presenting symptom of von Willebrand disease (VWD) or hereditary hemorrhagic telangiectasia (HHT), and is especially notable if it does not stop with pressure and requires either cautery or a visit to the emergency department.

Other bleeding episodes, whether spontaneous or provoked, should be elucidated. Bleeding into muscles and joints is characteristic of disorders of plasma clotting factors, whereas mucosal bleeding is seen more in disorders of primary hemostasis. Easy bruisability is a complaint voiced by many patients without underlying bleeding disorders, but certain historical features are worth noting. The new onset of bruising can herald a new thrombocytopenic disorder, such as idiopathic thrombocytopenic purpura or acute leukemia, or can point to acquired hemophilia. Bruising that only occurs over the hands and forearms suggests the presence of senile purpura.

Each individual surgical procedure undergone by the patient should be explored in depth. The details of bleeding, including timing (immediate or delayed), the need for transfusion, comments by the surgeon concerning the characteristics of the bleeding, any known anatomic sources of bleeding, etc., can shed immense light on the bleeding diathesis. Immediate bleeding may be more characteristic of a disorder of primary hemostasis, whereas delayed bleeding is seen more in patients with deficiencies in plasma clotting factors. Bleeding in patients with an underlying hemorrhagic condition is typically described as "diffuse oozing," without the readily identifiable bleeding source seen with a surgical mishap, such as a severed vessel. If a woman has bled with some procedures but not others, she should be asked whether she was on oral contraceptive pills (OCPs) or hormone replacement therapy (HRT) during the procedures in which she had good hemostasis, because OCPs and HRT can increase levels of von Willebrand factor (VWF), leading to normalization of hemostasis.

Women should be carefully questioned about their menstrual history. Duration and severity of flow are more important than the presence or severity of cramping. "How were your periods?" is likely to yield data insufficient to distinguish whether a bleeding diathesis is truly present or not. Although menorrhagia is medically defined as loss of more than 80 cc of blood per menstrual cycle, few if any women are capable of determining this with any degree of precision. Pad or tampon usage is imprecise as well, because the number of sanitary products used may vary with the degree of fastidiousness of each patient. To that end, pictorial assessments of blood loss (depicting pads or tampons with varying degrees of saturation) have been devised, with scores given for numbers of products used and their saturation. Scores have been correlated with the likelihood of an underlying bleeding disorder and have been found to have a sensitivity and specificity of approximately 85% [1,2]. An underlying bleeding disorder is found in between 10% and 30% of women who present for evaluation of menorrhagia [3–5].

Historical features correlated with a higher likelihood of an underlying bleeding disorder being found include:

- nighttime "flooding";
- passage of clots larger than a quarter;
- duration longer than 8 days; and
- the development of iron deficiency [6].

Whereas bleeding during pregnancy is less common in women with VWD and other bleeding disorders, postpartum hemorrhage is less rarely seen. This usually occurs 24–48 hours after delivery and can be markedly prolonged by weeks to months. Endometriosis and hemorrhagic ovarian cysts are seen with increased frequency in women with VWD [7].

A family history of bleeding should be carefully sought out. This may require several visits to fully document as familial memories are probed. A family history of bleeding with surgical procedures, bleeding requiring transfusions, and menorrhagia leading to hysterectomy at a young age should be queried. However, a negative family history does not rule out a congenital bleeding disorder. Approximately one-third of all cases of hemophilia A arise from spontaneous mutations [8]. Many of the rare coagulation disorders, including deficiencies of factors II, V, VII, X, Glanzmann thrombasthenia, and VWD type 2N, among others, are inherited in an autosomal recessive fashion, and other family members may be entirely asymptomatic.

Certain medications and herbal and dietary supplements increase the risk of bleeding. The use of these agents may precipitate a hemorrhage in those with milder bleeding disorders. The use of aspirin and non-steroidal anti-inflammatory agents impairs primary hemostasis, and their use should be avoided prior to surgery or prior to evaluation of the hemostatic system. Their inclusion in over-the-counter products seems ubiquitous, and careful attention to cold and flu remedy use is warranted. In some locations, aspirin-containing remedies are given names (such as Goody powders or BC powders) that disguise their content, and they are not viewed as medications. The use of these medications will likely not be volunteered and must be specifically queried.

The physical examination

The physical examination is an integral part of any diagnostic evaluation and may provide useful clues to the etiology of the patient's bleeding.

- Examining the skin may reveal petechiae, indicating thrombocytopenia, or the characteristic ecchymoses and lax skin seen with senile purpura. Patients with scurvy have characteristic perifollicular hemorrhages and "corkscrew hairs." Telangiectasia around the lips or on the fingertips may signal the presence of hereditary hemorrhagic telangiectasia syndrome. Bruising should be examined for:
- Their pattern and age; if they are all the same color and lividity, they may have all occured simultaneously.
- Is the pattern of distribution indicative of self-infliction, seen sometimes in patients with Munchausen's syndrome?

Oculocutaneous albinism is associated with several platelet disorders, including the Hermansky-Pudlak and Chediak-Higashi syndromes.

• Splenomegaly can be associated with thrombocytopenia and may indicate underlying cirrhosis. Other stigmata of liver disease, such as spider angiomata, gynecomastia, asterixis, and jaundice, also suggest that the patient may have liver coagulopathy.

• Joint hypermobility and skin hyper-elasticity may be found in Ehlers-Danlos syndrome, although not all patients with this disorder manifest the skin findings.

• A harsh systolic murmur may indicate severe aortic stenosis, which can cause an acquired type 2 VWD, with associated gastrointestinal bleeding from arteriovenous malformations [9].

• An enlarged tongue, carpal tunnel syndrome, and peri-orbital purpura may point to amyloidosis, which is associated with an acquired deficiency of many clotting proteins, including factors V and X, VWF, α2-antiplasmin, and plasminogen activator inhibitor 1. [10,11]

Laboratory evaluation

Introduction to coagulation laboratory testing

Although the history and physical examination can increase suspicion for the presence of a bleeding disorder, laboratory confirmation is required for precise diagnosis and treatment.

A negative bleeding history can be seen in individuals with mild bleeding disorders who have never been hemostatically challenged. Moreover, acquired disorders, such as acquired hemophilia, can present with no prior history of bleeding. On the other hand, laboratory evaluation should be guided by the history and physical examination. When used in this fashion, laboratory studies are most useful. A detailed description of each laboratory test can be found elsewhere in this book.

Clinicians must be aware that laboratory tests are affected by "pre-analytic variables." That is, preparation, handling, and sample characteristics will affect test results. The majority of coagulation studies are done on plasma samples isolated from blood anticoagulated with citrate.

• Tubes that are underfilled will have too much citrate for the plasma volume collected, and results may be erroneous. The ratio of citrate to plasma will also be altered in patients with a hematocrit value that is too high. In this case, too much of the blood volume is occupied by red cells, and the plasma volume is reduced.

• Samples can be contaminated with heparin when drawn from heparinized lines or from dialysis catheters.

• Samples should be processed as rapidly as possible to avoid: high temperatures, which can activate the clotting factors; contact with platelets, which can adsorb antiphospholipid antibodies; and prolonged contact with glass tubes, which can activate the contact factors.

• Tests of platelet function are altered by the method of collection. Drawing blood with vacutainer tubes or with needles of too small a gauge will cause shear stress and may activate platelets.

It is also important to note that there is no currently available test that serves as a screening test of global hemostasis. No test can include or exclude the presence of an underlying bleeding disorder. The bleeding time does not predict bleeding, as its name might suggest [12]. Screening tests may point to the presence of a factor deficiency or a defect in primary hemostasis, though more precise diagnoses will require more detailed testing. Finally, some patients and families have multiple abnormalities in their hemostatic systems, and finding a single abnormality should not halt the clinical evaluation if the laboratory abnormality fails to explain the entire clinical picture. For example, VWD has been reported in families with classical hemophilia A and B [13].

The prothombin time (PT) and the activated partial thromboplastin time (APTT)

The PT and the APTT are assays performed on citrated plasma that require enzymatic generation of thrombin on a phospholipid surface. Prolongation of the PT and the APTT can be seen in individuals with either deficiencies of, or inhibitors to, plasma clotting factors, although not all patients with prolongations of these assays will have bleeding diatheses.

The PT is designed to test components of the extrinsic and common pathways, including factors VII, V, X, II, and fibrinogen. It measures the time needed for formation of an insoluble fibrin clot once citrated plasma has been recalcified and thromboplastin has been added. Because thromboplastin from various sources and different lots can affect the rates of clotting reactions, the International Normalized Ratio (INR) was developed to avoid some of this variability in PT measurement. Each batch of thromboplastin reagent has assigned to it a numerical International Sensitivity Index (ISI) value. The INR is determined by the formula:

$$INR = (PT_{patient}/PT_{normal\ mean})^{ISI}$$

The INR is most properly used to measure anticoagulation in patients on vitamin K antagonists and is less predictive of bleeding in patients with liver disease. The INR can be inaccurate in patients with lupus anticoagulants that are strong enough to affect the PT.

The APTT tests the integrity of the intrinsic and the common clotting pathways, including factors XII, XI, IX, VIII, X, V, II, fibrinogen, high-molecular-weight kininogen, and prekallikrein. The reagents are described as a "partial thromboplastin" because hemophilic plasma gave a prolonged clotting that was not seen in assays such as the PT, which used "complete thromboplastins" [14]. Citrated plasma is recalcified, and phospholipids (to provide a scaffold for the clotting reactions) and an activator of the intrinsic system (such as kaolin, celite, or silica) are added. The reagents used show variable sensitivities to inhibitors such as lupus anticoagulants and heparin, and normal ranges will vary from laboratory to laboratory. APTT values that are vastly different from one lab to another should prompt suspicion of a lupus inhibitor.

The thrombin clotting time (TCT or TT) and reptilase time (RT)

The TCT measures the time needed for clot formation once thrombin is added to citrated plasma. Thrombin enzymatically cleaves fibrinopeptides A and B from the alpha and beta chains of fibrinogen, allowing for polymerization into fibrin. The TCT is prolonged in the presence of any thrombin inhibitor, such as heparin, lepirudin, or argatroban. Low levels of fibrinogen or structurally abnormal molecules (dysfibrinogenemias) also lead to TCT prolongation. Elevated levels of fibrinogen or fibrin degradation products can also prolong the assay by serving as nonspecific inhibitors of the reaction. Patients with paraproteins can have a

prolonged TCT because of the inhibitory effect of the paraprotein on fibrin polymerization.

Reptilase is a snake venom from *Bothrops atrox* that also enzymatically cleaves fibrinogen. Reptilase cleaves only fibrinopeptide A from the alpha chain of fibrinogen, but fibrin polymerization still occurs. The RT is not affected by heparin but may be more sensitive to the presence of a dysfibrinogenemia.

Mixing studies

Mixing studies are used to evaluate prolongations of the APTT (less commonly the PT or the TCT) and are useful in making the distinction between an inhibitor and a clotting factor deficiency. The patient's plasma is mixed 1:1 with normal control plasma, and the assay is repeated (with or without prolonged incubation at $37^{\circ}C$). Correction of the clotting test signifies factor deficiency, because the normal plasma will supply the deficient factor. Incomplete correction of the clotting test after mixing suggests the presence of an inhibitor; an inhibitor will prolong clotting in normal plasma, just as it does in the patient plasma. Incomplete correction can sometimes be seen with other nonspecific inhibitors, such as a lupus inhibitor, elevated fibrin split products, or a paraprotein. Less commonly, deficiencies of multiple clotting factors can lead to incomplete correction of the mixing study, because the mixing study was designed to correct deficiency of a single factor.

Specific clotting factor assays

Assays measuring the activity of specific clotting factors are done using a variant of the mixing study, in which patient plasma is mixed at different dilutions with reference plasma known to be deficient in the clotting factor of interest. Thus, the only source of the specific clotting factor will be the patient's plasma. The appropriate clotting assay (either PT or APTT) is performed, and the values are plotted against a standard curve to determine the factor activity in the sample. Ordering these assays should be guided by the clinical scenario and the results of screening assays.

The Bethesda assay

The Bethesda assay quantifies the strength of inhibitors to factor VIII and is used to detect and follow the clinical course of these inhibitors. Patient plasma is mixed and incubated with serial dilutions of normal control plasma, and the residual activity of FVIII is measured. The assay is controlled for normal decay of FVIII by performing the assay in tandem using control plasma diluted in buffer or in FVIII-deficient plasma (this is the Nijmegen modification). One Bethesda unit is the amount of antibody that inactivates 0.5 U of FVIII in normal plasma after incubation for 2 hours at 37°C. This assay can be adapted to test for inhibitors to other factors, such as FIX.

Assays for fibrinogen

Fibrinogen can be measured in a number of different ways. Clottable fibrinogen is measured by using a variant of the thrombin time, in which thrombin is added to citrated plasma. Either the rate at which clotting occurs is measured (Clauss method) or the total degree of clotting is assayed (Ellis method). Immunologic methods are used to determine the total amount of fibrinogen protein. Fibrinogen immunoelectrophoresis can be used to detect abnormal fibrinogen species.

Factor XIII

Factor XIII is activated by thrombin and serves to crosslink monomeric fibrin strands. Deficiency of FXIII leads to a severe bleeding diathesis but cannot be detected by standard clot-based assays (PT, APTT, or TCT). A simple assay to detect FXIII deficiency is based on the ability of a fibrin clot to resist lysis in a variety of solutions: either 5M urea, 1% chloracetic acid, or 2% acetic acid. Clots that dissolve in any of these solutions within 24 hours suggest a deficiency of FXIII. More specific functional assays as well as immunologic assays are available from reference laboratories.

Testing for VWD

VWF can be assessed by using either immunologic methods for detection of antigen or functional methods for detection of activity. Activity levels are assayed by determining either the ristocetin cofactor activity or the collagen-binding activity. Multimeric analysis requires electrophoresis in a denaturing agarose gel, followed by immunoblotting.

Assessment of the fibrinolytic system

Disorders of the fibrinolytic system, either congenital or acquired, can be associated with increased bleeding. The bleeding may be delayed, because a normal clot is formed at the time of injury, but breaks down more quickly than normal. Hyperfibrinolysis can be seen in conditions such as:

- envenomations;
- acute promyelocytic leukemia;
- overdoses of fibrinolytic agents;
- prostate and other uroepithelial cancers; and
- disseminated intravascular coagulation.

Fibrinolysis is typically assayed by measuring levels of fibrinogen and levels of breakdown products formed by lysing fibrin clot. Fibrin degradation products or fibrin split products are assayed by latex agglutination using polyclonal antibodies directed against fibrinopeptides D and E. Because this assay does not distinguish between breakdown products of fibrin and those of fibrinogen, it is not specific for disseminated intravascular coagulation (DIC) versus primary fibrinogenolysis. The D-dimer assay, however, is specific for breakdown products of cross-linked fibrin and uses a variety of immunologic techniques. Globally, hyperfibrinolysis can be assayed by use of the euglobulin clot lysis time (ECLT). Citrated plasma is treated to precipitate the euglobulin fraction, which contains fibrinogen and activators of plasminogen, as well as a portion of fibrinolytic inhibitors such as plasminogen activator inhibitor-1 (PAI-1). The euglobulin fraction is redissolved and the fibrinogen is clotted. Clot lysis time is then measured. Hyperfibrinolysis produces shortening of the ECLT. There are specific assays for inhibitors of the fibrinolytic system, including PAI-1 and α2-antiplasmin. Deficiencies of these proteins can be either congenital or acquired and can be the cause of rare bleeding conditions.

Tests of platelet function

This is an area that is reviewed elsewhere in greater detail in this book and is fraught with controversy [15,16]. Tests are poorly standardized and poorly reproducible. No test definitively assays all aspects of platelet function, and normal tests do not exclude a defect in platelet function.

The bleeding time

The bleeding time is an assay performed by making a small incision of standard size and depth on the forearm with a sphygmomanometer inflated to a pressure of 40 mm Hg on the upper arm. Blood is blotted away at standard intervals with a filter paper, and the time for bleeding cessation is measured. By blotting away

excess blood, primary hemostasis, rather than fibrin formation, is tested. The bleeding time will be prolonged in cases of:
- platelet dysfunction;
- von Willebrand disease;
- thrombocytopenia;
- severe anemia; and
- disorders of vascular contractility.

From a technical standpoint, it is affected by operator experience, cold exposure, vigorous exercise, anxiety, direction of the incision, and excessive wiping of the skin. Mild disorders of primary hemostasis may not, however, produce an abnormal bleeding time, making it less useful as a screening test.

Platelet Function Analyzer-100 (PFA-100)

The PFA-100 is another screening test for disorders of primary hemostasis and is performed on whole citrated blood, rather than on the skin of the patient. Citrated whole blood is aspirated through an aperture in a cartridge, where it contacts a membrane impregnated with a mixture of either collagen and epinephrine (Col/Epi) or collagen and adenosine diphosphate (Col/ADP). Contact with these agonists leads to platelet adhesion, aggregation, and activation, culminating in occlusion of the aperture and cessation of blood flow [17]. The time for aperture closure is known as the closure time (CT) and will be prolonged in patients with hematocrits below 30% and platelet counts below 100×10^9/L. The CTs are reliably prolonged in cases of severe platelet dysfunction and VWD. Milder cases of platelet dysfunction and mild type 1 VWD may not prolong the CT. Prolongation of the CT with Col/Epi but not Col/ADP should lead one to suspect aspirin ingestion or another defect in the thromboxane signaling pathway.

Platelet aggregation testing

Platelet-rich plasma is isolated from citrated blood, and platelet aggregation is tested in an aggregometer after exposure to a variety of platelet agonists. Exogenous platelet agonists include (but are not limited to) thrombin, collagen, epinephrine, arachidonic acid, ADP, the thromboxane receptor agonist U46619, and ristocetin. Platelet-aggregation tracings in response to weak agonists, such as epinephrine and low doses of ADP, show a primary wave of aggregation followed by a secondary wave once secretion of ADP within

platelet dense granules has occurred. Stronger agonists, such as thrombin and collagen, generally produce a single deep primary wave of aggregation because they do not require secretion. Platelets must be prepared freshly, and should be drawn with needles no smaller than 19–21 gauge, and into a syringe and not a vacutainer, in order to prevent platelet activation before the assay. When preparing PRP, red cell contamination should be avoided, because lysed red cells release ADP and lead to pre-activation of platelets [18].

Lumiaggregometry directly measures release of adenine nucleotides via bioluminescence, along with the extent of aggregation. It can be performed on whole blood or platelet-rich plasma. ADP released from dense granules is converted to ATP, which then reacts with luciferin, generating adenyl-luciferin, which becomes oxidized and emits light. Whole blood aggregometry measures the increase in impedance across electrodes placed in anticoagulated blood as they become accreted with activated platelets. Although whole blood aggregometry uses a smaller volume of blood and is therefore better suited for pediatric patients, it is not sensitive to secretion and therefore does not distinguish between primary and secondary waves of aggregation.

Platelets from patients with Glanzmann's thrombasthenia will not aggregate to any of the routinely used agonists but will agglutinate to ristocetin, whereas platelets from patients with Bernard-Soulier syndrome show the opposite findings. Patients with storage pool disease (SPD) have deficient secretion and may therefore fail to show a secondary wave of aggregation to weaker platelet agonists.

Electron microscopy

Ultrastructural analysis of platelets can help diagnose mild bleeding disorders due to SPD. Certain patients with mild SPD can have completely negative evaluation, including BT, PFA-100, and platelet aggregometry, but show abnormalities in granule number when evaluated by electron microscopy (EM) [19]. Additional disorders that can be diagnosed by EM include:
- Hermansky-Pudlak syndrome,
- May-Hegglin anomaly,
- Epstein syndrome,
- Fechtner syndrome, and
- Sebastian syndrome [20].

Final integration of clinical and laboratory data

The approach to the bleeding patient differs depending on the clinical scenario. Patients with active bleeding warrant an immediate, abbreviated evaluation, with clinical history aimed at determining whether the defect is congenital or acquired, and laboratory testing designed to look for gross perturbations of the hemostatic system. Acute bleeding can produce changes in the hemostatic system that make it difficult to detect minor defects. Evaluation of the patient who has had massive bleeding in the past but is now stable can be more detailed and thoughtful. Some patients present for pre-operative evaluation because of abnormal laboratory tests, and the clinician must determine whether the lab abnormality correlates with an underlying bleeding tendency. Other patients will present because a family member has been diagnosed with a bleeding diathesis, and in this case, the laboratory evaluation may be more truncated.

The next section will attempt to provide a useful framework for the patient with a suspected bleeding disorder (Fig. 6.1).

Prolongation of the PT with a normal APTT should be due to a deficiency in FVII. Congenital deficiency of FVII is a rare autosomal recessive disorder with variable manifestations, depending on the FVII activity level. Generally, 10% FVII activity is sufficient to pro-

vide adequate hemostasis. Inhibitors to FVII are rare but have been described [21]. Because FVII has the shortest clotting factor half-life, a systemic defect in coagulation can begin with a prolonged PT out of proportion to the APTT. These scenarios include DIC, liver disease, vitamin K deficiency, or warfarin use. Paraproteins and dysfibrinogenemias can also prolong the PT out of proportion to the APTT. In these latter two cases, the TCT and RT may also be prolonged. Recombinant activated FVII has been approved for treatment of this disorder (Fig. 6.2).

Congenital causes

Factor deficiencies in the intrinsic pathway that lead to bleeding include FXI, FIX, and VIII. Congenital deficiency of FXI is autosomal recessive and is seen with increased frequency in Ashkenazi Jews. This generally produces a milder bleeding disorder, and despite being due to a deficiency in a plasma clotting factor, FXI deficiency produces a mucocutaneous bleeding pattern, and the severity of bleeding is not strictly dependent on the level of FXI activity in plasma. Whether or not FXI-deficient patients bleed may depend on differences in their ability to generate thrombin, the ability to activate the thrombin-activatable fibrinolytic inhibitor, and/or the activity of the fibrinolytic system. Bleeding can be especially problematic from anatomic sites associated with high fibrinolytic activity (e.g. the oral cavity and urogenital tract). FXI deficiency is treated with either plasma or a plasma-derived FXI concentrate.

Factor VIII and FIX deficiency produce hemophilia A and B, respectively, and are the only two soluble clotting factor deficiencies that are inherited as X-linked recessive disorders. Several hundred distinct mutations in each gene have been reported [22]. These mutations result in mild, moderate, and severe forms of hemophilia, and the clinical manifestations of hemophilia A and B are, for all practical purposes, indistinguishable. In the severe form, both disorders are characterized by recurrent hemarthroses that result in chronic crippling hemarthropathy, most often affecting the ankles, knees, and elbows, unless treated by replacing the deficient factor on a prophylactic basis. Bleeding episodes may be "spontaneous," but on close questioning, bleeding can usually be related to trauma. Central nervous system hemorrhage is especially hazardous and remains one of the leading causes

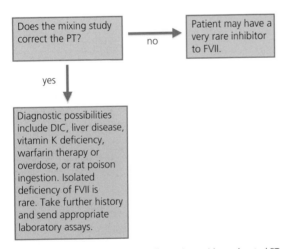

Figure 6.1 Diagnostic evaluation for patient with an elevated PT and normal APTT.

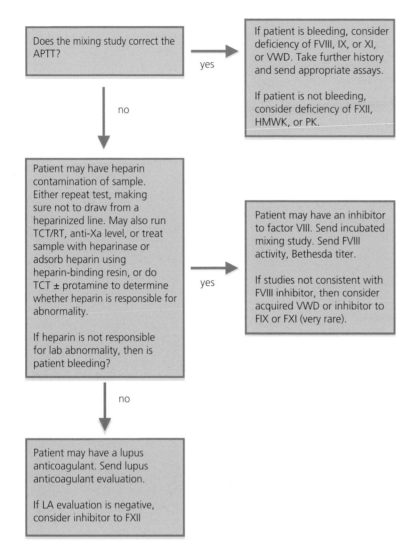

Does the mixing study correct the APTT?

yes →

If patient is bleeding, consider deficiency of FVIII, IX, or XI, or VWD. Take further history and send appropriate assays.

If patient is not bleeding, consider deficiency of FXII, HMWK, or PK.

no ↓

Patient may have heparin contamination of sample. Either repeat test, making sure not to draw from a heparinized line. May also run TCT/RT, anti-Xa level, or treat sample with heparinase or adsorb heparin using heparin-binding resin, or do TCT ± protamine to determine whether heparin is responsible for abnormality.

If heparin is not responsible for lab abnormality, then is patient bleeding?

yes →

Patient may have an inhibitor to factor VIII. Send incubated mixing study. Send FVIII activity, Bethesda titer.

If studies not consistent with FVIII inhibitor, then consider acquired VWD or inhibitor to FIX or FXI (very rare).

no ↓

Patient may have a lupus anticoagulant. Send lupus anticoagulant evaluation.

If LA evaluation is negative, consider inhibitor to FXII

Figure 6.2 Diagnostic algorithm for the patient with a normal PT and prolonged APTT.

of death. Mild hemophilia may present in adulthood with posttraumatic or surgical bleeding. Both plasma-derived and recombinant FVIII and FIX concentrates are available. Desmopressin can sometimes be helpful in the treatment of mild hemophilia A.

VWD is the most common inherited bleeding disorder, with low levels of VWF being found in 1% of the population. Symptomatic VWD likely affects approximately 1 in 1000 of the population. VWD is inherited in an autosomal fashion, with mild disease being dominantly transmitted and more severe disease being recessive. VWF protects FVIII from degradation in plasma, and FVIII levels can be low enough in VWD to cause slight prolongation of the APTT. Mild VWD produces mucocutaneous and postsurgical bleeding. Many women with VWD have significant menorrhagia, endometriosis, and postpartum hemorrhage and may suffer bleeding for more than a decade prior to diagnosis [7]. Type 2N VWD can be confused with mild hemophilia A. In this disorder, the site on VWD responsible for binding FVIII is mutated, and FVIII levels are usually between 10% and 20% of normal, with a normal FVIII gene. Desmopressin can be used for the treatment of mild type 1 VWD, but more severe bleeding and bleeding in patients with type 2 and 3 VWD typically requires infusion of VWF-containing FVIII concentrates.

Acquired causes

The most common cause of an acquired disorder that causes bleeding with an isolated APTT prolongation is an acquired inhibitor to FVIII. Patients with acquired hemophilia have a bimodal age distribution, with younger patients being female and older patients being male. This condition can be associated with the postpartum state, malignancies, or autoimmune conditions, but 50% of cases will be idiopathic. Patients have no prior history of bleeding, but the bleeding at the time of presentation can be severe. Unlike congenital hemophilia, bleeding tends to be mucocutaneous and multifocal, and hemarthroses are rare. The mixing study will fail to correct and will be further prolonged with incubation. Tests for the lupus inhibitor will be negative, and the Bethesda assay will show the presence of an inhibitor. There may be a small amount of residual FVIII activity in the plasma, but the bleeding will be out of proportion to the FVIII activity [23]. Treatment for acute bleeding episodes will require a bypassing agent (rFVIIa or an activated prothrombin complex concentrate) if the Bethesda titer is >5, but may be treated with higher doses of FVIII concentrates if the Bethesda titer is below 5. Patients may require immunosuppression to rid them of their inhibitor.

Acquired VWD is a rare condition that is typically associated with a lymphoproliferative disorder, although it can also be seen in the setting of hypothyroidism, myeloproliferative disorders, and severe aortic stenosis. Patients will have a prolonged APTT along with a prolonged bleeding time and PFA-100. Acquired inhibitors to FXI and FIX are rare and typically seen in association with other autoimmune conditions.

Heparin therapy will cause a prolonged APTT, more commonly with a normal PT, and can cause bleeding. The TCT will be prolonged, and the RT will be normal. Plasma cell dyscrasias can produce a heparin-like substance that will produce the same pattern of laboratory abnormalities (Fig. 6.3) [24].

Congenital causes

A deficiency of a factor in the common pathway will prolong both the PT and the APTT. Inherited deficiencies of factors V, X, II, and fibrinogen are autosomal recessive traits and are rare. Factor V deficiency produces

Do the mixing studies correct the PT and the APTT? — no → Is the TCT prolonged? — no → Patient may have a lupus anticoagulant. Send lupus anticoagulant evaluation.

Patient may have rare inhibitor to FII, FV, FX, or fibrinogen.

yes (from TCT) → Sample may be contaminated with heparin or patient may have a dysfibrinogenemia.

yes (from mixing studies) → Diagnostic possibilities include DIC, liver disease, vitamin K deficiency, warfarin therapy or overdose, or rat poison ingestion. Isolated deficiency of FVII is rare. Take further history and send appropriate laboratory assays.

Patient may have isolated deficiency of Factor FV, FX, FII, or fibrinogen. All are rare.

Patient may have combined deficiency of FV and FVIII or combined deficiencies of FII, FVII, FIX, and FX. Both are very rare.

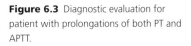

Figure 6.3 Diagnostic evaluation for patient with prolongations of both PT and APTT.

a bleeding disorder that is less severe than hemophilia A or B, even when FV levels are <1%. Bleeding times may be prolonged due to lack of platelet FV, which is reported to account for 20% of the FV in the body. It is treated with fresh frozen plasma. Factor X deficiency can be mild, moderate, or severe, with severe deficiency producing bleeding similar to that seen in classical hemophilia. Patients with bleeding can be treated with prothrombin complex concentrates (PCCs), and FX levels should not be raised above 50% to avoid thromboembolic complications. Inherited prothrombin deficiency is very rare and can also be treated with PCCs.

Fibrinogen gene mutations lead either to absence of fibrinogen (afibrinogenemia) or to production of a defective molecule (dysfibrinogenemia). Afibrinogenemia is very rare, leading to a severe bleeding disorder manifested by bleeding after trauma into subcutaneous and deeper tissues that may result in dissection. Bleeding from the umbilical stump is frequent. In addition to prolongation of the PT and the APTT, these patients also show a prolonged TCT and RT. The bleeding time is also prolonged due to the absence of fibrinogen in the platelet alpha granule. Treatment consists of transfusing cryoprecipitate to raise the fibrinogen level to the range of around 100 mg/dL. The majority of patients with dysfibrinogenemia are heterozygous for the disorder and show no evidence of either a hemorrhagic or a thrombotic state. Other dysfibrinogenemias, however, are associated with bleeding episodes, and a few may be associated with venous or arterial thrombosis. Bleeding patients should be treated with infusions of fibrinogen concetrates or cryoprecipitate.

Combined deficiency of multiple clotting factors can also be inherited, the most common conditions being combined deficiency of factors V and VIII and a combined deficiency of the vitamin K-dependent factors (prothrombin and factors VII, IX, X, and proteins C and S) [25,26]. A combined deficiency of factors V and VIII is inherited in an autosomal recessive fashion and is due to defects in one of two genes: the LMAN1 gene and a newly discovered gene called the "multiple clotting factor deficiency 2 (MCFD2) gene [26]. The products of both genes play an important role in the transport of factors V and VIII from the endoplasmic reticulum to the Golgi apparatus and are necessary for normal secretion of these factors. The disorder results

in a mild to moderate bleeding tendency with factor V and VIII levels ranging from 5% to 30% of normal. When both the PT and PTT are prolonged, and either factor V or VIII is found to be decreased, the combined deficiency should be suspected. Factor VIII is easily replaced using factor VIII concentrates, but the only readily available factor V replacement is fresh frozen plasma, which is limited in its ability to normalize the factor V level. In some cases, plasma exchange is necessary to raise the factor V to hemostatic levels.

Combined deficiencies of the vitamin K-dependent factors can be due to defects in either the gene for vitamin K-dependent carboxylase or the gene for vitamin K epoxide reductase [27]. This is an autosomal recessive disorder that may be associated with deficiencies of prothrombin, factors VII, IX, and X, as well as proteins C and S [26]. In this syndrome, both the PT and PTT are prolonged, and assays for the individual factors that influence these tests are necessary. Large doses of vitamin K may partially correct the hereditary defect in some but not all cases. Some bleeding episodes will require replacement with PCCs.

Acquired causes
Inhibitors to factor V are typically seen in patients who have undergone re-do vascular or cardiac surgery and are provoked by use of bovine thrombin. This hemostatic agent is contaminated with a small amount of bovine FV, and antibodies to bovine FV will cross-react with human FV. This condition may be self-limited, but bleeding can be treated with platelets, because platelet FV may be less susceptible to inhibitors in plasma.

Prothrombin antibodies can co-exist with the lupus inhibitor, and these inhibitors increase clearance of FII, causing an acquired deficiency, rather than neutralizing prothrombin function. Thus, the mixing studies for the PT will be normal.

Factor X deficiency can be seen in conjunction with amyloidosis, because the FX is adsorbed onto the amyloid protein. This can cause a severe hemorrhagic disorder that has been reported to respond to splenectomy. This condition will also produce a mixing study that normalizes the PT and the APTT.

Combined factor deficiencies can be seen in conditions such as vitamin K deficiency, disseminated intravascular coagulation, and severe liver disease. Severe liver disease can also lead to an acquired dysfibrinogenemia, which can produce a prolonged TCT and RT.

Anticoagulants such as heparin and coumadin can cause prolongation of both the PT and the APTT, especially when given in excess. Direct thrombin inhibitors such as lepirudin and argatroban will prolong the PT, the APTT, and the TCT.

Patients with bleeding, but normal PT and APTT

Congenital causes

Factor XIII deficiency is a rare autosomal recessive disorder that presents with severe bleeding. Prolonged bleeding from the umbilical stump is common, as is spontaneous intracranial hemorrhage. Treatment relies on cryoprecipitate, although FXIII concentrates are in clinical trials.

Congenital disorders of platelets include thrombocytopenic disorders, disorders of platelet surface glycoproteins, signaling pathway disorders, and storage pool and secretion disorders. They typically show prolongation of the bleeding time and the PFA-100. Platelet aggregation may show a typical pattern, but milder disorders may have normal platelet aggregation tracings. Mild thrombocytopathies may be missed by the bleeding time, the PFA-100, and platelet aggregation testing, and may require more specialized testing, such as flow cytometry or electron microscopy.

Congenital deficiencies of fibrinolytic inhibitors such as α2-antiplasmin and PAI-1 have been reported, and bleeding is typically delayed. The euglobulin lysis time can be shortened, and assays for these proteins can be performed but may not be helpful in the deficiency state, due to assay limitations.

VWD can present with normal APTT values, especially if the FVIII activity level is above 40–50%. Type 1 VWD is a quantitative deficit of VWF, and all multimeric forms are present. Mild type 1 VWD may be missed by the bleeding time and the PFA-100, making measurement of VWF antigen and activity levels necessary for proper diagnosis. Additionally, levels of VWF fluctuate in response to estrogens, stress, exercise, inflammation, and bleeding; and repeated assays are often required to make the diagnosis.

Hereditary HHT is an autosomal dominant disorder that is associated with arteriovenous malformations of the small vessels of the skin, oropharynx, lungs, gastrointestinal tract, and other tissues. The syndrome is often suspected by the presence of epistaxis, gastrointestinal bleeding, telangiectasia on the lips and fingertips, and iron deficiency anemia. Although bleeding does not occur at birth, it may begin in childhood, and by age 16, the majority of patients will experience hemorrhagic symptoms.

Ehlers-Danlos syndrome (EDS) is characterized by easy bruising and hemorrhage from ruptured blood vessels and is due to one of several genetic defects [28]. The classic EDS causing joint hypermobility and hyperextensibility of the skin may be associated with bruising but is not likely to result in massive bleeding. The vascular type IV EDS is the most likely to result in significant bruising and is due to a defect in type III collagen resulting from defects in the COL3A1 gene. In this type of EDS, bruising can be very extensive and vascular rupture can result in death. The skin may be thin and wrinkled, but hyperextensibility of the skin is not common. The bruising is sufficient to make one suspect a platelet disorder, but tests of platelet and coagulant function are normal. Diagnosis is dependent on demonstration of the genetic abnormality or the demonstration of abnormal type III collagen.

Acquired causes

Many drugs and herbs cause platelet dysfunction, and their use needs to be questioned extensively. Uremia, myeloproliferative disorders, and cardiac bypass will also cause a thrombocytopathy.

Amyloidosis has been reported in conjunction with acquired deficiencies of α2-antiplasmin and PAI-1. Inhibitors to FXIII have been reported and are rare.

Patients without bleeding history, but with abnormal coagulation testing

When doing pre-operative evaluations of these patients, it is important to recognize that many patients with mild bleeding disorders may have no known history of bleeding. Some may recall mild bleeding symptoms when carefully questioned, whereas some may not have had sufficient challenges to their hemostatic systems. Thus, some lab evaluation is required, depending on the severity of the surgery that is being planned.

Congenital causes

Deficiencies of high-molecular-weight kininogen, prekallikrein, and FXII will produce marked prolongation of the APTT without conferring an increased risk of abnormal bleeding. Some patients with FXI deficiency may have no bleeding symptoms, despite low levels of FXI. Patients with mild deficiency of FVII may also have no bleeding symptoms. Additionally, certain mutations in the FVII molecule affect its interaction with bovine but not human thromboplastin, and these mutations are not associated with clinical manifestations. Lastly, most dyfibrinogenemias are also associated with no clinical symptoms.

Acquired causes

Lupus anticoagulants prolong the APTT, and the mixing study fails to correct. Unless associated with acquired hypoprothrombinemia, lupus inhibitors confer no increased risk of bleeding. The majority of acquired FV antibodies are also asymptomatic and are self-limited. Although patients with severe liver disease may have a prolonged PT/INR, their bleeding symptoms may vary. These patients may clot and they are not "auto-anticoagulated," because they are deficient in many anticoagulant proteins as well.

Conclusion

Evaluation of the bleeding patient requires a careful history and physical examination. Laboratory workup should be tailored to the clinical presentation and the pretest probability of finding an underlying bleeding diathesis. Many of the laboratory tests are best conducted at a tertiary center with expertise in hemostasis. Accurate diagnosis allows for rational, intelligent treatment and prophylaxis of bleeding.

References

1 Higham JM, O'Brien PM, Shaw RW. Assessment of menstrual blood loss using a pictorial chart. *Br J Obstet Gynaecol* 1990;97(8):734–9.

2 Rodeghiero F, Kadir RA, Tosetto A, James PD. Relevance of quantitative assessment of bleeding in haemorrhagic disorders. *Haemophilia* 2008;14(Suppl 3):68–75.

3 Philipp CS, Faiz A, Dowling N, et al. Age and the prevalence of bleeding disorders in women with menorrhagia. *Obstet Gynecol* 2005;105(1):61–6.

4 Trasi SA, Pathare AV, Shetty SD, Ghosh K, Salvi V, Mohanty D. The spectrum of bleeding disorders in women with menorrhagia: a report from Western India. *Ann Hematol* 2005;84(5):339–42.

5 Woo YL, White B, Corbally R, et al. von Willebrand's disease: an important cause of dysfunctional uterine bleeding. *Blood Coagul Fibrinolysis* 2002;13(2): 89–93.

6 Lee CA. Women and inherited bleeding disorders: menstrual issues. *Semin Hematol* 1999;36(3 Suppl 4): 21–7.

7 James AH. More than menorrhagia: a review of the obstetric and gynaecological manifestations of bleeding disorders. *Haemophilia* 2005;11(4):295–307.

8 Gitschier J. Molecular genetics of hemophilia A. *Schweiz Med Wochenschr* 1989;119(39):1329–31.

9 Sucker C. The Heyde syndrome: proposal for a unifying concept explaining the association of aortic valve stenosis, gastrointestinal angiodysplasia and bleeding. *Int J Cardiol* 2007;115(1):77–8.

10 Sucker C, Hetzel GR, Grabensee B, Stockschlaeder M, Scharf RE. Amyloidosis and bleeding: pathophysiology, diagnosis, and therapy. *Am J Kidney Dis* 2006;47(6):947–55.

11 Mumford AD, O'Donnell J, Gillmore JD, Manning RA, Hawkins PN, Laffan M. Bleeding symptoms and coagulation abnormalities in 337 patients with AL-amyloidosis. *Br J Haematol* 2000;110(2):454–60.

12 Lind SE. The bleeding time does not predict surgical bleeding. *Blood* 1991;77(12):2547–52.

13 O'Brien SH, Ritchey AK, Ragni MV. Combined clotting factor deficiencies: experience at a single hemophilia treatment center. *Haemophilia* 2007;13(1):26–9.

14 Langdell RD, Wagner RH, Brinkhous KM. Effect of antihemophilic factor on one-stage clotting tests; a presumptive test for hemophilia and a simple one-stage antihemophilic factor assy procedure. *J Lab Clin Med* 1953;41(4):637–47.

15 Shah U, Ma AD. Tests of platelet function. *Curr Opin Hematol* 2007;14(5):432–7.

16 Michelson AD, Frelinger AL 3rd, Furman MI. Current options in platelet function testing. *Am J Cardiol* 2006;98(10A):4N–10N.

17 Favaloro EJ. Clinical application of the PFA-100. *Curr Opin Hematol* 2002;9(5):407–15.

18 Zhou L, Schmaier AH. Platelet aggregation testing in platelet-rich plasma: description of procedures with the aim to develop standards in the field. *Am J Clin Pathol* 2005;123(2):172–83.

19 Lorez HP, Richards JG, Da Prada M, et al. Storage pool disease: comparative fluorescence microscopical,

cytochemical and biochemical studies on amine-storing organelles of human blood platelets. *Br J Haematol* 1979;43(2):297–305.

20 White JG. Use of the electron microscope for diagnosis of platelet disorders. *Semin Thromb Hemost* 1998;24(2):163–8.

21 Mullighan CG, Rischbieth A, Duncan EM, Lloyd JV. Acquired isolated factor VII deficiency associated with severe bleeding and successful treatment with recombinant FVIIa (NovoSeven). *Blood Coagul Fibrinolysis* 2004;15(4):347–51.

22 Stenson PD, Ball EV, Mort M, et al. Human Gene Mutation Database (HGMD): 2003 update. *Hum Mutat* 2003;21(6):577–81.

23 Ma AD, Carrizosa D. Acquired factor VIII inhibitors: pathophysiology and treatment. *Hematol Am Soc Hematol Educ Program* 2006:432–7.

24 Torjemane L, Guermazi S, Ladeb S, et al. Heparin-like anticoagulant associated with multiple myeloma and neutralized with protamine sulfate. *Blood Coagul Fibrinolysis* 2007;18(3):279–81.

25 McMillan C, Roberts H. Congenital combined deficiency of coagulation factors II, VII, IX and X. *N Engl J Med* 1966;274:1313–5.

26 Zhang B, Ginsburg D. Familial multiple coagulation factor deficiencies: new biologic insight from rare genetic bleeding disorders. *J Thromb Haemost* 2004;2(9):1564–72.

27 Li T, Chang CY, Jin DY, Lin PJ, Khvorova A, Stafford DW. Identification of the gene for vitamin K epoxide reductase. *Nature* 2004;427(6974):541–4.

28 De Paepe A, Malfait F. Bleeding and bruising in patients with Ehlers-Danlos syndrome and other collagen vascular disorders. *Br J Haematol* 2004;127(5):491–500.

7 Hemophilia A and B

Rhona M. Maclean and Michael Makris

Introduction

Hemophilia A and B are bleeding disorders inherited in an X-linked recessive fashion, caused by deficiencies in factor VIII (FVIII) and factor IX (FIX), respectively. The first description of hemophilia is thought to be a passage describing bleeding following circumcision in the Babylonian Talmud of the 2nd century AD, "It was taught by the Tana'im: If she circumcised her first son and he died, and a second son and he died, she must not circumcise a third one."

It was initially thought that hemophilia was caused by abnormalities of the vascular system, and it was not until the late 1800s and early 1900s that a deficiency of a component of the blood was thought to be responsible.

All racial groups are equally affected by hemophilia with an incidence of 1 in 5000 live male births for hemophilia A, and 1 in 30,000 live male births for hemophilia B. The clinical symptoms and signs of these two disorders are identical in presentation, and specific clotting factor assays are required to distinguish them. With modern management and the ready availability of clotting factors, children with hemophilia today can look forward to a normal life expectancy [1].

Factor VIII gene and protein

In the two decades since the FVIII protein was first purified (1983) and the gene cloned (1982–4), advances in molecular biology and protein biochemistry have led to a greatly improved understanding of the structure and function of both the FVIII gene and the protein. The crystal structure of FVIII was recently published [2].

The FVIII gene (F8) is situated in the most distal band of the long arm of the X chromosome at Xq28, spans 186,000 base pairs (bp) of DNA, contains 26 exons, and is transcribed from the telomeric to centromeric direction to produce a mature mRNA of approximately 9 kb. The precursor protein (2351 amino acids) is predominantly synthesized in hepatocytes and has a molecular weight of approximately 293,000 Da.

After cleavage of the secretory leader sequence, the FVIII protein has a mature sequence of 2332 amino acids with the domain structure A1-a1-A2-a2-B-a3-A3-C1-C2. The domain structure of FVIII is very similar to that of coagulation factor V, and its A domains are homologous with ceruloplasmin. As the FVIII protein is very susceptible to proteolysis after secretion, the majority of circulating FVIII comprises heavy chains (the A1 and A2 domains with variable lengths of the B domain) noncovalently linked to light chains (A3, C1, and C2 domains). The B domain is unnecessary for FVIII procoagulant activity. FVIII exerts its procoagulant activity by accelerating the activation of coagulation factor X by factor IXa. FVIII circulates bound to and is stabilised by von Willebrand factor (VWF), with a ratio of approximately 1 molecule of FVIII to 50 molecules of VWF.

Mutations in F8

There are many F8 gene defects listed on the online hemophilia A mutation database (http://europium.csc.mrc.ac.uk). These can be categorised as (1) gross gene rearrangements, (2) insertions or deletions of genetic sequence, or (3) single base substitutions (leading to missense, nonsense, or splicing defects). All types of mutation can lead to severe disease, but the most clinically important defect, responsible for 40–45% of cases of severe hemophilia A, is the F8 intron 22 inversion. This inversion mutation virtually always occurs in male germ cells during spermatogenesis; in more than 95% of hemophiliacs with the intron 22 inversion, their mothers were demonstrated to be carriers.

The majority of point mutations have been reported only once; however, there are some recurrent mutations, often with variable clinical phenotype and FVIII activity. This suggests that there are other factors, in addition to the F8 gene defect, responsible for the clinical severity of the disease.

Overall, mutations are now identifiable in over 90% of individuals with hemophilia A (see Chapter 3 for further information regarding molecular defects in hemophilia A and their detection).

Factor IX gene and protein

The FIX gene (F9) is centromeric to F8 on the X chromosome at Xq27, and the gene is predominantly expressed in the liver. It is considerably smaller than F8, spanning 34 kb of DNA and containing only 8 exons (a–h), which code for an mRNA of 2.8 kb that translates into a protein of 415 amino acids. After entry into the endoplasmic reticulum, the 18-amino-acid prepeptide (encoded by the first exon, a) is cleaved off. The FIX protein is a member of the serine protease family, and its domain structure is similar to that of FVII, FX, and protein C. As with the other serine proteases, it requires posttranslational γ-carboxylation of its glutamyl (Glu) residues by a vitamin-K-dependent process.

Mutations in F9

There are many different mutations reported in F9, and a very useful resource is the hemophilia B mutation database (http://www.kcl.ac.uk/ip/petergreen/hemBdatabase.html). The majority of mutations in F9 are point mutations (~80%), with the remainder being splice site, frameshift, or gross deletions/rearrangements (~3–4% each). (See Chapter 3 for further information regarding the molecular genetics and diagnostics of hemophilia B.)

Table 7.1 Classification of severity of hemophilia.

Classification of severity	Concentration of coagulation factor
Severe	<0.01 IU/mL or <1% of normal
Moderate	0.01–0.05 IU/mL or 1–5% of normal
Mild	>0.05 IU/mL or >5% of normal

Severity and symptoms

Hemophilia is classified as severe, moderate, or mild on the basis of assayed plasma coagulation factor levels. This laboratory classification largely correlates with the clinical bleeding risk (Table 7.1), thus allowing a prediction to be made about individual bleeding risk and outcome. Approximately 50% of patients with hemophilia have severe disease, 10% moderate, and 40% mild hemophilia.

Severe disease

Those with severe disease develop spontaneous joint and muscle hematomas, in addition to bleeding after minor injuries, accidents, and surgical procedures. Most patients with severe hemophilia A are diagnosed within the first year of life, either due to testing around the time of birth, in those with a family history, or because of abnormal bruising/bleeding. Thereafter, in the first 6–9 months of life, cutaneous bruising or oral bleeding (due to teething or cuts in the oral cavity) can occur. Once the baby becomes more mobile (rolling, crawling, toddling, cruising), bruising and joint bleeds can occur. Although bruising can be prominent in young children (it resolves once they start prophylaxis), it is not a feature of adult severe hemophilia.

Moderate disease

Those with moderate disease do not tend to bleed spontaneously, but develop muscle and joint hematomas after mild trauma. They also bleed excessively after surgery and dental extractions.

Mild disease

Individuals with mild hemophilia do not bleed spontaneously. They do, however, bleed after surgery, significant trauma, or dental extractions.

Inheritance

Both hemophilia A and B are X-linked recessive inherited disorders and therefore affect males almost exclusively. It is not uncommon, however, for carrier females to have reductions in FVIII or FIX levels to the extent that they may experience menorrhagia or will require treatment prior to any invasive procedure or following major trauma.

Where the female is a carrier, there is a 50:50 chance that a son will be affected by hemophilia or that a daughter will be a carrier. When the children are from a hemophilic male and a normal female, all sons will be unaffected, but all daughters will be obligate carriers.

Approximately one-third of cases of hemophilia are 'sporadic,' that is, due to the occurrence of a new mutation, with no family history of the disease.

Mosaicism occurs when a proportion of the cells of the body contain a mutation, whereas the majority do not. Gonadal mosaicim, in which the mutation is confined to the gonadal tissue, has been reported in both hemophilia A and B [3]. Should gonadal mosaicim be present, the risk of passing on the disease to any future children will be higher than the risk in the general population. Care must therefore be taken when counseling women who do not appear to be carriers, yet have a child with hemophilia.

Females with markedly reduced FVIII/IX levels

This is possible in the following rare circumstances:
• With extreme lyonization of F8 or F9 in hemophilia carriers (resulting in most of the expression deriving from the hemophilic X chromosome); rarely carriers can have levels <10%.
• If there is hemizygosity of the X chromosome [e.g. in Turner (XO) syndrome].
• A female can be affected if she is the offspring of a hemophilic male and a carrier female.
• In females with the Normandy variant of von Willebrand disease (Type 2N VWD; FVIII deficiency only).
• In females with acquired hemophilia due to autoantibody development.

Carrier testing

All females who are obligate or possible carriers of hemophilia should be offered genetic counseling to provide them with the information necessary to make informed reproductive choices and for the optimal management of their pregnancies. The majority of individuals with hemophilia A and B now have an identifiable mutation. If the mutation within the family is known, it is straightforward to screen the potential carrier and confirm the carrier status in obligate carriers. If the mutation is not known, then linkage analysis using informative genetic polymorphisms is usually successful (if sufficient family members are available for testing). If neither of these approaches is suitable, then direct mutation detection can be performed (see Chapter 3). All carriers of hemophilia A or B should have their factor VIII/IX levels checked to evaluate their personal risk of bleeding.

Prenatal diagnosis

Although the treatment of hemophilia has greatly improved over the last 10–20 years, many carriers of hemophilia (often those who have grown up with a family member who had complications of the disease, such as inhibitors or viral infections) will request prenatal diagnosis. Chorionic villus sampling is the most widely used method of prenatal diagnosis, and can be performed at 10–12 weeks' gestation, allowing for first trimester termination if desired. Alternatively, amniocentesis can be performed at 16 weeks. The risks of these procedures are low in experienced centers, with a miscarriage rate of 0.5–1%. Fetoscopy to allow for fetal blood sampling is rarely performed as it can only be performed after 20 weeks' gestation and has a higher risk of fetal death (1–6%). Following the discovery of fetal DNA in maternal blood, PCR-based techniques have been developed to detect specific Y-chromosomal sequences in maternal blood samples. Although not yet available in many centers, it is now possible to determine the sex of a fetus from as early as 7 weeks' gestation [4].

Embryo selection: Preimplantation Genetic Diagnosis

Preimplantation Genetic Diagnosis involves the genetic testing of an embryo prior to implantation and before pregnancy occurs. It is used in conjunction with in vitro fertilization, and only embryos found to be free of a specific genetic disorder are transferred into a woman for pregnancy. The advantage of this approach is that the trauma of termination of pregnancy can be avoided [5].

Delivery of an at-risk pregnancy

All carriers of hemophilia should have an ultrasound scan at around 20 weeks' gestation to identify the fetal sex (if other prenatal diagnostic tests have not been performed). Should the baby be male, then care should be taken to minimize the risk of bleeding at delivery; for example, vacuum (ventouse) extraction, rotational forceps, and invasive monitoring techniques, including placement of scalp electrodes, should be avoided. The mode of delivery should be for obstetric reasons and need not be by cesarean mode. The choice between vaginal and cesarean delivery is hotly debated.

A cord sample should be sent from all male infants born to known carriers for FVIII/IX estimation. Vitamin K should be given orally until it is definitely known that the baby is not affected by hemophilia.

Making the diagnosis

Immediately following the birth of a male infant to a known carrier of hemophilia, the following tests should be performed on the cord blood:
• Prothrombin time (PT);
• Activated partial thromboplastin time (APTT);
• Fibrinogen level;
• FVIII or FIX activity; and
• Where there is no family history, if the FVIII level is low, VWF assays for antigen and activity should be performed.

The APTT of an affected infant will usually be prolonged when compared with a gestation-specific normal range. FVIII levels in infants are comparable with those of adults, allowing for an accurate diagnosis. Although FIX levels in infants are considerably lower than those in adults, if the FIX level is less than 1%, a diagnosis of severe hemophilia B can be made. All neonates given a diagnosis of hemophilia on testing a cord blood sample should have this confirmed on a venous blood sample. Those with equivocal results should have a repeated test at 6 months of age.

Approximately one-third of individuals with hemophilia have no family history of a bleeding disorder. A diagnosis of hemophilia should be suspected if a child has a history of excessive bruising or bleeding or presents with a swollen painful joint or muscle hematoma.

The majority of children with moderate or severe hemophilia will present by 4–5 years of age. Where there is no family history, it is important to exclude the diagnosis of VWD, as the Normandy variant of VWD is phenotypically identical to mild/moderate hemophilia A (although with autosomal inheritance). If this is suspected, a VWF–FVIII binding assay or mutation analysis of exons 18–25 of the VWF gene should be undertaken to establish the correct diagnosis (see Chapter 6).

The neonate with hemophilia

The neonatal period is defined as the first 28 days after delivery, irrespective of gestation. Most bleeding episodes in neonates with hemophilia are due to birth trauma. It has been estimated that 3.5–4% of neonates with severe hemophilia have intracranial hemorrhages, most associated with the presence of an extracranial hemorrhage, the risk being greater if the delivery was traumatic/vacuum-assisted [6]. As yet there is no consensus as to whether routine cranial ultrasound should be performed after delivery in neonates known to have hemophilia, or whether prophylactic factor concentrate should be given after delivery. Most clinicians would give prophylactic coagulation factor concentrate if the delivery was traumatic, instrumental, or in the presence of prematurity.

Bleeding episodes in the neonate with hemophilia occurring in the first week of birth are usually due to heel pricks performed for blood sampling, intramuscular injections of vitamin K, or after circumcision.

Clinical manifestations and their treatment

Bleeding episodes

General principles

Bleeding episodes are treated by increasing the appropriate coagulation factor to hemostatic levels. For mild hemophilia, it is often possible to use desmopressin (DDAVP) for this purpose; an infusion of DDAVP 0.3 μg/kg will increase the FVIII levels (and VWF levels) three- to five-fold. For those with moderate or severe hemophilia A or those with hemophilia B, infusions of coagulation factor concentrates are required. Pharmacokinetic studies have shown that 1 U FVIII/kg body weight increases the FVIII level on average 0.02 IU/mL (2%), whereas 1 U FIX/kg body weight increases the FIX level 0.01 IU/mL (1%).

Calculating the quantity of FVIII required

Units of FVIII to be infused = [(desired FVIII level −actual FVIII level) × patient weight]/2.

For example, if a 70-kg man with severe hemophilia A (FVIII <1%) has a muscle hematoma and the desired FVIII level is 50% of normal, then:

Units of FVIII to be infused

$$= [(50 - 0) \times 70]/2 = 1750\,\text{U}.$$

Calculating the FIX required

Units of FIX to be infused = (desired level FIX −actual level FIX) × weight in kg.

Recombinant FIX has a 30% lower recovery in comparison with plasma-derived FIX. If the product to be used is recombinant FIX, then the result of the above equation should be multiplied by 1.4.

Joint bleeds

Joints are the most common sites of spontaneous bleeding in those with severe hemophilia A and B (Fig. 7.1 & Plate 7.1). The affected joint is painful, warm, swollen, occasionally erythematous, and tends to be held in a flexed position. It must be appreciated that early on there may be no abnormal physical signs of a hemarthrosis, but patients often know if a bleed is starting. If treated promptly, levels of 30–50% will usually suffice to treat a minor bleed, together with paracetamol (acetaminophen) for pain. Occasionally,

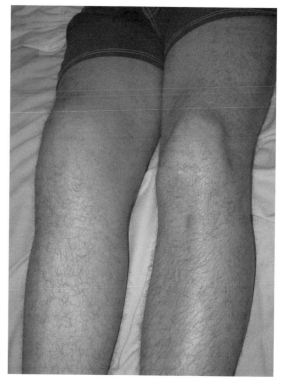

Figure 7.1 Right knee hemarthrosis in a severe hemophilia A patient. Bleeds such as this are unusual in countries where patients have home treatment with clotting factor concentrates. Usually there are no physical signs, and the only symptoms are pain and limitation of joint movement.

a second dose (8–12 hours after the first) may be required. With severe bleeding, several days of treatment with opiate analgesia may be required. Table 7.2 shows the distribution of spontaneous bleeds in severe hemophiliacs.

Physiotherapy is important from an early stage to ensure that muscle atrophy does not occur and to

Table 7.2 Joints most frequently affected by spontaneous bleeds in severe hemophilia.

Knee	45%
Elbow	25%
Ankle	15%
Shoulder	5%
Hip	5%
Other joints	5%

CHAPTER 7

prevent the development of joint flexures. Recurrent joint bleeds usually benefit from regular coagulation factor infusions (secondary prophylaxis) in order to prevent the development of hemophilic arthropathy. In some patients, "target" joints develop (repeated bleeding into a joint, without a return to "normal" between bleeds) with chronic synovitis. Regular coagulation factor prophylaxis, physiotherapy, anti-inflammatory drugs, intra-articular steroids, or synovectomy (whether surgical, radioisotopic, or chemical) may be required to halt the cycle of recurrent bleeds and inflammation [7].

Despite the above, a number of patients will need joint replacement surgery; it is expected that the need for this should diminish with the increasing use of prophylaxis.

Muscle bleeds
Muscle bleeds within closed fascial compartments can be limb-threatening because of blood vessel and nerve compression. Bleeding into the iliopsoas muscle and retroperitoneum is not uncommon, and patients present with:
• groin pain;
• hip flexion; and
• internal rotation.

Blood loss can be significant and femoral nerve compression can occur, resulting in permanent neurologic deficit. Pelvic ultrasound or CT scanning will confirm the diagnosis, and treatment is required to raise the coagulation factor level to 100% for several days.

Intracranial hemorrhage
This is the most common cause of death from bleeding in hemophiliacs and can occur spontaneously as well as after trauma (Fig. 7.2). If suspected, or if thought to be possible following head trauma, coagulation factor concentrates should be immediately administered to raise the coagulation factor level to 100% prior to any diagnostic tests.

Hematuria
Spontaneous hematuria is relatively common in severe hemophiliacs. It tends to be painless and is usually self-limiting, unless clots form within the ureters. Treatment of the hematuria predominantly consists of maintaining adequate hydration and analgesia if required. If the hematuria fails to settle within a few

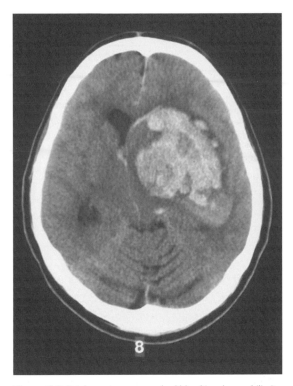

Figure 7.2 Fatal spontaneous cerebral bleed in a hemophilia B patient.

days, it may be necessary to raise coagulation factor levels to 50% of normal. Antifibrinolytic agents should never be given, as these increase the likelihood of intraureteric clot formation and clot colic. The etiology of this hematuria is usually unknown, but other causes, such as infection, renal calculi, and neoplastic disease in the older hemophiliac, should be considered. One of the HIV protease inhibitor drugs (indinavir) induces crystalluria and calculus formation, which can lead to hematuria.

Gastrointestinal bleeding
Gastrointestinal bleeding tends to be caused by anatomical lesions rather than coagulation factor deficiency and should be fully investigated. Raising the coagulation factor level to >50% is usually sufficient. Antifibrinolytics are helpful in mucosal bleeding.

Pseudotumors
Repeated, inadequately treated bleeding episodes at a single site result in the development of an

encapsulated hematoma. This progressively enlarges, erodes, and invades surrounding structures, hence the name pseudotumour (Plate 7.2). Surgical removal is difficult and is associated with a significant morbidity/mortality. These are now rare in countries with ready availability of clotting factor concentrates [8].

Dental treatment

Minor dental work (scaling and polishing) can be performed without factor replacement, but inferior dental nerve blocks or extractions require factor concentrates or desmopressin administered as appropriate. Antifibrinolytic agents (such as tranexamic acid as a mouthwash) should be provided for 3–5 days after any dental extractions.

Surgery

For major surgical procedures, coagulation factor levels should be maintained at 50–100% for 7–10 days to ensure adequate hemostasis and wound healing. This can be achieved either by bolus injections, with an initial bolus dose to bring the factor level to 100% followed by once daily FIX or twice daily FVIII injections, or by continuous infusion after the initial bolus dose, as guided by coagulation factor assays.

Continuous infusions have the advantage of:
• eliminating the "peaks and troughs" seen with bolus factor administration;
• less factor concentrate consumption for the same procedure;
• less cost; and
• more convenient for staff to administer.

One disadvantage is that these infusions tend to cause venous irritation, but this can be reduced by an infusion of saline in tandem through the same cannula. Intramuscular injections and nonsteroidal anti-inflammatory drugs should be avoided.

Primary prophylaxis

Primary prophylaxis was first introduced in Sweden (by Professor Inga Marie Nilsson) in the late 1950s and early 1960s. The rationale was that moderate hemophiliacs do not have spontaneous hemarthroses, and they also have significantly less joint arthropathy compared with those with coagulation factor levels of <1% [9].

It has since been shown that converting a severe hemophiliac to one with moderate disease by regular infusions of coagulation factor concentrate reduces the number of spontaneous joint bleeds, reduces the resulting joint damage [10], and is now recommended for all children with severe disease.

In the UK, prophylaxis tends to be introduced after one or two spontaneous joint bleeds, and the dose and frequency of administration is titrated to prevent spontaneous bleeding events. FVIII (20–40 IU/kg) is given ideally three times weekly (or alternate days) by intravenous infusion, whereas FIX (25–40 IU/kg) usually only needs to be given twice weekly.

Initially, prophylaxis is given by staff based at the hemophilia center, while training the parents (and later the child) to take over this role. In many children, it is possible to manage with peripheral venous access, but in some, it is necessary to use central venous access devices (e.g. Port-A-Caths). Some centers found that the use of play therapists significantly increased the proportion of children managing with peripheral venous access. More recently, internal arteriovenous fistulae in the forearm, such as those used for hemodialysis, have been used for venous access because of complications of infection and thrombosis associated with central venous access devices.

Treatment

Clotting factor replacement

A landmark in the treatment of patients with bleeding disorders was the introduction of fresh frozen plasma in the 1940s, which, because it contained all clotting factors, could be used to treat all clotting factor deficiencies. Over the last 70 years, the number of different products, as well as their purity, has increased significantly; and in the last 15–20 years, molecular technology has produced both FVIII and FIX as recombinant proteins [11].

Plasma-derived concentrates

Human plasma-derived concentrates are made from pools, with each containing up to 30,000 plasma donations. Table 7.3 lists currently available concentrates.

Transfusion-transmitted infection was the major potential complication of plasma-derived clotting factor concentrates. Because of this, all plasma-derived concentrates undergo viral inactivation by at least one, and preferably two, different viral inactivation

Table 7.3 Currently available clotting factor concentrates.

Factor concentrate	Type available
Fibrinogen	Plasma-derived
Factor VII	Plasma-derived and activated recombinant
Factor VIII	Plasma-derived and recombinant
Porcine FVIII	Recombinant (in trials)
VWF	Plasma-derived and recombinant (in trials)
Factor IX	Plasma-derived and recombinant
Factor XI	Plasma-derived
Factor XIII	Plasma-derived and recombinant (in trials)
Prothrombin complex	Plasma-derived
Activated prothrombin complex	Plasma-derived

procedures. Table 7.4 lists some of the currently used viral inactivation procedures. Although in the past some of the procedures were not very effective in eliminating all pathogenic viruses, the currently used ones are highly efficient in this respect.

Recombinant products

Recombinant clotting factors are produced by the insertion of the relevant gene into a cell line [either Chinese Hamster ovary (CHO) or Baby Hamster Kidney (BHK)]. Following cell culture, the clotting factor is secreted into and harvested from the culture medium. Recombinant concentrates are currently available for factors VIII, IX, and VII (as activated FVII), and recombinant FXIII is in clinical trials.

Table 7.4 Viral inactivation and removal techniques.

Heat treatment
    Dry heat at 80°C for 72 hours
    Heat in solution at 60°C for 10 hours (pasteurization)
    Vapour heat at 60°C for 10 hours, 1160 mb pressure
Solvent detergent treatment
    TNBP and Tween
    Triton X-100
    Cholate
Nanofiltration
Chromatographic purification
    Monoclonal antibody
    Heparin affinity
    Ion exchange

Early preparations of recombinant concentrates contained human albumin as a stabilizer and used animal proteins during the manufacturing process (first-generation products). Second-generation recombinant clotting factors are stabilized without the addition of human albumin but have albumin in the cell culture medium. In third-generation products, human and animal proteins have been removed from the culture media. As for plasma-derived products, all recombinant clotting factor concentrates also undergo viral inactivation.

Other hemostatic agents

Cryoprecipitate and fresh frozen plasma

Hemophilia care should be delivered from hemophilia centers with access to plasma-derived, virally inactivated clotting factor concentrates. In underdeveloped countries and in developed countries in an emergency (if FVIII concentrate is unavailable), cryoprecipitate can be used as the source of FVIII, but it must be appreciated that each cryoprecipitate unit contains only 80–100 IU of FVIII, and it is not virally inactivated. In the absence of FIX concentrates, fresh frozen plasma (preferably virally inactivated) should be used for hemophilia B patients.

Desmopressin (DDAVP)

DDAVP is a vasopressin analogue that can release stored VWF from endothelial cells and results in a secondary increase in FVIII levels. It can be given intravenously (0.3 µg/kg as an infusion over 30 minutes), subcutaneously (0.3 µg/kg), or intranasally. It is useful in the management of mild hemophilia A, type 1 VWD and some patients with platelet function defects. DDAVP administration can be repeated over a short period, but efficacy will then decrease because of tachyphylaxis. However, a few days later, the endothelial stores are replenished, and original efficacy is reestablished.

Common adverse effects include a mild headache, flushing, and fluid retention, so patients should be advised to reduce their fluid intake in the subsequent 12–24 hours. Because of the problem with fluid retention, DDAVP should be avoided in children under the age of 2 years.

Tranexamic acid

Tranexamic acid is an antifibrinolytic agent that can be given orally or intravenously. It is very useful where there is mucosal bleeding and should be routinely administered to hemophiliacs having dental extractions.

Complications of treatment

Despite the success of concentrate treatment, a number of complications occur; these are summarized in Table 7.5 [12].

Inhibitor development

Allo-antibodies develop in up to 30% of children with severe hemophilia A who receive treatment with FVIII concentrate. Although uncommon, they can also occur in patients with mild or moderate hemophilia A after treatment with factor VIII; in some instances, cross-reacting with autologous factor VIII. They are rare in hemophilia B patients (<3%). These antibodies (inhibitors) are more likely to develop:

Table 7.5 Complications of clotting factor therapy.

Allo-antibody formation – inhibitor development
Infections
  HIV
  Hepatitis A, B, C, D, G
  Parvovirus B19
  vCJD
Immune modulation
Thrombosis
Anaphylaxis

- before the age of 5 years;
- within the first 50 treatment days;
- in those of African descent;
- where there is a family history of inhibitor development; or
- in patients with FVIII/IX gene deletions.

They are usually suspected when a previously effective treatment is no longer sufficient to achieve hemostasis. The prolonged APTT does not normalize in vitro after the addition of normal plasma, and confirmation is made with the Bethesda assay [13].

The treatment of acute bleeding in hemophiliacs with inhibitors is difficult and expensive. It depends on the level of the inhibitor and whether it is a low- or a high-responding one.

High-responding patients develop a rapidly increasing antibody level each time they are exposed to human FVIII. The two main types of treatment of acute bleeding in these patients are:

1 Activated prothrombin complex concentrates, such as FEIBA; and
2 Recombinant FVIIa (NovoSeven).

A recent comparative study found that the two products are equally effective, but some patients respond better to one versus the other [14]. Other than through clinical response, there is currently no reliable widely used method to monitor treatment with these products in the laboratory; although global assays, such as thrombin generation, thromboelastometry, and thromboelastography, are showing promise.

Porcine FVIII concentrate is also useful in patients without a cross-reacting antibody to porcine FVIII. Although currently not widely available, studies of recombinant porcine FVIII are underway.

In every patient with an inhibitor, the possibility of elimination through immune tolerance should be considered. There are three immune tolerance protocols available:

1 *High-dose protocol:* administers FVIII daily;
2 *Low-dose protocol:* alternate daily administration; or
3 *Malmo protocol:* FVIII is combined with intravenous immunoglobulin, cyclophosphamide, and immunoadsorption or plasmapheresis.

The reported success rates from small series are 30–80%. Once an inhibitor has been eliminated, the chance of it recurring is 15%. An international immune tolerance induction study in patients with severe hemophilia A and inhibitors is underway comparing low- and high-dose immune tolerance regimens (http://www.itistudy.com). Rituximab (a monoclonal anti-CD20 antibody) treatment has been tried in some hemophilia patients with inhibitors with varying success [15].

Infections

The viral inactivation of concentrates introduced in 1985 was highly effective in eliminating most transfusion-transmitted viruses. The risk of infection in patients treated prior to 1985 was 25–70% for HIV, 100% for hepatitis C, and 50% for hepatitis B.

Human immunodeficiency virus (HIV)

The transmission of HIV infections by plasma-derived concentrates in the early 1980s has had a devastating effect in the lives of hemophiliacs. Approximately two-thirds of the HIV-infected hemophiliacs have now died, but in those still alive, the use of highly active antiretroviral therapy (HAART) has allowed near normal existence with immune reconstitution and a dramatically reduced mortality.

Hepatitis C

• 15% of patients infected cleared the virus naturally (antibody-positive but PCR-negative).
• 85% were chronically infected (persistence more than 6 months).
• Approximately 20–30% of infected patients have evidence of cirrhosis.
• 5–10% have developed liver failure or hepatocellular carcinoma.

  Factors accelerating liver disease progression include:
• time since infection;
• older age at infection;
• HIV coinfection; and
• higher alcohol consumption.

  Treatment with pegylated interferon and ribavirin achieves cure of hepatitis C in 30–40% of those infected with HCV genotype 1 and 70% of those infected with genotype 2 or 3.

Hepatitis B

Approximately 50% of hemophiliacs treated with pooled plasma products prior to viral inactivation were infected with hepatitis B virus, but most cleared the virus spontaneously; less than 5% of these patients show active chronic hepatitis B virus infection. All non-immune and non-infected hemophiliacs should be vaccinated against this virus.

Parvovirus B19

This causes fifth disease in childhood, and most adults show evidence of past infection. Although the disease itself is relatively minor, its importance lies in the fact that the virus is resistant to all currently used viral inactivation techniques. The implication of this is that unknown viruses can theoretically be transmitted by all currently available plasma-derived clotting factor concentrates, and this is one of the main reasons for the introduction of recombinant concentrates in countries where alternative "safe" plasma-derived concentrates exist.

Variant Creutzfeldt–Jakob disease (vCJD)

vCJD is a prion disease that is the human equivalent of the bovine spongiform encephalopathy, which was endemic in the British cow population in the late 1980s and early 1990s. vCJD can be transmitted through transfusion of fresh cellular components. A significant number of UK hemophiliacs have been exposed to plasma from donors who subsequently developed vCJD. Although no hemophiliac has ever developed clinical vCJD, in February 2009 it was reported that vCJD related priors were identified in the spleen of a hemophiliac who died from an unrelated cause. This patient was treated with FVIII prepared from a donor who subsequently developed vCJD.

Immune modulation

In vitro, it is possible to show that concentrates exert an immunosuppressive effect. This has been observed and reported in hemophiliacs, but this phenomenon could have been a result of the chronic hepatitis C affecting the hemophiliacs studied.

Thrombosis

Thrombosis is a rare complication that was well recognized when prothrombin complex concentrates were used to cover surgery in patients with hemophilia B, prior to the addition of antithrombin and heparin to the product. It is still seen in patients treated with activated prothrombin complex concentrates, especially when the daily dosage exceeds 200 IU/kg.

Anaphylaxis

Allergic reactions to concentrates are now very rare because of the higher purity of the products. Although it used to occur with the administration of porcine plasma-derived FVIII, this is not currently available. Anaphylaxis remains a problem with recombinant factor IX concentrate in severe hemophilia B patients, especially those with FIX gene deletions. The first 20 treatments of newly diagnosed hemophilia B patients should be administered in a hospital or at a location with resuscitation facilities.

Acquired hemophilia A

Acquired hemophilia is a rare bleeding disorder caused by the development of specific autoantibodies that are capable of inhibiting the action of naturally occurring FVIII. Its incidence is 1.5 per million population per year. It is largely a disease of the elderly. Patients with malignancy or autoimmune disorders are more likely to be affected. Less than 10% of all cases occur in the postpartum period [16].

Patients present with prominent subcutaneous hematomas as well as bleeding elsewhere (Fig. 7.3 and Plate 7.1). Unlike classic hemophilia, hemarthroses are rare. There is prolongation of the APTT, which does

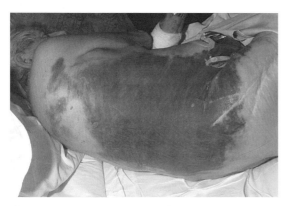

Figure 7.3 Extensive spontaneous subcutaneous hematoma in a patient with acquired hemophilia A. In contrast to congenital hemophilia, these patients often present with extensive subcutaneous bleeds and rarely have hemarthroses.

not correct following the in vitro addition of normal plasma. The FVIII level is reduced but rarely to <2%. The Bethesda assay demonstrates an inhibitor, but the degree of bleeding is often more severe than suggested by the inhibitor level.

Treatment is aimed at stopping the acute bleeding and eliminating the inhibitor. Acute bleeds are treated with activated prothrombin complex concentrates or recombinant FVIIa. The efficacy of these two treatments is similar. DDAVP and high doses of FVIII concentrate are rarely helpful in acquired hemophilia. The most common method used to eliminate the inhibitor is through immunosuppression with the use of high-dose steroids (1 mg/kg/day) with or without low-dose cytotoxic therapy (cyclophosphamide or azathioprine). Other treatments, such as cyclosporine, mycophenolate, and intravenous immunoglobulin (0.4 mg/kg/day for 5 days), may be useful in nonresponsive patients.

Recently, the monoclonal anti-CD20 antibody, rituximab, has been shown to be effective in the elimination of acquired inhibitors, but its precise role in practice remains to be established. There are no clinical trials comparing its effectiveness prospectively to standard therapy with steroids.

Over 80% of patients achieve remission from the disease, but 20% of these relapse. Most patients with acquired hemophilia die within 1–2 years of diagnosis, from comorbid conditions rather than bleeding, which is actually a rare cause of death in this condition, occurring in <10% of patients. In acquired hemophilia, more patients die from the complications of immunosuppression than from the disease itself [16].

The future

Undoubtedly, hemophilia care in the western world is currently the best it has ever been, and the clotting factor concentrates have never been safer. A number of advances are currently under development and are likely to enter clinical practice and perhaps become routinely available within the next decade, including:
• Recombinant clotting factors with no human or animal proteins used in the manufacturing process.
• Recombinant factors for the rarer deficiencies, e.g. FV, FX, FXI, and FXIII.

- Modified recombinant clotting factors with longer half-lives.
- Recombinant porcine FVIII for use in inhibitor patients.
- Recombinant VWF concentrate.
- Agents to be coadministered with DDAVP to improve its efficacy (e.g. interleukin 11).
- Embryo selection in hemophilia carriers to exclude implantation of affected embryos.
- Gene therapy where a normal FVIII or FIX gene is introduced in patients with hemophilia.

References

1 Mannucci PM, Tuddenham EG. The hemophilias: from royal genes to gene therapy. *N Engl J Med* 2001;344:1773–9.

2 Shen BW, Spiegel PC, Chang CH, et al. The tertiary structure and domain organization of coagulation FVIII. *Blood* 2008;111:1240–7.

3 Leuer M, Oldenburg J, Lavergne JM, et al. Somatic mosaicism in hemophilia A: a fairly common event. *Am J Hum Genet* 2001;69(1):75–87.

4 Lee CA, Chi C, Pavord SA, et al. The obstetric and gynaecological management of women with inherited bleeding disorders: review with guidelines produced by a taskforce of UK Haemophilia Centre Doctors Organization. *Haemophilia* 2006;12:301–36.

5 Michaelides K, Tuddenham EG, Turner C, Lavender B, Lavery SA. Liver birth following the first mutation specific preimplantation genetic diagnosis for haemophilia A. *Thromb Haemost* 2006;95:373–9.

6 Ljung RC. Intracranial haemorrhage in haemophilia A and B. *Br J Haematol* 2008;140(4):378–84.

7 Llinas A. The role of synovectomy in the management of a target joint. *Haemophilia* 2008;14(Suppl 3): 177–80.

8 Rodriguez-Merchan EC. Haemophilic cysts (pseudotumours). *Haemophilia* 2002;8:393–401.

9 Ljung R. Paediatric care of the child with hemophilia. *Haemophilia* 2002;8:178–82.

10 Manco-Johnson MJ, Abshire TC, Shapiro AD, et al. Prophylaxis versus episodic treatment to prevent joint disease in boys with severe hemophilia. *N Engl J Med* 2007;357:535–44.

11 Keeling D, Tait R, Makris M. Guideline on the selection and use of therapeutic products to treat haemophilia and other hereditary bleeding disorders. *Haemophilia* 2008;14:671–84.

12 Mannucci PM. Hemophilia and related bleeding disorders: a story of dismay and success. *Hematology (Am Soc Hematol Educ Program)* 2002:1–9.

13 Hay CR, Brown S, Collins PW, Keeling DM, Liesner R. The diagnosis and management of factor VIII and IX inhibitors: a guideline from the UK Haemophilia Centre Doctors' Organization. *Br J Haematol* 2006;133: 591–605.

14 Astermark J, Donfield DM, DiMichele DM, et al. A randomised comparison of bypassing agents in hemophilia complicated by an inhibitor: the FEIBA Novo-Seven comparative (FENOC) study. *Blood* 2007;109: 546–57.

15 Franchini M, Mengoli C, Lippi G, et al. Immune tolerance with rituximab in congenital haemophilia with inhibitors: a systematic literature review based on individual patients' analysis. *Haemophilia* 2008;14:903–12.

16 Collins PW, Hirsch S, Baglin TP, et al. Acquired haemophilia A in the United Kingdom: a 2 year national surveillance study of the United Kingdom Haemophilia Centre Doctors' Organisation. *Blood* 2007;109:1870–7.

8 Von Willebrand disease

Giancarlo Castaman, Alberto Tosetto, and Francesco Rodeghiero

Introduction: the von Willebrand factor

Von Willebrand disease (VWD) is caused by a deficiency and/or abnormality of von Willebrand factor (VWF) and represents the most frequent inherited bleeding disorder [1]. VWF is synthesized by endothelial cells and megakaryocytes. Its gene includes about 178 kilobases with 52 exons and is located at chromosome 12p13.2. A non-coding homologous pseudogene has been identified in chromosome 22, which spans the gene sequence from exon 23 to 34 [2]. The primary product of the VWF gene is a 2813-amino-acid protein comprising a signal peptide of 22 amino acids (also called pre-peptide), a large pro-peptide of 741 amino acids (also called pro-peptide), and a mature VWF subunit of 2050 amino acids. Four types of repeated molecular domains (D1, D2, D', D3, A1, A2, A3, D4, B, C1, C2) of cDNA are responsible for the different binding functions of the molecule. The building block of VWF multimers is a dimer made by two single-chain pro-VWF molecules, joined through disulphide bonds within their C-terminal region. This reaction occurs after the cleavage of the signal peptide and the subsequent translocation and glycosylation of the precursor molecules into the endoplasmic reticulum. The pro-VWF dimers are then transported to the Golgi apparatus, where, after further post-translational modifications, including processing of high mannose oligosaccharides, they are polymerized into very large molecules up to a molecular weight of $20,000 \times 10^3$ through disulphide bonds connecting the two N-terminal ends of each dimer. After polymerization, pro-VWF multimers move to the trans-Golgi network, where the pro-peptide (also called VWAgII), is cleaved off by a paired amino acid-cleaving enzyme (PACE or furin), and remains, at least within the cell, noncovalently associated with VWF [3].

VWF is secreted from the cell via a constitutive and a regulated pathway. The latter is used for a rapid stimuli-induced release (e.g. by desmopressin through its binding to vasopressin V2 receptor of endothelial cells) from specialized storage organelles of endothelial cells known as Weibel-Palade bodies. Only Weibel-Palade bodies or α-granules in platelets contain fully processed and functional VWF with "unusually large" multimers. These large multimers are usually not found in the circulation. Indeed, a specific plasma protease acts on VWF multimers released from the cell, cleaving the VWF subunit at the bond between Tyr 1605 and Met 1606 (Tyr 842 and Met 843 of the mature subunit), thus creating the full spectrum of circulating VWF species, ranging from the single dimer to multimers made of up to 20 dimers in each VWF multimer [4].

In addition to endothelial cells, megakaryocytes, and platelets, VWF is present in the subendothelial matrix, where it is bound through specific regions in its A1 and A3 domains to different types of collagen.

Physiological role of VWF

VWF is essential for platelet–subendothelium adhesion and platelet-to-platelet cohesion and aggregation in vessels with elevated shear stress [5]. This function is partially explored in vivo by measuring the bleeding time. Adhesion is promoted by the interaction of a region of the A1 domain of VWF with platelet GpIb. It is thought that high shear stress is able to activate the A1 domain of the collagen-bound VWF by stretching VWF multimers into a filamentous form. The interaction between GPIb and VWF can be mimicked by the addition of the antibiotic ristocetin, which promotes the binding of VWF to GPIb present on fresh or formalin-fixed platelet suspensions. Aggregation of platelets within the growing hemostatic plug is promoted by the interaction with a second receptor on platelets, the GPIIb-IIIa (or integrin $\alpha_{IIb}\beta_3$), which after activation binds to VWF and fibrinogen, recruiting more platelets into a stable plug. Both of these binding activities of VWF are highest in the largest VWF multimers.

VWF is the carrier of factor VIII (FVIII) in plasma. VWF protects FVIII from proteolytic degradation, prolonging its half-life in the circulation and efficiently localizing it at the site of vascular injury [6]. Each monomer of VWF has one binding domain, located in the first 272 amino acids of the mature subunit (D' domain), that is able to bind one FVIII molecule. In vivo, however, only 1–2% of available monomers are occupied by FVIII. This explains why high-molecular-weight multimers are not essential for the carrier function of FVIII, although one would expect that molecules of the highest molecular weight should be most effective in localizing FVIII at the site of vascular injury. In any case, any change in plasma VWF level is usually associated with a concordant change in FVIII plasma concentration.

Classification of VWD

The current nomenclature of the factor VIII/VWF complex, as recommended by the International Society on Thrombosis and Hemostasis, is summarized in Table 8.1 [7]. The current revised classification of

Table 8.1 Recommended nomenclature of FVIII/VWF complex.

Factor VIII	
Protein	VIII
Antigen	VIII:Ag
Function	VIII:C
Von Willebrand factor	
Mature protein	VWF
Antigen	VWF:Ag
Ristocetin cofactor activity	VWF:RCo
Collagen binding capacity	VWF:CB
FVIII binding capacity	VWF:FVIIIB

Table 8.2 Classification of VWD (modified from Sadler et al. [7]).

Quantitative deficiency of VWF
- **Type 1**: Partial quantitative deficiency of VWF
- **Type 3**: Virtually complete deficiency of VWF

Qualitative deficiency of VWF
- **Type 2**: Qualitative deficiency of VWF
  - **Type 2A**: Qualitative variants with decreased platelet-dependent function associated with the absence of high- and intermediate-molecular-weight VWF multimers
  - **Type 2B**: Qualitative variants with increased affinity for platelet GPIb, with the absence of HMW VWF multimers
  - **Type 2M**: Qualitative variants with decreased platelet-dependent function not caused by the absence of HMW VWF multimers
  - **Type 2N**: Qualitative variants with markedly decreased affinity for FVIII

VWD identifies two major categories, characterized by quantitative (type 1 and 3) or qualitative (type 2) VWF defects (Table 8.2). Partial quantitative deficiency of VWF in plasma and/or platelets identifies type 1 VWD, whereas type 3 VWD is characterized by total absence or trace amounts of VWF in plasma and platelets. Type 1 is easily distinguished from type 3 by its milder VWF deficiency (usually in the range of 20–40%), the autosomal dominant inheritance pattern, and the presence of milder bleeding symptoms. Among type 2 variants, four subtypes have been identified reflecting different pathophysiological mechanisms. Classical type 2A is characterized by the absence of high- and intermediate-molecular-weight (HMW) multimers of VWF in plasma. Type 2B is characterized by an increased affinity of VWF for platelet GpIb, causing removal of HMW multimers from plasma. As a consequence, ristocetin-induced platelet aggregation (RIPA) in platelet-rich plasma from these patients occurs at low ristocetin concentrations. The identification of variants with decreased platelet-dependent function and the presence of normal multimers on gel electrophoresis have required the addition of a new subtype, called 2M. Type 2N (Normandy) shows a full array of multimers because the defect lies in the N-terminal region of the VWF, where the binding domain for FVIII resides. This subtype is phenotypically identified only by tests exploiting FVIII–VWF binding.

Genetics and molecular biology of VWD

The first mutations observed in patients with VWD were detected in exon 28 of the VWF gene, which codes for the A1 and A2 domains of mature VWF, responsible for the interaction with platelet receptor GPIb. Most type 2A cases are due to missense mutations in the A2 domain. In particular, R1597W or Q or Y and S1506L represent about 60% of cases. Expression experiments have demonstrated two possible mechanisms [8]. Group I mutations show impaired secretion of HMW multimers, due to secondary defective intracellular transport. Group II mutations show normal synthesis and secretion of a VWF that is probably more susceptible to in vivo proteolysis.

The vast majority of type 2B cases are due to missense mutations in the A1 domain. About 90% of cases are due to R1306W, R1308C, V1316M, and R1341Q mutations [9]. A peculiar mutation (P1266L) is responsible for the type 2B New York/Malmö phenotype. These patients show an enhanced RIPA, but HMW multimers are present in plasma and no thrombocytopenia occurs after stress situations. The majority of patients with the P1266L mutation have additional nucleotide substitutions, all matching the VWF pseudogene sequence. This finding has been attributed to a mechanism of gene conversion between the VWF gene and its pseudogene [10]. Usually type 2A and 2B are autosomal dominant disorders with high penetrance and expressivity.

A few heterogeneous mutations (C1315C, G1324S/A, R1374C/H, etc.) are responsible for type 2M [9].

Missense mutations in the FVIII-binding domain located at the N terminus of VWF are responsible for type 2N. The R854Q mutation is the most frequent mutation observed, found in about 2% of the Dutch population. This mutation may cause symptoms only in the homozygous or compound heterozygous state. Type 2N mutation is suspected in the presence of a marked reduction of FVIII in comparison to VWF, and is confirmed by assessing FVIII–VWF binding. Its identification is important for genetic counseling, to exclude hemophilia A carriership in affected females [10].

Type 1 VWD is usually an autosomal dominant disorder, with variable expressivity and penetrance [11]. However, three distinct groups pointing to a different genetic background can be identified (Table 8.3). Group A includes cases displaying high penetrance and expressivity: linkage with a VWF allele is usually clear [12]. In this group, missense mutations have been described, resulting in a dominant-negative mechanism. In this model, mutant-wild type heterodimers are retained in the endoplasmic reticulum and only wild type homodimers are released into the circulation [13]. An additional illustrative variant is represented by VWD Vicenza, formerly included among type 2M VWD cases, but now included in type 1 VWD group [7]. These patients are characterized by severely reduced plasma FVIII and VWF levels, the presence of ultra-large VWF multimers in plasma, a normal platelet VWF content, a marked increase of FVIII and VWF after desmopressin, but with a rapid disappearance from the circulation ("Increased Clearance") [14,15]. In vivo studies have demonstrated decreased cellular secretion, and a common genetic background has been identified (R1205H in the D3 domain of VWF). Group

Table 8.3 Type 1 VWD: heterogeneity of clinical and laboratory phenotype.

	Group A	Group B	Group C
Symptoms	Manifest bleeding	Intermediate bleeding	Mild or dubious bleeding
Cosegregation with low VWF/VWF haplotype	Invariable; VWF gene mutations usually detected	Variable	Inconsistent
VWF level	About 10% in all affected	About 30% in most affected; propositus may have lower values	40–50%
Diagnosis	Easy, often increased VWF clearance	Repeated testing needed	Not always possible; blood group-adjusted range?

B is characterized by intermediate reduction of VWF, with variable penetrance and expressivity. This heterogeneity may indeed be explained in some cases by the inheritance of two different VWD alleles. For example, coinheritance of the R854Q mutation with a null mutation increases the severity of bleeding within a given family, so that simple heterozygotes show only minor bleeding symptoms and greater VWF levels [17]. Null alleles may be caused by frameshifts, nonsense mutations, or deletions that overlap with those identified in type 3 VWD. Group C comprises cases with borderline VWF levels and mild symptoms. In some of these families, linkage studies failed to establish a relationship of the phenotype with a given VWF allele. Therefore, it is assumed that gene(s) outside the VWF gene, and perhaps other nongenetic factors, contribute to the expression of a bleeding phenotype.

In 2007, the results of two large multicenter studies (The European MCMDM1-VWD and the Canadian studies) provided illuminating results about the genetic background of type 1 VWD [18,19]. Overall, these studies demonstrated that most of the mutations responsible for type 1 are indeed missense mutations, that the likelihood to detect a mutation was highest in patients with the lowest VWF, and that the linkage to the VWF gene was very high in these patients [20,21]. However, in about 40% of cases, no mutation in the VWF gene was evident, suggesting that the phenotype of VWD could be modified by other genes,

or by the effect of the ABO blood group. The likelihood of finding a VWF gene mutation was clearly related to the plasma levels of VWF (Table 8.4). Recently, the UK Haemophilia Centres Doctors' Organization reported the results of a National study on type 1 VWD [22]. VWF mutations were detected in 17/32 index cases (53%), a rate which was similar to those reported in the MCMDM-1VWD (55%) and the Canadian study (63%). Furthermore, three additional families carried the R924Q mutation, which was considered a common polymorphism in the UK population because it was detected also in 8/121 (6.6%) of a reference-panel DNA. This mutation was, however, considered causative in the MCMDM-1VWD (type 1 as a single mutation and type 3 in compound heterozygosity) and the Canadian study (8 index cases reported), but no population prevalences for these studies have been provided. In the UK study, 8/17 mutations were represented by the Y1584C mutation, which was considered a polymorphism. Of interest, VWF:Ag in these subjects ranged from 21 to 74 IU/dL, and almost all were of blood group O. Both blood group O and Y1584C are associated with increased proteolysis of VWF by ADAMTS13, and they interact in lowering VWF levels in plasma. Heterozygosity for Y1584C segregated with VWD in three families, did not segregate in an additional three families, and the results were equivocal in two families. Thus, this mutation shows incomplete penetrance and

Table 8.4 Association between the presence of mutations and VWF level in index cases in the MCMDM-1VWD Study.

VWF level in IC	Mutation	No mutation	OR (95% CI)*
VWF:Ag (IU/dL)			
>45	27	27	1[†]
31–45	24	11	2.2 (0.90–5.3)
16–30	30	6	5.0 (1.81–4.0)
0–15	23	1	23.0 (2.9–182.6)
VWF:RCo (IU/dL)			
>45	23	25	1[†]
31–45	24	12	2.2 (0.89–5.3)
16–30	17	6	3.1 (1.04–9.2)
0–15	40	2	21.7 (4.7–100.3)

*OR, odds ratio; CI, confidence interval.
[†]Reference category.

does not consistently segregate with VWD. As previously demonstrated in the Canadian study [19], a founder effect is also likely to occur in the UK families. The Y1584C mutation alone was identified in 10 index cases [22], and in compound heterozygosity in an additional 3 cases of the MCMDM-1VWD cohort (8% of the whole index cases), with the same wide range of VWF levels [18]. Notwithstanding these gray areas that still require further studies, great progress has been made in elucidating the molecular bases of a large proportion of patients with type 1 VWD.

About 60% of the variation in VWF plasma is due to genetic factors, with VWF level 25–35% lower in type-O subjects than in non-O individuals [23]. Blood group plays a major role in subjects with VWF levels at the lower end of the normal range, in whom heritability is less predictable.

In type 3 VWD, in addition to mechanisms shared with some type 1 cases (see above), partial or total gene deletions have also been reported [24]. Notably, homozygosity for gene deletion may be associated with the appearance of neutralizing antibodies against VWF, which may render replacement therapy ineffective and stimulate anaphylactic reaction upon treatment. In general, mutations may be scattered over the entire gene, but some mutations (e.g. 2680delC or R2535X) are particularly recurrent in Northern Europe. Several stop codon mutations, either in homozygotes or compound heterozygotes, have also been reported.

Prevalence and frequency of subtypes of VWD

Until the late 1980s, estimates of the prevalence of VWD were based on the number of patients registered at specialized centers, with figures ranging from 4 to 10 cases/100,000 inhabitants. It is generally assumed that the number of persons with symptomatic VWD, requiring specific treatment, is at least 100 per million.

A few studies estimated the prevalence of VWD by screening small populations using formal, standardized criteria. A prevalence approaching 1% has been demonstrated, without ethnic differences [25]. However, the large majority of cases diagnosed by population studies appear to have a mild disease, and most of these subjects were never referred for detailed

hemostatic evaluation. It remains unknown what proportion of these cases is the effect of a gene(s) outside the VWF gene influencing the circulating level of VWF [26].

About 70% of VWD cases appear to have type 1 by Center series. These estimates are obviously biased because it is expected that many type 1 cases without major symptoms are not referred for evaluation, whereas almost all severe type 3 cases are followed at a specialized center. Indeed, recent results from the MCMDM-1 VWD study demonstrated by an accurate VWF multimeric evaluation that many of the patients previously identified as type 1 VWD had subtle multimeric abnormalities that suggested type 2 VWD [27]. However, for most of them, this evidence did not affect their treatment because they showed complete response to desmopressin administration.

In contrast to the above-reported percentages, almost all cases were represented by type 1 in population studies.

Clinical manifestations

Clinical expression of VWD is usually mild in type 1, with increasing severity in type 2 and type 3. However, in some families, variable severity of bleeding manifestations is evident, underlying the different molecular basis responsible for the diverse phenotypes of this disorder and its variable penetrance. In general, the severity of bleeding correlates with the degree of the reduction of FVIII:C, but not with the magnitude of BT prolongation or with ABO blood type of the patient. Mucocutaneous bleeding (epistaxis, menorrhagia, easy bruising) is a typical, prominent manifestation of the disease and may affect the quality of life. VWD may be highly prevalent in patients with isolated menorrhagia. Females with VWD may require treatment with antifibrinolytics, iron supplementation, or an estroprogestinic pill to control heavy menses. Bleeding after dental extraction is the most frequent postoperative bleeding manifestation. Because FVIII:C is usually only mildly reduced, manifestations of a severe coagulation defect (hemarthrosis, deep muscle hematoma) are rarely observed in type 1 VWD and are mainly posttraumatic. On the contrary, in type 3 VWD, the severity of bleeding may sometimes be similar to that of hemophilia. Bleeding after delivery in type 1 is rarely observed because FVIII/VWF levels tend to correct at the end of pregnancy in mild type 1 cases. A few cases, however, fail to have their FVIII/VWF levels normalized and need prophylaxis with DDAVP or FVIII/VWF concentrates before delivery. Type 2A and 2B and type 3 females usually need replacement therapy postpartum to prevent immediate or delayed bleeding. Postoperative bleeding may not occur even in more severely affected type 1 patients, whereas in type 3, prophylactic treatment is always required.

Usually, the distribution of different types of bleeding (apart from joint bleeding) is similar among the different subtypes. However, the severity of bleeding manifestations (e.g. menorrhagia or gastrointestinal bleeding) is clearly more prominent in type 3 VWD, often requiring substitution therapy. Heterozygous carriers of type 3 VWD may experience bleeding depending on their actual circulating FVIII [28].

Diagnosis of VWD

The diagnosis of VWD, and in particular of type 1, may require several clinical and laboratory assessments [9]. The diagnostic workup of VWD can be divided into three steps: (1) the identification of patients suspected of having VWD, on the basis of data from personal and family clinical history and results of laboratory screening tests of hemostasis; (2) diagnosis of VWD with identification of its type; and (3) characterization of the subtype. Table 8.5 summarizes a practical approach for diagnosing and typing VWD.

Bleeding history

A history of mucocutaneous bleeding symptoms may be considered the hallmark of VWD, and it could therefore be considered a necessary requirement before a full laboratory assessment is initiated. It is recommended that a thorough clinical investigation on type and frequency of bleeding symptoms is collected in all prospective patients. A bleeding history could, however, be absent in those patients without any prior hemostatic challenges, as in very young subjects; in these patients, screening for VWD is recommended only when there is a strong clinical suspicion (e.g. one ore more relatives with a diagnosis of VWD). A bleeding history may be considered to be suggestive for VWD when the patient has at least three different hemorrhagic symptoms or when the bleeding score is greater than 3 in males or greater than 5 in

Table 8.5 Practical approach to the diagnosis of VWD

1. VWD diagnosis should be considered within the context of an appropriate personal and/or familial bleeding history.
2. Other common hemostatic defects should be excluded by performing BT, platelet count, APTT, PT.
3. If personal and/or familial bleeding history is significant, VWF:RCo assay should be carried out at this stage. If not possible, VWF:Ag assay or VWF:CB assay should be performed. VWF:Ag <3 U/dL suggests type 3 VWD.
4. If any of these tests is below 0.4 IU/mL, the diagnosis of VWD should be considered.
5. In mild deficiencies, the assay should be repeated on a second occasion to confirm the diagnosis or to increase the sensitivity of the procedure in case of normal test in a patient with a high diagnostic suspicion.
6. Other family members with possible bleeding history should be evaluated. Finding another member with bleeding and reduced VWF strongly confirms the diagnosis.
7. VWF:Ag and VWF:RCo and FVIII:C should be measured on the same sample to assess the presence of reduced ratio VWF:RCo/VWF:Ag (a ratio <0.7 suggests type 2 VWD) or FVIII:C/VWF:Ag (a ratio <0.7 suggests type 2N VWD, to be confirmed by binding study of FVIII:C to patient's VWF).
8. Aggregation of patient platelet-rich plasma in presence of increasing concentration of ristocetin (0.25, 0.5, 1.0 mg/mL, final concentration) should be assessed. Aggregation at low concentration (≤0.5 mg) suggests type 2B VWD.
9. Multimeric pattern using a low-resolution gel should be evaluated. Lack of HMW multimers suggests type 2A and/or 2B. Presence of full complement of multimers suggests type 1 (or 2N, 2M). Absence of multimers in type 3.
10. If bleeding history is clinically significant, carry out a test-infusion with desmopressin. FVIII/VWF measurements should be evaluated at baseline, 60, 120, and 240 from the start of intravenous infusion or subcutaneous injection. Bleeding time (or PFA-100 if available) should be measured at 60 and 240 minutes.

Table 8.6 Grades of bleeding severity used to compute the bleeding score in the International Multicenter Study [29].

Symptom	Score			
	0	1	2	3
Epistaxis	No or trivial	Present	Packing, cauterization	Blood transfusion or replacement therapy
Cutaneous	No or trivial	Petechiae or bruises	Hematomas	Consultation
Bleeding from minor wounds	No or trivial	Present (1–5 episodes/year)	Consultation	Surgical hemostasis
Oral cavity	No or trivial	Present	Consultation only	Surgical hemostasis/blood transfusion
GI bleeding	No or trivial	Present	Consultation only	Surgery/blood transfusion
Tooth extraction	No or trivial	Present	Suturing or packing	Blood transfusion
Surgery	No or trivial	Present	Suturing or resurgery	Blood transfusion
Menorrhagia	No or trivial	Present	Consultation, pill use, iron therapy	Blood transfusion, hysterectomy, Dilatation & Currettage
Postpartum hemorrhage	No or trivial	Present, iron therapy	Blood transfusion, dilatation and curretage, suturing	Hysterectomy
Muscle hematomas	No or trivial	Present	Consultation only	Blood transfusion, surgery
Hemarthrosis	No or trivial	Present	Consultation only	Blood transfusion, surgery

females [29,30]. The bleeding score is a summative index accounting for both the number and the severity of bleeding symptoms that is generated by summing the severity of all bleeding symptoms reported by a subject, and graded according to an arbitrary scale (Table 8.6).

Laboratory evaluation

In VWD patients, the platelet count is usually normal, but mild thrombocytopenia may occur in patients with type 2B. The bleeding time (BT) is usually prolonged but may be normal in patients with mild forms of VWD, especially when platelet VWF content is normal. The prothrombin time (PT) is normal, whereas the partial thromboplastin time (PTT) may be prolonged to a variable degree, depending on the plasma FVIII levels. Whatever the results of these screening tests, VWD diagnosis always requires the demonstration of reduced VWF antigen and/or activity.

VWF antigen (VWF:Ag) is unmeasurable in type 3 VWD (below 3% or 0.03 IU/mL), whereas it is decreased in type 1 and low–normal in type 2 VWD. The assay for ristocetin cofactor activity (VWF:RCo)

explores the interaction of VWF with the platelet glycoprotein Ib/IX/V complex, and it is still the standard method for measuring VWF platelet-dependent activity. It is based on the property of the antibiotic ristocetin to agglutinate formalin-fixed normal platelets in the presence of VWF. In type 1 VWD patients, concomitantly reduced levels of VWF:RCo and VWF:Ag are observed, because in these patients, circulating VWF has a normal structure. Both VWF:Ag and VWF:Rco have wide variation in normal subjects, with blood group O individuals having VWF:Ag and VWF:Rco levels as low as 40% (0.40 IU/dL). However, VWD should be strongly suspected only when VWF:Ag and VWF:RCo are below this cut-off, and the likelihood of VWD is particularly high only for values below 30% (0.30 IU/mL). A new ELISA test exploiting the interaction of VWF with plate-immobilized Gp Ib in the presence of ristocetin seems to be very promising as a replacement for VWF:RCo, although it has not yet been fully validated. FVIII:C plasma levels are very low (1–5%) in patients with type 3 VWD. In patients with type 1 or type 2 VWD, FVIII may be decreased to a variable extent but sometimes is normal.

Additional tests used in VWD diagnosis include the Closure Time (CT) and assays of VWF activity based on binding to collagen (VWF:CB). The evaluation of CT with PFA-100 (Platelet Function Analyzer) allows rapid and simple determination of VWF-dependent platelet function at high-shear stress. This system was demonstrated to be sensitive and reproducible when screening for severe VWD, even though the CT is normal in type 2N VWD. Its use in the clinical setting, however, remains to be demonstrated. Assays for VWF:CB are also available, and the ratio of VWF:CB to VWF:Ag levels appears to be useful for distinguishing between types 1 and 2 VWD. These relatively new assays have not been properly standardized yet and are not officially recommended by the Scientific Standardization Committee of the International Society of Thrombosis and Haemostasis. Tables 8.7 and 8.8 summarize the diagnostic tests and their significance.

Characterization of the subtype

For a more precise diagnosis, other assays are necessary to define specific subtypes of VWD [9]. RIPA is performed by mixing increasing concentrations of ristocetin and patient platelet-rich plasma in the aggregometer. Results are expressed as the concentration of ristocetin (mg/mL) that induces 30% of maximal agglutination. Most VWD types and subtypes are characterized by hypo-responsiveness to ristocetin, at variance with type 2B, which is characterized by hyper-responsiveness to ristocetin, due to a higher than normal affinity of VWF for platelet GP Ib/IX/V complex. VWF multimeric analysis with low-resolution agarose gels distinguishes VWF multimers, which are conventionally indicated as high, intermediate, and low molecular weight. In type 1 VWD, all multimers are present, whereas in types 2A and 2B, high and intermediate or high multimers, respectively,

Table 8.7 Basic and discriminating laboratory assays for the diagnosis of VWD.

Test	Pathophysiological significance	Diagnostic significance
Ristocetin cofactor (VWF:RCo), using formalin-fixed platelets and fixed ristocetin concentration (1 mg/mL)	VWF-Gp Ib interaction as mediated by ristocetin in vitro (ristocetin, normal platelets, patient's plasma)	"Functional test"; most sensitive screening test
Immunological assay with polyclonal antibody (VWF:Ag)	Antigen concentration	Correlates with VWF:RCo in type 1; reduced VWF:RCo/VWF:Ag (<0.7) suggests type 2 VWD; level <3 U/dL suggests type 3 VWD
FVIII:C level (one-stage assay)	FVIII-VWF interaction	Not specific, but useful for patient management; disproportionately reduced compared with VWF in type 2N VWD
Bleeding time (Ivy method)	Platelet-vessel wall VWF-mediated interaction	Not specific; correlates with platelet VWF content in type 1 VWD
RIPA using patient platelets	Threshold ristocetin concentration inducing patient's platelet-rich plasma aggregation	Allows the discrimination of type 2B, characterized by reduced threshold; absent in type 3 at every ristocetin concentration
Multimeric analysis (low-resolution gel)	Multimeric composition of VWF	Presence of full range of multimers in type 1; high- and intermediate-molecular-weight multimers absent in type 2A and high in type 2B; multimers absent in type 3
Platelet VWF	Reflects endothelial stores	Useful to predict responsiveness to desmopressin in type 1
Binding of VIII:C to VWF	Interaction of normal FVIII with patient plasma VWF	Allows the identification of type 2N, characterized by low binding values

Table 8.8 Other tests proposed for VWD diagnosis.

Test	Pathophysiological significance	Diagnostic significance
Binding of VWF to collagen	VWF–collagen interaction	Correlates with VWF:RCo in type 1 VWD; some collagen preparations more sensitive to HMW multimers; not yet well standardized
Closure time PFA-100	Simulates primary hemostasis after injury to a small vessel	More sensitive than BT in screening for VWD; not tested in bleeding subjects without specific diagnosis; specificity unknown; more data needed before recommendation for clinical laboratory
Monoclonal antibody-based ELISA	Moab against an epitope of VWF involved in the interaction with GpIb	Correlation with VWF:RCo not confirmed; not to be used in place of VWF:RCo
ELISA-based "VWF:RCo"	Measures interaction between VWF and captured rGp Ibα fragment in the presence of ristocetin	Promising new test proposed as a substitute for VWF:RCo; validation on larger patient series required
Propeptide assay	Measures the amount of VWFpp released in plasma	Increased VWFpp/VWF:Ag ratio identifies patients with shortened VWF survival after desmopressin; still for research purposes

are missing. Multimeric analysis with high-resolution agarose gels can allow better identification of type 1 and type 2 VWD subtypes.

Platelet VWF plays an important role in primary hemostasis, because it can be released from alpha granules directly at the site of vascular injury. On the basis of its measurement, type 1 VWD may be classified into three subtypes: type 1 "platelet normal," with a normal content of functionally normal VWF; type 1 "platelet low," with low concentrations of functionally normal VWF; and type 1 "platelet discordant," containing dysfunctional VWF in platelets. Factor VIII binding assay measures the affinity of VWF for FVIII. This assay allows type 2N VWD to be distinguished from mild to moderate hemophilia A.

In general, a proportionate reduction of VWF:Ag and VWF:RCo levels with a RCo/Ag ratio >0.7 suggests diagnosis of type 1 VWD. If the VWF:RCo/Ag ratio is <0.7, a type 2 VWD might be present. According to the RIPA method, type 2B VWD can be diagnosed by an enhanced RIPA (<0.8 mg/mL), whereas type 2A and 2M are characterized by reduced RIPA (>1.2

mg/mL). Multimeric analysis in plasma is necessary to distinguish between type 2A VWD (lack of the largest and intermediate multimers) and type 2M VWD (all multimers present as in normal plasma). Type 2N VWD can be suspected in cases with discrepant values between FVIII and VWF:Ag (ratio $<0.7–1$), and the diagnosis is confirmed by a specific test of VWF:factor VIII binding capacity (VWF:FVIIIB). In type 1 VWD, the ratio between FVIII and VWF:Ag is always ≥ 1, and the severity of the type 1 VWD phenotype can usually be evaluated by performing platelet VWF measurements.

VWF propeptide and increased VWF clearance

The level of VWF in plasma is the result of the ratio between its production and clearance. The VWF propeptide (VWFpp) noncovalently associates with mature VWF multimers from which it dissociates after secretion into plasma. The half-life of VWFpp is around 2–3 hours, whereas normal VWF has a half-life of 8–12 hours. An increased clearance of VWF from plasma has been reported as a novel mechanism for type 1 VWD. Patients with R1205H (VWD Vicenza) show a shortened VWF survival after desmopressin (1–2 hours only), in contrast to the VWFpp half-life, which is normal [16]. Thus, an increased ratio of steady-state plasma VWFpp to VWF:Ag has been demonstrated to identify patients with increased VWF clearance. Typically, they show a severe VWF reduction at baseline and a marked but short-lived VWF increase after desmopressin. In addition to R1205H, other mutations have been convincingly associated with increased clearance (C1130F, W1144G, S2179F) [31,32]. Thus, the measurement of VWFpp in plasma by an ELISA could help to identify the pathopysiological mechanism responsible for low VWF in a given patient, predicting his/her response to desmopressin. The assay is still used for research purposes, but it is likely that it could soon be widely available to all labs dealing with the diagnosis of VWD.

Management of patients with VWD

Desmopressin and transfusional therapy with blood products represent the two treatments of choice in VWD [33]. Other forms of treatment can be considered as adjunctive or alternative to these two modalities.

Desmopressin

Desmopressin (1-deamino-8-D-arginine vasopressin; DDAVP) is a synthetic analog of vasopressin originally designed for the treatment of diabetes insipidus. DDAVP increases FVIII and VWF plasma concentrations without relevant side effects when administered to healthy volunteers or patients with mild hemophilia A and VWD. DDAVP has become widely used for the treatment of these diseases. It is relatively inexpensive and carries no risk of transmitting blood-borne viruses. DDAVP is usually administered intravenously at a dose of 0.3 μg/kg diluted in 50–100 mL saline infused over 30 minutes. The drug is also available in concentrated form for subcutaneous or intranasal administration, which can be convenient for home treatment. This treatment increases plasma FVIII/VWF 3 to 5 times above basal levels within 30–60 minutes. In general, high FVIII/VWF concentrations last for 6–8 hours. Because the responses in a given patient and

within his/her family are consistent on different occasions, a test dose of DDAVP administered at the time of diagnosis helps to establish the individual response pattern and will permit planning future treatment. Infusions can be repeated every 12–24 hours depending on the type and severity of the bleeding episode. However, most patients treated repeatedly with DDAVP become less responsive to therapy.

Side effects of DDAVP may include mild tachycardia, headache, and flushing. These symptoms are attributed to the vasomotor effects of the drug and can often be attenuated by slowing the rate of infusion. Hyponatremia and volume overload due to the antidiuretic effects of DDAVP are relatively rare complications. A few cases have been described, mostly in young children who received closely repeated infusions. Even though no thrombotic episodes have been reported in VWD patients treated with DDAVP, this drug should be used with caution in elderly patients with atherosclerotic disease, because a few cases of myocardial infarction and stroke have occurred in hemophiliacs and uremic patients given DDAVP.

Patients with type 1 VWD, especially those who have normal VWF in storage sites (type 1, "platelet normal"), are the best candidates for DDAVP treatment. In these patients, FVIII, VWF, and the BT are usually corrected within 30 minutes and remain normal for 6–8 hours. Response to DDAVP is assessed at least after 1 hour (peak) following the infusion and is defined as an increase of at least three-fold over baseline levels of FVIII:C and VWF:RCo, reaching plasma levels of at least 30 U/dL. FVIII:C and VWF:RCo plasma levels should also be assessed at 4 hours post-DDAVP infusion to assess the pattern of clearance of these moieties and to identify patients with increased clearance who are possible candidates for alternative treatments [32,33].

In other VWD subtypes, responsiveness to DDAVP is variable. In type 2A, FVIII levels are usually increased by DDAVP, but the BT is shortened in only a minority of cases. Desmopressin is best avoided in type 2B, because of the transient appearance of thrombocytopenia. However, there have been reports on the clinical usefulness of DDAVP in some 2B cases. In any case, platelet count should be checked during test infusion to unravel possible nonclassical type 2B cases with thrombocytopenia occurring after infusion. In type 2N, relatively high levels of FVIII are observed following DDAVP, but released FVIII circulates for a shorter time period in patient plasma because the stabilizing effect of VWF is impaired. Patients with type 3 VWD are usually unresponsive to DDAVP, although in some patients, an increase of FVIII:C to effective hemostatic levels may occur, despite no change in the BT [34].

Other nontransfusional therapies for VWD

Two other types of nontransfusional therapies are used in the management of VWD: antifibrinolytic amino acids and estrogens. Antifibrinolytic amino acids are synthetic drugs that interfere with the lysis of newly formed clots by saturating the binding sites on plasminogen, thereby preventing its attachment to fibrin and making plasminogen unavailable within the forming clot. Epsilon aminocaproic acid (50 mg/kg four times a day) and tranexamic acid (15–25 mg/kg three times a day) are the most frequently used antifibrinolytic amino acids. Both medications can be administered orally, intravenously, or topically and are useful alone or as adjuncts in the management of oral cavity bleeding, epistaxis, gastrointestinal bleeding, and menorrhagia. They carry a potential risk of thrombosis in patients with an underlying prothrombotic state. They are also contraindicated in the management of urinary tract bleeding. Estrogens increase plasma VWF levels, but the response is quite variable and unpredictable, so they are not widely used for therapeutic purposes. It is common clinical experience that the continued use of oral contraceptives is very useful in reducing the severity of menorrhagia in women with VWD, even in those with type 3, despite the fact that FVIII/VWF levels are not modified.

Transfusional therapies

Transfusional therapy with blood products containing FVIII/VWF is currently the treatment of choice in patients who are unresponsive to DDAVP [33]. Cryoprecipitate has been the mainstay of VWD therapy for many years. However, at present, its role remains significant only in the emerging countries, and it should preferably be prepared from virus-inactivated plasma using simple physical methods, such as methylene blue inactivation. In Western countries, virus-inactivated concentrates, originally developed for the treatment of hemophilia A, are the treatment of choice for VWD patients unresponsive to DDAVP. Concen-

trates obtained by immunoaffinity chromatography on monoclonal antibodies (FVIII >2000 IU/mg) contain very small amounts of VWF and are therefore unsuitable for VWD management. Recently, a chromatography-purified concentrate particularly rich in VWF and with a very low content of FVIII has also been produced, and it has been called very-high-purity VWF concentrate. This concentrate was effective when tested in a small cohort of type 3 VWD cases, but it is not yet available in North America. The very low content in FVIII of this concentrate necessitates the infusion of a single supplemental dose of purified FVIII concentrate for the treatment of acute bleeding episodes and for emergency surgeries to ensure hemostasis. Thereafter, infused VWF stabilizes endogenously synthesized FVIII with normalization of FVIII levels after 6–8 hours, so that no further infusion of FVIII containing concentrates is necessary. The dosages of concentrates recommended for the control of bleeding episodes are summarized in Table 8.9. Because commercially available intermediate and high-purity FVIII/VWF concentrates contain large amounts of FVIII and VWF, high post-infusion levels of these moieties are consistently obtained. Moreover, there is a sustained rise in FVIII lasting for up to 24 hours, higher than predicted from the doses infused. This pattern is due to the stabilizing effect of exogenous VWF on endogenous FVIII, which is synthesized at a normal rate in these patients. The cumulation of exogenous FVIII infused with the concentrates together with that endogenously synthesized and stabilized by infused VWF causes very high FVIII levels when multiple infusions are given for severe bleeding episodes or to cover major surgery. Recently, episodes of deep vein thrombosis have been reported in patients with VWD receiving repeated infusions of FVIII/VWF concentrates for maintaining clinical hemostasis, especially following surgery.

These FVIII/VWF products are not always effective in correcting the BT [35]. No concentrate contains a completely functional VWF, as tested in vitro by evaluating the multimeric pattern, because VWF proteolysis occurs during purification due to the action of platelet and leukocyte proteases contaminating the plasma used for fractionation. Despite their limited and inconsistent effect on the BT, FVIII/VWF concentrates are successfully used for the treatment of VWD patients unresponsive to DDAVP, especially

Table 8.9 Doses of FVIII-VWF concentrates recommended in VWD patients unresponsive to desmopressin.

Type of bleeding	Dose FVIII (IU/kg)	Number of infusions	Objective
Major surgery	50	Once a day or	Maintain FVIII >50 U/dL
	50	every other day	for at least 7 days
Minor surgery	30	Once a day or	FVIII >30 U/dL
	30	every other day	for at least 5–7 days
Dental extractions	20–40	Single	FVIII >30 U/dL
			for up to 6 hours
Spontaneous or posttraumatic bleeding	20–40	Single	

for soft-tissue and postoperative bleeding. A number of retrospective studies on Haemate P®, Alphanate®, and Fanhdi® showed excellent or good hemostasis in 96% of cases on the day of surgery, and 100% efficacy over the next few days. The VWF/FVIII concentrate Haemate P/Humate P® has been used in VWD patients since the early 1980s. Two prospective studies have documented safety and efficacy in acute spontaneous bleeding (excellent/good results in 98% of the cases) and surgical events (excellent/good results in 100% of the cases) [33]. A recent prospective study evaluated the choice of doses in the management of surgical patients through a careful PK analysis of 29 cases with VWD undergoing elective surgery and showed that serial dosing decisions based on preoperative median values were efficacious and safe [36]. This study demonstrated for the first time that the incremental recovery is constant over a wide range of doses of VWF/FVIII concentrate (dose linearity relationship) and that the pretreatment PK results can be used to decide the plan of treatment in these patients.

When the BT remains prolonged and bleeding persists despite replacement therapy, other therapeutic options are available. DDAVP, given after cryoprecipitate, further shortened or normalized the BT in patients with type 3 VWD in whom cryoprecipitate failed to correct the BT. Platelet concentrates (given before or after cryoprecipitate, at doses of 4–5 × 10^{11} platelets) achieved similar effects in patients unresponsive to cryoprecipitate alone, both in terms of BT correction and bleeding control. These data emphasize the important role of platelet VWF in establishing and maintaining primary hemostasis. For the rare patients with type 3 VWD who develop anti-VWF alloantibodies after multiple transfusions, the infusion of VWF concentrates may not only be ineffective, but may also cause post-infusion life-threatening anaphylaxis due to the formation of immune complexes.

Figure 8.1 summarizes a practical approach to VWD treatment.

Secondary long-term prophylaxis

Patients with severe forms of VWD (i.e. FVIII:C levels <5 U/dL) may suffer from recurrent hemarthroses or gastrointestinal bleeding, which may also affect patients with type 2 and the loss of HMW multimers, and may therefore benefit from secondary long-term prophylaxis. Even children with frequent epistaxis could represent ideal candidates. The largest experience on secondary prophylaxis in VWD has been collected in Sweden in 35 patients with severe VWD, with excellent results [37]. Secondary prophylaxis was also retrospectively evaluated in a cohort of 12 Italian VWD patients, who underwent 17 long-term secondary prophylaxis periods to prevent recurrent gastrointestinal or joint bleeding, with clinical responses rated as excellent or good in 100% of cases [38]. However, more prospective trials are needed to better evaluate the cost-effectiveness of this approach versus on-demand therapy. An International Project is ongoing to clarify this issue.

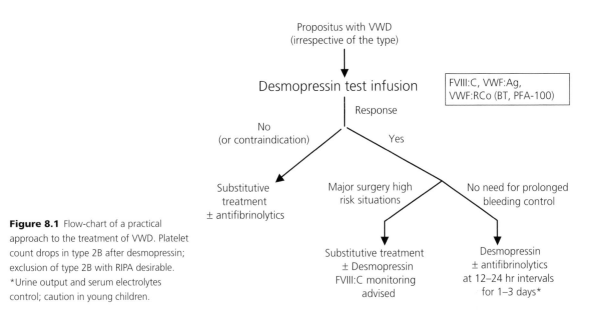

Propositus with VWD
(irrespective of the type)

Desmopressin test infusion

FVIII:C, VWF:Ag,
VWF:RCo (BT, PFA-100)

Response

No
(or contraindication)

Yes

Substitutive
treatment
± antifibrinolytics

Major surgery high
risk situations

No need for prolonged
bleeding control

Substitutive treatment
± Desmopressin
FVIII:C monitoring
advised

Desmopressin
± antifibrinolytics
at 12–24 hr intervals
for 1–3 days*

Figure 8.1 Flow-chart of a practical approach to the treatment of VWD. Platelet count drops in type 2B after desmopressin; exclusion of type 2B with RIPA desirable. *Urine output and serum electrolytes control; caution in young children.

Treatment of women with VWD

Women with VWD in childbearing age may suffer from special therapeutic problems related to physiological events, such as pregnancy and parturition [39]. Women with VWD may also be affected more frequently than normal women by an array of other gynecological ailments (such as bleeding at ovulation), and hysterectomy is more frequently performed than in normal women. Pregnant women with VWD are at increased risk of postpartum hemorrhage if untreated (16–29% in the first 24 hours and 22–29% after 24 hours compared with 3–5% in the general population). In patients with VWD types 1 or 2, the levels of VWF and FVIII rise two- to three-fold during the second and third trimester but fall to baseline levels after delivery. Patients with the frequent VWD Vicenza and C1130F mutations show only a slight increase of these moieties during pregnancy, so that treatment with desmopressin is required at delivery [40,41]. Patients with type 2N associated with the common R854Q mutation show a complete normalization of FVIII:C, and no treatment is usually required [42]. In VWD type 2B, the increase of the abnormal VWF can cause or worsen thrombocytopenia. In general, VWD patients should be monitored for VWF:RCo and FVIII:C levels once during the third trimester of pregnancy and within 10 days of the expected delivery date. The risk of bleeding is minimal when FVIII:C and VWF:RCo levels are higher than 30 U/dL. In type 1 VWD pregnant women with FVIII:C levels <30 U/dL, desmopressin on the day of villocentesis, amniocentesis, and parturition, and for a couple of days thereafter, is advisable. In order to prevent late bleeding, VWF:RCo and FVIII:C levels should be checked and women monitored clinically for at least 2 weeks postpartum. In type 3 VWD women, VWF and FVIII do not increase during pregnancy, and thus VWF/FVIII concentrates are required to cover delivery or cesarean section. The latter should be reserved only for the usual obstetric indications. There is no apparent increased bleeding risk for neonates with VWD.

Conclusions

VWD is the most frequent inherited bleeding disorder. Definite diagnosis and characterization usually requires an array of tests and should be reserved for patients with a significant bleeding history. For subjects belonging to Group C, as reported in Fig. 8.1, the benefit of a definite diagnosis of VWD versus the social burden of receiving the stigmata of a congenital disorder and the related anxiety should be carefully weighed. For these cases, simply reassuring the patient that she/he does not have a severe bleeding disorder, and offering the possibility of consultation in case of need, is the preferred choice. Today, several safe and effective therapeutic options are easily available to prevent or control bleeding episodes, which rarely persistently affect the quality of life.

References

1 Rodeghiero F, Castaman G, Dini E. Epidemiological investigation of the prevalence of von Willebrand's disease. *Blood* 1987;69:454–9.

2 Mancuso DJ, Tuley EA, Westfield LA, et al. Human von Willebrand factor gene and pseudogene: structural analysis and differentiation by polymerase chain reaction. *Biochemistry* 1991; 30:253–69.

3 Wagner DD. Cell biology of von Willebrand factor. *Annu Rev Cell Biol* 1990;6:217–46.

4 Furlan M, Robles R, Lammle B. Partial purification and characterization of a protease from human plasma cleaving von Willebrand factor to fragments produced by in vivo proteolysis. *Blood* 1996;87:4223–34.

5 Ruggeri ZM. Structure of von Willebrand factor and its function in platelet adhesion and thrombus formation. *Clin Haematol* 2001;14:257–79.

6 Vlot AJ, Koppelman SJ, Bouma BN, Sixma JJ. Factor VIII and von Willebrand Factor. *Thromb Haemost* 1998;79:456–65.

7 Sadler JE, Budde U, Eikenboom JC, et al. Update on the pathophysiology and classification of von Willebrand disease: a report of the Subcommittee on von Willebrand Factor. *J Thromb Haemost* 2006;4:2103–14.

8 Lyons SE, Bruck ME, Bowie EJW, Ginsburg D. Impaired cellular transport produced by a subset of type IIA von Willebrand disease mutations. *J Biol Chem* 1992;267:4424–30.

9 Castaman G, Federici AB, Rodeghiero F, Mannucci PM. Von Willebrand's disease in the year 2003: towards the complete identification of gene defects for correct diagnosis and treatment. *Haematologica* 2003;88:94–108.

10 Baronciani L, Federici AB, Castaman G, Punzo M, Mannucci PM. Prevalence of type 2b 'Malmö/New York' von Willebrand disease in Italy: the role of von Willebrand factor gene conversion. *J Thromb Haemost* 2008;6:887–90.

11 Rodeghiero F, Castaman G. Congenital von Willebrand disease type I: definition, phenotypes, clinical and laboratory assessment. *Best Pract Res Clin Haematol* 2001;14:321–35.

12 Castaman G, Eikenboom JCJ, Missiaglia E, Rodeghiero F. Autosomal dominant type 1 von Willebrand disease due to G3639T mutation (C1130F) in exon 26 of von Willebrand factor gene: description of five Italian families and evidence for a founder effect. *Br J Haematol* 2000;108:876–9.

13 Eikenboom JC, Matsushita T, Reitsma PH, et al. Dominant type 1 von Willebrand disease caused by mutated cysteine residues in the D3 domain of von Willebrand factor. *Blood* 1996;88:2433–41.

14 Mannucci PM, Lombardi R, Castaman G, et al. von Willebrand disease "Vicenza" with larger-than-normal (supranormal) von Willebrand factor multimers. *Blood* 1988;71:65–70.

15 Schneppenheim R, Federici AB, Budde U, et al. Von Willebrand disease type 2 M "Vicenza" in Italian and German patients: identification of the first candidate mutation (G3864A; R1205H) in 8 families. *Thromb Haemost* 2000;83:136–40.

16 Casonato A, Pontara E, Sartorello F, et al. Reduced von Willebrand factor survival in type Vicenza von Willebrand disease. *Blood* 2002;99:180–4.

17 Eikenboom JCJ, Reitsma PH, Peerlinck KMJ, et al. Recessive inheritance of von Willebrand's disease type I. *Lancet* 1993;341:982–6.

18 Goodeve A, Eikenboom J, Castaman G, et al. Phenotype and genotype of a cohort of families historically diagnosed with type 1 von Willebrand disease in the European study, Molecular and Clinical Markers for the Diagnosis and Management of Type 1 von Willebrand Disease (MCMDM-1VWD). *Blood* 2007;109:112–21.

19 James PD, Notley C, Hegadorn C, et al. The mutational spectrum of type 1 von Willebrand disease: Results from a Canadian cohort study. *Blood* 2007;109:145–54.

20 Eikenboom J, Van Marion V, Putter H, et al. Linkage analysis in families diagnosed with type 1 von Willebrand disease in the European study, molecular and clinical markers for the diagnosis and management of type 1 VWD. *J Thromb Haemost* 2006;4:774–82.

21 James PD, Paterson AD, Notley C, et al. Genetic linkage and association analysis in type 1 von Willebrand disease: results from the Canadian type 1 VWD study. *J Thromb Haemost* 2006;4:783–92.

22 Cumming A, Grundy P, Keeney S, et al. An investigation of the von Willebrand factor genotype in UK patients diagnosed to have type 1 von Willebrand disease. *Thromb Haemost* 2006;96:630–41.

23 Mohlke KL, Ginsburg D. von Willebrand disease and quantitative variation in von Willebrand factor. *J Lab Clin Med* 1997;130:252–61.

24 Eikenboom JCJ. Congenital von Willebrand disease type 3: clinical manifestations, pathophysiology and molecular biology. *Clin Haematol* 2001;14:365–79.

25 Rodeghiero F, Castaman G. von Willebrand disease: epidemiology. In: Lee CA, Berntorp EE, Hoots WK,

eds. *Textbook of Hemophilia*. Oxford: Blackwell, 2005; 265–71.

26 Castaman G, Eikenboom JCJ, Bertina R, Rodeghiero F. Inconsistency of association between type 1 von Willebrand disease phenotype and genotype in families identified in an epidemiologic investigation. *Thromb Haemostas* 1999;82:1065–70.

27 Budde U, Schneppenheim R, Eikenboom J, et al. Detailed von Willebrand factor multimer analysis in patients with von Willebrand disease in the European study, molecular and clinical markers for the diagnosis and management of type 1 von Willebrand disease (MCMDM-1VWD). *J Thromb Haemost* 2008;6:762–71.

28 Castaman G, Rodeghiero F, Tosetto A, et al. Hemorrhagic symptoms and bleeding risk in obligatory carriers of type 3 von Willebrand disease: an International, multicenter study. *J Thromb Haemost* 2006;4:2164–9.

29 Rodeghiero F, Castaman G, Tosetto A, et al. The discriminant power of bleeding history for the diagnosis of type 1 von Willebrand disease: an international, multicenter study. *J Thromb Haemost* 2005;3:2619–26.

30 Tosetto A, Rodeghiero F, Castaman G, et al. Impact of plasma von Willebrand factor levels in the diagnosis of type 1 von Willebrand disease: results from a multicenter European study (MCMDM-1VWD). *J Thromb Haemost* 2007;5:715–21.

31 Castaman G, Lethagen S, Federici AB, et al. Response to desmopressin is influenced by the genotype and phenotype in type 1 von Willebrand disease (VWD): results from the European Study MCMDM-1VWD. *Blood* 2008;111:3531–9.

32 Haberichter SL, Castaman G, Budde U, et al. Identification of type 1 von Willebrand disease patients with reduced von Willebrand factor survival by assay of the VWF propeptide in the European study: molecular and clinical markers for the diagnosis and management of type 1 VWD (MCMDM-1VWD). *Blood* 2008;111:4979–85.

33 Rodeghiero F, Castaman G. Treatment of von Willebrand disease. *Semin Hematol* 2005;42:29–35.

34 Castaman G, Lattuada A, Mannucci PM, et al. Factor VIII:C increases after desmopressin in a subgroup of patients with autosomal recessive von Willebrand disease. *Br J Haematol* 1995;89:147–51.

35 Mannucci PM, Tenconi PM, Castaman G, Rodeghiero F. Comparison of four virus-inactivated plasma concentrates for treatment of severe von Willebrand disease: a cross-over randomized trial. *Blood* 1992;79: 3130–7.

36 Lethagen S, Kyrle PA, Castaman G, et al. von Willebrand factor/factor VIII concentrate (Haemate P) dosing based on pharmacokinetics: a prospective multicenter trial in elective surgery. *J Thromb Haemost* 2007;5:1420–30.

37 Berntorp E, Petrini P. Long-term prophylaxis in von Willebrand disease. *Blood Coagul Fibrinolysis* 2005;16:S23–6.

38 Federici AB, Castaman G, Franchini M, et al. Clinical use of Haemate P in inherited von Willebrand disease: a cohort study on 100 Italian patients. *Haematologica* 2007;92:944–51.

39 Kouides PA. Females with von Willebrand disease: 72 years as the silent majority. *Haemophilia* 1998;4:665–76.

40 Castaman G, Eikenboom JCJ, Contri A, Rodeghiero F. Pregnancy in women with type 1 von Willebrand disease caused by heterozygosity for von Willebrand factor mutation C1130F. *Thromb Haemostas* 2000;84:351–2.

41 Castaman G, Federici AB, Bernardi M, Moroni B, Bertoncello K, Rodeghiero F. Factor VIII and von Willebrand factor changes after desmopressin and during pregnancy in type 2M von Willebrand disease Vicenza: a prospective study comparing patients with single (R1205H) and double (R1205H-M740I) defect. *J Thromb Haemost* 2006;4:357–60.

42 Castaman G, Bertoncello K, Bernardi M, Rodeghiero F. Pregnancy and delivery in patients with homozygous or heterozygous R854Q type 2N von Willebrand disease. *J Thromb Haemost* 2005;3:391–2.

The rarer inherited coagulation disorders

Paula Bolton-Maggs and Jonathan Wilde

Introduction

The inherited coagulation disorders hemophilia A and B (described in Chapter 7) and von Willebrand disease (described in Chapter 8) are well characterized. However, inherited abnormalities of all the other coagulation factors have been recognized but are not so well known. All are inherited autosomally and generally, with the exception of factor XI, are associated with few or no symptoms in heterozygote individuals. Most of the factor deficiencies are caused by abnormalities in the gene encoding for the particular factor. There are three interesting exceptions.

1 Combined FV and FVIII deficiency is caused by a defect in a protein involved in processing of proteins within the hepatic cells.

2 Combined deficiency of the vitamin K-dependent factors is a disorder caused by mutations in genes encoding enzymes involved in vitamin K-dependent carboxylation.

3 A third syndrome has recently been described where FVII and FX are both affected by abnormalities (deletions or translocations) in chromosome 13, where both genes are located, and usually associated with other abnormalities, such as mental retardation, microcephaly, cleft palate [1].

As all these disorders are rare (Table 9.1), most hematologists and pediatricians will have limited experience, and it is essential that the affected individuals are registered with a hemophilia center.

The annual report from the UKHCDO national database [2] (data for 2006) shows that factor XI deficiency (9%) is more common than hemophilia B (7%), demonstrating that this should perhaps no longer be considered a "rare" bleeding disorder. The other disorders to be considered in this chapter are all

rare, making up a total of 6% of patients in the UK register. The World Federation of Hemophilia (WFH) performs annual global surveys via the national patient organizations in about 100 countries. Since 2004, the survey reports some information about the rare disorders and confirms the variation in distribution in different parts of the world, with higher prevalence of these disorders in countries where consanguineous marriage is common. The global surveys can be viewed on the WFH Web site (http://www.wfh.org).

Rare bleeding disorders have certain features in common that can be considered together.

Genetics

These disorders are autosomal recessive conditions and most commonly occur in individuals whose parents are related, so therefore are much more common in ethnic groups in which consanguineous marriage is customary, such as in many Asian and Arabic communities. Factor XI deficiency (not recessive as symptoms occur in a proportion of heterozygotes) is particularly common in Ashkenazi Jews.

Clinical features

As autosomal disorders, both males and females are affected; menorrhagia is a common feature of all these disorders, and many are associated with hemorrhage related to childbirth. Bleeding at ovulation or from corpus luteum cysts is also reported and can be very severe [3].

Severely deficient infants with these disorders (except factor XI) are particularly at risk for intracranial hemorrhage (ICH) and need to be identified quickly

Table 9.1 Prevalence and chromosomal location of affected gene in the rare inherited coagulation disorders (modified from [26]).

Deficiency	Estimated prevalence of severe deficiency (factor level <10%)	Gene on chromosome
Factor VIII	133:1,000,000 males*	X
Factor IX		
Fibrinogen	1:1,000,000	4
Prothrombin	1:2,000,000	11
Factor V	1:1,000,000	1
Combined V and VIII	1:1,000,000	18
Factor VII	1:500,000	13
Factor X	1:100,000	13
Factor XI	1:1,000,000[†]	4
Factor XIII	1:2,000,000	6 [subunit A]
		1 [subunit B]

*Data from WFH, combined factor VIII and IX, all severity.
[†]Higher in Ashkenazy Jews, where the prevalence of severe deficiency is estimated to be 1 in 190, and 8.1% of the population are heterozygotes [27].

so that appropriate treatment is rapidly available for serious bleeding.

In general, bleeding manifestations in these disorders tend to be more variable and less predictable than in hemophilia A and B (and the classification by factor level used for mild, moderate, and severe hemophilia is not applicable to these other disorders). Some of the deficiencies (factor VII, fibrinogen) are associated with thrombosis, probably as a consequence of particular molecular defects, although in some instances this may be due to coinheritance of a prothrombotic disorder.

Treatment products for most of these conditions are generally not licensed and are not stocked in most hospitals. If fresh frozen plasma (FFP) is used, either because it is the only treatment option or in an emergency while awaiting a specific concentrate, it should preferably be virally inactivated (either by solvent-detergent or methylene blue treatment). As plasma products are used for treatment in most of these disorders, affected individuals should be vaccinated against both hepatitis A and B using the subcutaneous route in order to avoid the risk of muscle hematoma associated with the intramuscular route [4].

Antifibrinolytic therapy, such as tranexamic acid, is a useful adjunct to blood products, particularly for mucous membrane bleeding, but must be used with caution in those disorders with an associated risk of thrombosis.

Guidelines covering treatment products have been published and recently revised. These guidelines should be consulted for further information [5]. The WFH updated its monograph on coagulation factor concentrates in 2008 [6].

Pregnancy

Pregnancy and delivery should be carried out in an obstetric unit with an associated hemophilia center, or at least in close liaison with a hemophilia center specialist. Women with severe deficiency of fibrinogen and factors VII, X, and XIII are at risk of miscarriage if not treated prophylactically during pregnancy. Good communication is essential between obstetric, hemophilia unit, and pediatric staff in order to optimize treatment for the mother and to rapidly identify and plan replacement therapy for an affected neonate.

Investigation

Accurate laboratory testing is important in the identification of these disorders. Sampling of neonates and young infants can be particularly difficult. It is vital to establish that a sample has been properly taken in order to interpret the results. The use of appropriate normal ranges for infants is also essential [7]. Vitamin K deficiency will affect the levels of factors II, VII, IX, and X. This may need to be taken into account in interpretation of results. Normal adult population ranges should be defined for each assay by the local laboratory. The lower limit of normal for many of these factors is higher than the frequently quoted 50 U/dL.

Individual deficiencies

Fibrinogen
Hereditary defects of the fibrinogen gene result in three phenotypes:
1 Impaired production: hypofibrinogenemia or afibrinogenemia, depending on severity.

2 Synthesis of abnormally structured molecules: dysfibrinogenemia.

3 Reduced production of an abnormal molecule: rare (hypodysfibrinogenemia).

Afibrinogenemia

This defect is associated with a bleeding tendency, although variable, and people with severe deficiency may have infrequent bleeding, whereas others have marked mucosal and intramuscular bleeding. Neonates may present with umbilical cord bleeding, and they may have ICH. Wound healing may be impaired. Women are at risk of recurrent miscarriage and both ante- and postpartum hemorrhage. Paradoxically, thrombosis has also been reported in severe deficiency not in relation to therapy or other provoking events. Individuals with hypofibrinogenemia are also at risk of bleeding with less severe manifestations, such as bleeding after surgery rather than spontaneous events. The diagnosis of afibrinogenemia depends on demonstrating absence of fibrinogen by both functional and antigenic assays.

Dysfibrinogenemia

This is a collection of disorders with variable clinical features (over 300 variants have been described). About 25% of patients have a mild bleeding disorder. In roughly another 25%, the specific molecular defects are associated with thrombosis [8]. The diagnosis may be difficult, although generally there is a significant discordancy between fibrinogen antigen and activity values. Family studies may be extremely informative, as many dysfibrinogenemias are inherited in an autosomal dominant manner. The personal and family history of bleeding and thrombosis will help in guiding management.

Treatment

Fibrinogen concentrates are available in some countries [6]. These are preferred to cryoprecipitate as they are treated to reduce risks of viral transmission. The half-life of fibrinogen is 3–5 days, and a level of more than 0.5 g/L is associated with a reduced risk of bleeding.

Prothrombin

Prothrombin deficiency is extremely rare. It has recently been reviewed in detail [9]. Complete deficiency is not recorded and is probably incompatible with life (analogous to the situation in prothrombin "knockout" mice). The two phenotypes are:
• quantitative (hypoprothrombinemia); and
• qualitative (dysprothrombinemia).

Individuals with hypoprothrombinemia may suffer from joint and muscle bleeds and also mucosal bleeding. It is notable that about 70% of patients with prothrombin disorders are of Latin country origin. Heterozygotes may be missed as the prothrombin time may be normal.

Treatment can be given with three-factor (II, IX, X) or four-factor (II, VII, IX, X) concentrates (prothrombin complex concentrates, originally developed for FIX deficiency). Prothrombin has a long half-life, so that treatment may be given every 2–3 days.

Factor V deficiency

Factor V deficiency presents in childhood with bruising and mucous membrane bleeding. Infants with severe deficiency are at risk of ICH, which may occur antenatally. Reported cases appear to have a high risk of inhibitor development associated with replacement therapy. Affected children should also have a factor VIII assay performed to exclude combined deficiency (see below).

Treatment is with FFP. Large volumes may be required leading to a risk of fluid overload. The minimum level of FV required for hemostasis is at least 15 U/dL.

Combined deficiency of factors V and VIII

This interesting disorder is caused by defects in the gene for a protein responsible for intracellular transport (LMAN1) [10,11]. Levels of both factors are most commonly between 5 and 20 IU/dL. Spontaneous bleeding is relatively uncommon; bleeding after surgery is a risk. Parents have normal levels of both factors.

Treatment is with both factor VIII concentrate (principles as for hemophilia A) and FFP (as for FV deficiency).

Factor VII deficiency

This is the most common of the rare disorders (excluding FXI). It has recently been reviewed in detail [9]. People with mild deficiency (heterozygotes) do not usually have a bleeding problem. Generally, bleeding is confined to individuals with very low levels (<2 IU/dL), but the correlation of level with bleeding is not close; that is, some individuals with very low levels do not bleed, whereas those with higher levels do.

Mucous membrane bleeding is particularly common. Menorrhagia is common in women. Thrombosis has also been reported. Neonates with severe deficiency are at risk of ICH [12]. The molecular defects are heterogeneous. It is also important to note that the the factor VII level can vary depending on the source of the thromboplastin used in the laboratory assay and may be related to particular molecular abnormalities (e.g. factor VII Padua). People formerly diagnosed as FVII-deficient using rabbit brain thromboplastin have been shown to have normal FVIIC levels with recombinant human thromboplastin [13]. Girolami notes that different mutations may give similar phenotypes, and conversely, patients with the same mutation may have different phenotypes, thus the genotype–phenotype relationships are complex [9].

The recommended treatment is with recombinant activated factor VII (rVIIa) or with a plasma-derived concentrate. The half-life of factor VII is particularly short (6 hours), but despite this, prophylaxis (where indicated) one to three times a week may be sufficient.

Factor X deficiency

Severe factor X deficiency (FX <1 IU/dL) is associated with a significant risk of ICH in the first weeks of life. Umbilical stump bleeding also occurs. Mucosal hemorrhage is a particular feature, with severe epistaxis being common at any level of deficiency. Menorrhagia occurs in half of affected females. Severe arthropathy may occur as a result of recurrent joint bleeds. Mild deficiency is defined by FX levels of 6–10 IU/dL; these individuals are often diagnosed incidentally but may experience easy bruising or menorrhagia. A number of clinical variants have been described, and assay by more than one method is recommended in order not to miss some variants [13–15].

Antifibrinolytic medication is particularly useful for mucous membrane bleeding. Factor X is present in prothrombin complex concentrates, which are therefore the recommended treatment. The half-life of factor X is 20–40 hours. Caution is required because of the known prothrombotic properties of these concentrates. Therefore, factor X levels should be monitored.

In those children with recurrent joint bleeds, prophylaxis has been successfully admitted either every third day, or once a week. Experience with FFP suggests that, in severe deficiency, an FX level of 20–35 IU/dL is sufficient for hemostasis postoperatively in severe deficiency, but it is likely that levels lower than this (e.g. down to 5 IU/dL) may be sufficient.

Factor XI deficiency

The role of factor XI in the coagulation mechanism is debated; there is some evidence that factor XI is physiologically activated by traces of thrombin and serves to potentiate the propagatory pathway once coagulation has been initiated via the tissue factor pathway. However, this view has been challenged [16]. Bleeding risk may be more related to increased fibrinolysis because of the reduction in generation of the thrombin activatable fibrinolysis inhibitor secondary to a low factor XI. FXI is a serine protease that is unique in being a dimer. Although factor XI deficiency is particularly common in Ashkenazi Jews, it is found in all ethnic groups. The mutations in Jewish patients are restricted with two being particularly common [17]. Overall, the prevalence of severe deficiency is 1 in 1 million, but mild deficiency is much more common. In the UK, mild factor XI deficiency is currently being reported more often than hemophilia B. This is partly because current activated partial thromboplastin time (APTT) reagents are sensitive to mild FXI deficiency and there is a greater readiness to investigate these mildly prolonged APTT levels.

Factor XI deficiency is unlike most of the other rare coagulation disorders in that heterozygotes may have a significant bleeding tendency that is poorly predicted by the factor XI level [18]. Spontaneous bleeding is extremely rare, even in those with undetectable FXI levels; bleeding is provoked by injury and surgery, particularly in areas of high fibrinolytic activity (mouth, nose, and genitourinary tract). Women with both severe and mild deficiency may suffer menorrhagia and bleeding in relation to childbirth. The bleeding tendency varies within both a family and an individual at different times. This may be related to mild variation in other factors, such as von Willebrand factor. These factors make the management of surgery in FXI deficiency more complicated. Babies with severe deficiency do not bleed spontaneously (ICH and other serious bleeding is not reported). Male babies are at risk of excessive bleeding at circumcision. UK guidelines recommend that the factor XI level should be checked, and if less than 10 IU/dL at birth, circumcision should be delayed and the level checked at 6 months. If still less than 10 IU/dL, the procedure should be performed in hospital with FFP or concentrate cover (see below), and the religious requirements discussed with the family. If the level is more than 10 IU/dL, tranexamic acid alone can be given.

Oral antifibrinolytic therapy is very useful for the management of mucosal bleeding (menorrhagia) and is sufficient for the management of dental extractions, even in people with severe deficiency. The management of other types of surgery depends, to some extent, on whether it is in an area of high fibrinolytic activity (such as tonsillectomy) when factor XI replacement is indicated, as opposed to other types of surgery (e.g. herniorrhaphy) where replacement therapy may be more parsimonious [19] .

Two factor XI concentrates are available, but both have been associated with thrombotic events in some individuals, particularly those with additional risk factors, such as older age, the presence of cardiovascular disease, or malignancy. Because of this, antifibrinolytic drugs should not accompany them, and peak levels of more than 100 IU/dL should be avoided. FFP can be used, but in people with severe deficiency it is difficult to produce a sufficient rise (to about 20 to 30 IU/dL) without the risk of fluid overload.

The management of subjects with heterozygous deficiency and a bleeding history (FXI of about 20–60 IU/dL) is more difficult and is dependent on the bleeding history of the individual patient, the presence or absence of associated factor deficiencies, and the nature of the hemostatic challenge.

Inhibitors can develop in severe deficiency [20]; activated recombinant factor VII (rVIIa) has been used successfully. It may also be useful in patients without inhibitors but has been associated with thrombosis in this setting.

Factor XIII deficiency

Factor XIII cross-links and stabilizes fibrin. Severe deficiency, with undetectable factor XIII, is associated with:

• a serious bleeding disorder, usually presenting in infancy;
• bleeding from the umbilical stump in 80%;
• ICH;

• joint and muscle bleeds;
• miscarriages and bleeding after delivery or surgery; and
• delayed wound healing.

For these reasons, usually once severe deficiency is detected, an individual is treated with prophylaxis for life. Individuals with levels of 1–4 U/dL are also likely to have bleeding symptoms, and rarely bleeding is reported in people with levels above 5 U/dL. For a review of factor XIII deficiency, see Anwar and Miloszewski [21]. There is some data emerging suggesting a bleeding diathesis in some heterozygous individuals.

The diagnosis is suspected when the coagulation screen is normal. Clot solubility in urea or acetic acid will be abnormal, and the defect is confirmed by a factor XIII assay. Inconsistent results in the screening tests were noted in the UK NEQAS exercises [22]. Because this is not a routine in most laboratories, it is advisable to send the sample to a specialist center.

Plasma-derived concentrates are the treatment of choice but a recombinant FXIII concentrate is in clinical trials. Factor XIII has a long half-life of 7–10 days, and in practice, dosing at 4–6 weekly intervals has proved effective. It is suggested that levels of 4–10 U/dL are sufficient to prevent hemorrhage.

In the emergency situation, for example, when presented with an infant with a serious bleeding diathesis, once blood has been taken for testing, either FFP or cryoprecipitate is effective treatment.

Combined deficiencies of the vitamin K-dependent factors: II, VII, IX, and X

Combined deficiency of all the vitamin K-dependent factors is a rare but important bleeding disorder to recognize. By 2008, only 29 cases from 24 families had been reported. The inheritance is autosomal recessive and is caused by defective function of either gamma-carboxylase or vitamin K 2-3 epoxide reductase. Mucocutaneous and postsurgery-related bleeding has been reported. Severe cases may present with ICH or umbilical cord bleeding in infancy [23,24]. The clinical picture and response to vitamin K is variable, some responding to low-dose oral vitamin K and others nonresponsive even to high-dose intravenous replacement. In those nonresponsive to vitamin K, prothrombin complex concentrates are the product of choice. Levels of the factors range from less than 1 to 50 IU/dL. Some individuals have associated skeletal abnormalities (probably related to abnormalities in bone vitamin K-dependent proteins, such as osteocalcin). Genetic defects have been reported in the enzymes associated with vitamin K metabolism (e.g. in γ-glutamyl carboxylase).

Illustrative case histories

Case 1

A 13-month-old infant presented with a 2-cm diameter swelling on his head and a swollen thigh caused by running into a door 2 weeks previously. He was thought to be suffering from nonaccidental injury and was admitted. Ultrasound examination confirmed a muscle hematoma. Coagulation screening demonstrated a prolonged prothrombin time (PT) of 25.4 seconds (NR 11.5–15) and APTT of 80 seconds (NR 27–39). His factor X level was <1 U/dL. Both parents (who were unrelated) had prolonged coagulation tests and low factor X levels. Both were asymptomatic. He was treated for the acute bleed with an intermediate purity factor IX (prothrombin complex) concentrate with monitoring of factor X levels. Over the next 3 years, he had repeated muscle and joint bleeds and is now being treated with once weekly prophylaxis. His concentrate dose is determined by regular dose–response and half-life analysis.

Comment

This case illustrates a picture similar to severe hemophilia A. Nonaccidental injury is unfortunately more common than bleeding disorders, so that, unless appropriate investigations are undertaken, diagnosis may be delayed or missed.

Case 2

A baby boy developed massive bilateral cephalhematomas 24 hours after spontaneous vaginal delivery. He was otherwise well with normal, unrelated parents. Blood tests showed a profound anemia (Hb 7.0 g/dL) and incoagulable blood with undetectable fibrinogen. Liver disease was excluded and he was not septic. Cranial ultrasound confirmed that there was no evidence of ICH. Both parents and both maternal grandmothers were noted to have low fibrinogen levels and prolonged thrombin times. He was transfused with red cells and treated with regular cryoprecipitate until fibrinogen concentrate could be obtained. He

was treated prophylactically, requiring a central venous access device, but by 9 months of age, was noted to have subclavian vein thrombosis related to this. MR scanning demonstrated extensive thrombosis of the upper body venous system. It was not possible to determine whether therapy had contributed to the thrombotic risk. Prophylaxis was stopped for 5 months, during which time he had several bruises and was treated for minor bumps to the head, but had no serious bleeding. When he began to walk and fall, his mother was anxious for regular prophylaxis to be resumed. It is unclear whether this is necessary in the long term.

Comment

In the absence of mutation detection, it was impossible to be sure that this child did not have compound heterozygosity for hypo- and dysfibrinogenemia, which might have increased his risk of thrombosis. Mutation detection can be helpful in predicting the clinical picture in fibrinogen disorders, and will probably also prove useful in factor VII and X deficiency where the clinical picture can be variable.

Case 3

A 12-year-old girl was admitted after a heavy third menstrual period. She had been bleeding for 10 days, fainted at school, and on admission was found to have severe anemia with Hb 6.0 g/dL. Coagulation testing demonstrated a normal APTT and a PT of 41 seconds. Her factor VII level was 2.2 IU/dL (2.2%). She had been adopted and had no other bleeding problems; she had not bled excessively after being bitten by a dog, requiring open reduction of a fracture of the forearm, nor after being knocked down by a car. Once her periods had become established and controlled with hormone therapy, she did not have any other bleeding problems, and by the age of 18, had defaulted from follow-up.

Comment

This case illustrates that individuals with severe factor VII deficiency may have very few problems and contrasts with the next case.

Case 4

An Asian baby with parents who were first cousins was delivered by cesarean section. He was noted to have nasal bleeds twice on day 3 and a bloodstained discharge from the umbilical cord on day 5. He was admitted with irritability on day 18 and collapsed on admission with Hb 8 g/dL, PT 32 seconds, APTT 39 seconds. CT scanning of the head showed ICH in the posterior fossa. His FVII level was 4 IU/dL. He was treated initially with FFP (which did not shorten the PT) until a FVII concentrate was available. He was treated symptomatically over this acute event. However, further episodes of ICH occurred over the next 2 months, leading to cerebral atrophy and predictable developmental delay. He was started on prophylaxis twice a week at the age of 6 months via a venous access device. At 4.5 years, he had a mental age of 2.5, epilepsy, no speech, and no vision on the R side as a consequence of his previous ICHs. At the age of 5.5 years, he was noted to have severe iron deficiency (Hb 6.9 g/dL, MCV 59), common in children of Asian origin (dietary), compounded by developmental problems and his bleeding disorder.

Comment

Where ICH occurs in relation to a severe congenital factor deficiency, it needs to be recognized and treated early and intensively to try to avoid long-term developmental problems. Iron deficiency is very common in the Asian community due to dietary deficiency.

Case 5

A Pakistani child with related parents was referred at the age of 1 year. She had easy bruising and bleeding from minor cuts, which lasted several hours. Her PT was 45 seconds and the APTT was 92 seconds. Factor V was <1 U/dL. At the age of 15 and 18 months, she had recurrent mouth bleeds from trauma associated with walking and was treated prophylactically twice weekly with FFP. At 2 years, she had a retroperitoneal hemorrhage. At 3 years, there were concerns about her neurological development, and at 5.5 years, imaging supported the occurrence of a possible ICH in the past. At 3 years, there was evidence of a factor V inhibitor and regular FFP infusions were stopped. She had recurrent muscle bleeds leading to shortening and wasting, and the necessity for tendon-lengthening surgery at the age of 7 years, by which time her inhibitor had disappeared. She continued to have recurrent muscle and joint bleeds treated symptomatically with FFP infusions (the inhibitor having resolved). Menarche occurred at age 13, and her periods have not been heavy.

Comment

Factor V deficiency is difficult to manage and may be associated with the development of inhibitors, as in this case.

Conclusion

The rare coagulation disorders may present with serious and life-threatening bleeding. Prompt investigation and recognition of these disorders is essential so that the appropriate treatment can be instigated. ICH is a serious risk in many of these disorders and may have catastrophic consequences. Hematologists need to work closely with pediatricians to recognize these disorders. In communities where consanguinity is common, there needs to be a heightened awareness of the risk of these potentially serious bleeding disorders. Mutation analysis can be very helpful, as it offers the potential for subsequent antenatal diagnosis in families with severe bleeding disorders.

Acknowledgments

This chapter is based on guidelines published by members of the Rare Haemostatic Disorders Working Party of the United Kingdom Haemophilia Centre Doctors' Organization [25].

References

1 Girolami A, Ruzzon E, Tezza F, Scandellari R, Scapin M, Scarparo P. Congenital FX deficiency combined with other clotting defects or with other abnormalities: a critical evaluation of the literature. *Haemophilia* 2008;14(2):323–8.

2 UKHCDO. *National Haemophilia Database:* Annual Report for 2007, annual returns for 2006. Manchester, UKHCDO, 2007.

3 Gupta N, Dadhwal V, Deka D, Jain SK, Mittal S. Corpus luteum hemorrhage: rare complication of congenital and acquired coagulation abnormalities. *J Obstet Gynaecol Res* 2007;33(3):376–80.

4 Makris M, Conlon CP, Watson HG. Immunization of patients with bleeding disorders. *Haemophilia* 2003;9(5):541–6.

5 UKHCDO. Guidelines on the selection and use of therapeutic products to treat haemophilia and other hereditary bleeding disorders. *Haemophilia* 2003;9(1): 1–23.

6 Brooker M. *Registry of Clotting Factor Concentrates.* Montreal: WFH, April 2008.

7 Williams MD, Chalmers EA, Gibson BE. The investigation and management of neonatal haemostasis and thrombosis. *Br J Haematol* 2002;119(2):295–309.

8 Haverkate F, Samama M. Familial dysfibrinogenemia and thrombophilia. Report on a study of the SSC Subcommittee on Fibrinogen. *Thromb Haemost* 1995;73(1):151–61.

9 Girolami A, Scandellari R, Scapin M, Vettore S. Congenital bleeding disorders of the vitamin K-dependent clotting factors. *Vitam Horm* 2008;78:281–374.

10 D'Ambrosio R, Santacroce R, Di Perna P, Sarno M, Romondia A, Margaglione M. A new case of combined factor V and factor VIII deficiency further suggests that the LMAN1 M1T mutation is a frequent cause in Italian patients. *Blood Coagul Fibrinolysis* 2007;18(2): 203–4.

11 Ginsburg D, Nichols WC, Zivelin A, Kaufman RJ, Seligsohn U. Combined factors V and VIII deficiency–the solution. *Haemophilia* 1998;4(4):677–82.

12 Perry DJ. Factor VII deficiency. *Br J Haematol* 2002;118(3):689–700.

13 Bolton-Maggs PH, Hay CR, Shanks D, Mitchell MJ, McVey JH. The importance of tissue factor source in the management of Factor VII deficiency. *Thromb Haemost* 2007;97(1):151–2.

14 Peyvandi F, Mannucci PM, Lak M, et al. Congenital factor X deficiency: spectrum of bleeding symptoms in 32 Iranian patients. *Br J Haematol* 1998;102(2): 626–8.

15 Uprichard J, Perry DJ. Factor X deficiency. *Blood Rev* 2002;16(2):97–110.

16 Pedicord DL, Seiffert D, Blat Y. Feedback activation of factor XI by thrombin does not occur in plasma. *Proc Natl Acad Sci U S A* 2007;104(31):12855–60.

17 Hancock JF, Wieland K, Pugh RE, et al. A molecular genetic study of factor XI deficiency. *Blood* 1991;77(9):1942–8.

18 Bolton-Maggs PH, Patterson DA, Wensley RT, Tuddenham EG. Definition of the bleeding tendency in factor XI-deficient kindreds: a clinical and laboratory study. *Thromb Haemost* 1995;73(2):194–202.

19 Salomon O, Steinberg DM, Seligshon U. Variable bleeding manifestations characterize different types of surgery in patients with severe factor XI deficiency enabling parsimonious use of replacement therapy. *Haemophilia* 2006;12(5):490–3.

20 Salomon O, Zivelin A, Livnat T, et al. Prevalence, causes, and characterization of factor XI inhibitors in patients with inherited factor XI deficiency. *Blood* 2003;101(12):4783–8.

21 Anwar R, Miloszewski KJ. Factor XIII deficiency. *Br J Haematol* 1999;107(3):468–84.

22 Jennings I, Kitchen S, Woods T, Preston F. Problems relating to the laboratory diagnosis of FXIII deficiency: A UK NEQAS study. *J Thromb Haemost* 2003;1(12): 2603–8.

23 Brenner B. Hereditary deficiency of vitamin K-dependent coagulation factors. *Thromb Haemost* 2000; 84(6):935–6.

24 Oldenburg J, von Brederlow B, Fregin A, et al. Congenital deficiency of vitamin K dependent coagulation factors in two families presents as a genetic defect of the vitamin K-epoxide-reductase-complex. *Thromb Haemost* 2000;84(6):937–41.

25 Bolton-Maggs PH, Perry DJ, Chalmers EA, et al. The rare coagulation disorders–review with guidelines for management from the United Kingdom Haemophilia Centre Doctors' Organisation. *Haemophilia* 2004;10(5):593–628.

26 Peyvandi F, Duga S, Akhavan S, Mannucci PM. Rare coagulation deficiencies. *Haemophilia* 2002;8(3): 308–21.

27 Seligsohn U, Peretz H. Molecular genetics aspects of factor XI deficiency and Glanzmann thrombasthenia. *Haemostasis* 1994;24(2):81–5.

10 Quantitative platelet disorders

Jeremy D. Robertson, Victor S. Blanchette, and Walter H.A. Kahr

Introduction

Thrombocytopenia is defined as a platelet count of less than 150×10^9/L (the normal range is 150–400 $\times$ 10^9/L). Increased bleeding purely as a result of a reduction of platelets does not usually occur until the count drops below 50×10^9/L. Platelet counts of less than 20×10^9/L increase the risk of life-threatening bleeding (e.g. central nervous system or gastrointestinal). However, several prospective studies have revealed that hemorrhagic risk was similar using a 10×10^9/L or 20×10^9/L threshold for prophylactic platelet transfusions, suggesting that life-threatening bleeding increases significantly only when the platelet count drops below 10×10^9/L [1]. Furthermore, the bleeding risk at any given platelet count is partly dependent on the underlying etiology.

The differential diagnosis of thrombocytopenia varies with the age of onset, severity, clinical features, and presence or absence of other hematologic abnormalities. For example, the most probable cause of thrombocytopenia in a newborn infant is different from that of an older child or adult, or that of a pregnant woman. Ranking of the most likely causes of a low platelet count will also depend on whether the patient is systemically well or not. This chapter focuses on a practical approach in the assessment and management of inherited and acquired quantitative platelet disorders. Qualitative platelet disorders are covered in Chapter 11.

Platelet production

Platelets are shed from megakaryocytes through the action of thrombopoietin (TPO) and other cy-tokines to a lesser extent, which collectively stimulate pluripotent hematopoietic stem cells to form mature megakaryocytes in bone marrow [2]. The TPO receptor (c-Mpl, TPO-R) is expressed on the surface of megakaryocytes, platelets, and primitive (pluripotent) stem cells and mediates its action via a signal transduction pathway similar to that of erythropoietin [3]. Thrombopoietin is synthesized predominantly in the liver and released into circulation at a constant rate, where it is largely cleared by binding to TPO-R on platelets. TPO levels are increased up to 20-fold in bone marrow failure states, are only slightly elevated in immune thrombocytopenia (ITP), and are low in liver failure.

The average life span of human platelets is 7–10 days. Older platelets are removed from circulation by reticulo-endothelial cells, although little is known about the mechanisms through which these senescent platelets are identified. A daily turnover of approximately 40×10^9 platelets/L blood is required to maintain a constant platelet count. Aspirin (ASA) inhibits platelets irreversibly; thus, at least 7 days are required to remove ASA-exposed platelets from the circulation.

Newly formed platelets are thought to be more functional in hemostasis than older platelets. However, some antibodies observed in neonatal alloimmune thrombocytopenia (NAIT) may impede platelet function of young platelets by inactivating interaction with the fibrinogen receptor glycoprotein (GP) IIb/IIIa. The higher incidence of serious bleeding in NAIT compared with ITP (antibody binding to GPIIb/IIIa and other platelet surface receptors) at equivalent low platelet counts suggests that the function of platelets in ITP is not impaired.

Mechanisms of thrombocytopenia in children and adults

Thrombocytopenia can be classified according to whether it is explained by increased platelet sequestration, the presence of decreased platelet production, or accelerated platelet destruction (Table 10.1). In addition, dilutional thrombocytopenia following massive transfusion is a common iatrogenic mechanism in which platelet concentration is reduced but total platelet mass is preserved. Artefactual (false) thrombocytopenia is another important consideration in the initial diagnostic evaluation, particularly when an asymptomatic individual is unexpectedly found to have a severely reduced platelet count. This most often results from anticoagulant-dependent platelet clumping ex vivo (pseudothrombocytopenia) or the formation of small clots in the specimen tube following traumatic collection (e.g. heelprick collection in neonates). A diagnostic strategy for evaluating thrombocytopenia in a "well" child or adult is shown in Fig. 10.1.

Platelet sequestration

In healthy individuals, splenic pooling (sequestration) accounts for approximately one-third of the total platelet mass, but may be as high as 90% in individuals with massive splenomegaly. The platelet count does not always correlate directly with splenic size, and the underlying mechanisms of platelet trapping within the extravascular splenic pool remain poorly understood. Preferential diversion of platelets through the splenic cords (by virtue of their small size) as well as binding to receptors on splenic macrophages may play a role in pathophysiology.

Decreased platelet production

Platelets originate from megakaryocytes in the bone marrow. Megakaryoctes protrude extensions (proplatelets) into blood vessels, where flowing blood shear forces facilitate platelet shedding into the circulation [4]. Reduction of total megakaryocyte mass or functional impairment results in underproduction of platelets and subsequent thrombocytopenia.

Table 10.1 Causes of thrombocytopenia in children and adults.

Increased platelet sequestration
Hypersplenism

Decreased platelet production
Aplastic anemia (idiopathic or drug-induced)
Myelodysplastic syndrome
Marrow infiltrative process
Infection (bacterial; viral: HIV, CMV, HCV)
Osteopetrosis
Nutritional deficiencies (iron, folate, vitamin B_{12})
Drug or radiation-induced (see Table 10.3)
Hereditary platelet disorders (see Table 10.2)

Increased platelet destruction
Immune-mediated thrombocytopenias
Acute and chronic ITP
Autoimmune diseases with ITP (SLE, Evans syndrome, autoimmune lymphoproliferative disorders, lymphoma, antiphospholipid antibody syndrome)
Infection-related (viral, bacterial, fungal, protozoan)

Alloimmune (e.g. NAIT)
Post-transfusion purpura
Drug-induced (immune or nonimmune)
Nonimmune-mediated thrombocytopenias
Disseminated intravascular coagulation
Kasabach–Merritt syndrome
Thrombotic thrombocytopenic purpura
Hemolytic uremic syndrome
Catheters, prostheses, cardiopulmonary bypass
Familial hemophagocytic lymphohistiocytosis
Hereditary platelet disorders (see Table 10.2)

Miscellaneous
Liver disease, renal disease, thyroid disease
Massive transfusions, exchange transfusions, extracorporeal circulation
Allogeneic bone marrow transplantation, graft-versus-host disease
Heat or cold injury

Abbreviations: HIV, human immunodeficiency virus; CMV, cytomegalovirus; HCV, hepatitis C virus; SLE, systemic lupus erythematosus.

Drug-associated marrow suppression is the most common cause; however, some agents preferentially affect megakaryocytes (see below). Excess alcohol is also directly toxic to megakaryocytes, and thrombocytopenia in this setting may be exacerbated by other factors, such as nutritional deficiencies and chronic liver

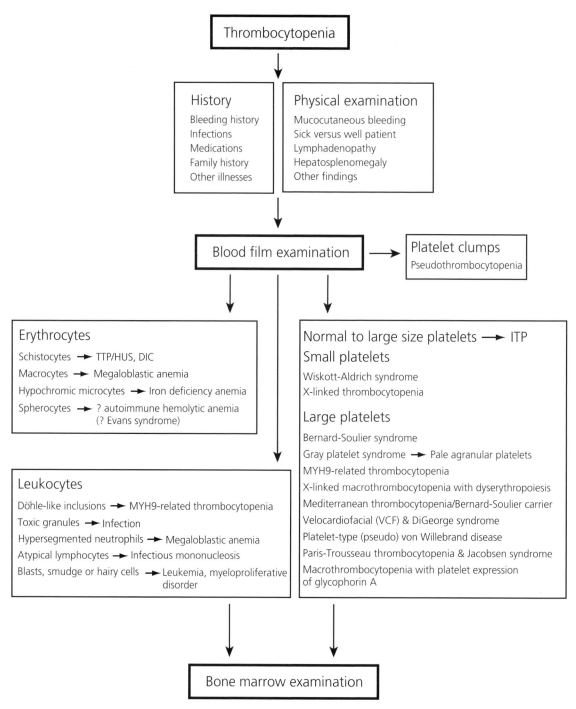

Figure 10.1 Diagnostic strategy for evaluating thrombocytopenia in a "well" child or adult.

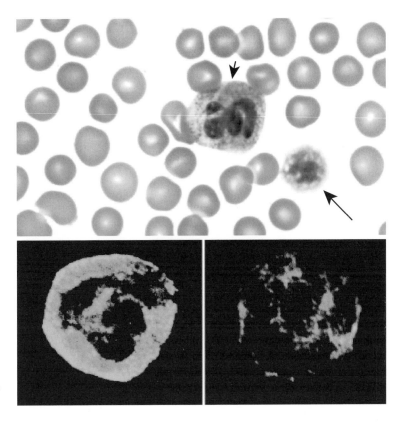

Figure 10.2 May-Grünwald-Giemsa stained blood film (top) demonstrating giant platelet (arrow) and neutrophil inclusion (arrowhead). Immunofluorescent visualization of non-muscle myosin heavy chain IIA aggregates (bottom): normal homogenous cytoplasmic staining (lower left), abnormal variable speckled cytoplasmic staining (lower right). See also colour plate 10.1.

disease. A number of viruses also cause thrombocytopenia by inhibition of megakaryopoiesis, including measles, human immunodeficiency virus (HIV), varicella, mumps, Ebstein-Barr virus (EBV), rubella, cytomegalovirus (CMV), parvovirus, and dengue infection. Thrombocytopenia resulting from marrow suppression usually recovers once the offending agent has been removed.

Marrow infiltration (myelophthisis) by leukemia, solid tumors, storage diseases, fibrosis, and disseminated Langerhans' cell histiocytosis causes thrombocytopenia through displacement of normal hemopoietic cells, including megakaryocytes. Pancytopenia is more common than isolated thrombocytopenia in this context. Acquired or inherited bone marrow failure (e.g. aplastic anemia, Fanconi anemia) is characterized by progressive pancytopenia in association with a hypocellular marrow. However, isolated thrombocytopenia with megakaryocytic hypoplasia can occur early in the course of these disorders. Thrombocytopenia resulting from hereditary platelet disorders may

be caused either by inadequate platelet production (megakaryocyte defect) or by the increased clearance of platelets because of inherent structural defects.

Ineffective megakaryocytopoiesis results in thrombocytopenia, despite normal or increased megakaryocyte mass. This typically accompanies megaloblastic anemia (B_{12} or folate deficiency) but may also be a prominent feature of some myelodysplastic syndromes.

Increased platelet destruction

Accelerated platelet destruction is the most common cause of thrombocytopenia and is usually immune-mediated, although nonimmune (consumptive) mechanisms are well characterized (Table 10.1). Antibodies against epitopes on the platelet surface are frequently implicated, although T cell- and dendritic cell-mediated immunological mechanisms are also thought to play a role [5]. The bone marrow in destructive thrombocytopenias typically reveals megakaryocytic hyperplasia, although ITP is sometimes accompanied by suboptimal megakaryopoiesis for reasons that are still being elucidated (see below).

Patient history

Immediate (rather than delayed) bleeding is typical of thrombocytopenia, similar to other disorders of primary hemostasis, including platelet function defects and von Willebrand disease (VWD). Distinctive features include:

- petechiae,
- mucocutaneous bleeding,
- epistaxis, and
- menorrhagia.

Conversely, hemarthroses and intramuscular hematomas are rare in contrast to defects of secondary hemostasis, such as hemophilia. A careful history assessing the response to trauma, surgical challenges (including circumcision, dental extraction, and tonsillectomy), menses, and postpartum hemorrhage can be useful in defining the presence of a primary hemostatic defect.

Bleeding since birth or early childhood is suggestive of an inherited condition, whereas symptoms in older patients are more likely to be caused by an acquired defect.

Family history

A family history of bleeding and thrombocytopenia suggests an inherited condition. Table 10.2 lists some hereditary thrombocytopenias and their mode of inheritance [6,7]. A preponderance to autoimmune disease, including ITP, is also observed in some families. A diagnosis of NAIT may be foreshadowed by a history of a previous child (sibling or cousin) affected by intracranial hemorrhage (ICH) or thrombocytopenia during the neonatal period.

Medication history

A careful medication history is important because many drugs can cause thrombocytopenia, as shown in Table 10.3 [8,9]. Platelet-inhibiting drugs, such as ASA and other nonsteroidal anti-inflammatory drugs (NSAIDs), ticlopidine, clopidogrel, dipyridamole, and GPIIb/IIIa antagonists (abciximab, tirofiban, eptifibatide), should also be identified when evaluating a thrombocytopenic patient, as these agents may exacerbate the bleeding. Particular attention should be paid to whether the patient is receiving heparin (including exposure to heparin in line flushes) because heparin-induced thrombocytopenia (HIT; see below) needs to be excluded. Nonprescription (e.g. herbal) medications should also be documented, as they may contribute to thrombocytopenia and/or platelet dysfunction. For instance, patients and physicians may not be aware that tonic water (as in "gin and tonic") contains quinine, an extract from cinchona tree bark that can be associated with thrombocytopenia.

Medical history

Infection

One of the most common causes of thrombocytopenia is infection. Infectious causes of thrombocytopenia include HIV, hepatitis C virus (HCV), influenza, varicella zoster virus, rubella virus, EBV, CMV, hantavirus, mycoplasma, mycobacteria, malaria, trypanosomiasis, *Rickettsiae*, and *Ehrlichiae*. Patients at risk for HIV and HCV infection, such as intravenous drug users and individuals who practice high-risk sexual activities (e.g. unprotected sex with multiple partners) warrant particular attention, as virus-associated thrombocytopenia is common in these diseases (see below). Transient thrombocytopenia may be observed in children receiving live viral vaccines, although a direct causative role has not been established. *Helicobacter pylori* infection can be associated with ITP, and antimicrobial therapy may improve platelet counts in these patients. Infection-associated hemolytic uremic syndrome (HUS) caused by *Escherichia coli* (serotype O157:H7), *Shigella*, *Salmonella*, and *Campylobacter jejuni* can follow an acute diarrheal illness and is characterized by thrombocytopenia with schistocytes seen on a blood film. Meningococcemia should always be considered in any unwell child found to have thrombocytopenia. Severe sepsis resulting from bacterial infection leading to disseminated intravascular coagulation (DIC) results in thrombocytopenia and

Table 10.2 Hereditary thrombocytopenias (adapted from Balduini et al. [6] and Drachman [7]).

Disorder	Gene (chromosome)	Pertinent features
X-linked disorders		
Wiskott–Aldrich syndrome (WAS)	*WAS* (Xp11.23-p11.22)	Moderate–severe thrombocytopenia; small platelets; immunodeficiency; eczema; absent WAS protein in lymphocytes detected by Western blot
X-linked thrombocytopenia (XLT)	*WAS* (Xp11.23-p11.22)	As for WAS, except mild/absent immunodeficiency/eczema
X-linked macrothrombocytopenia with dyserythropoiesis	*GATA1* (Xp11.23)	Dysmegakaryocytopoiesis and dyserythropoiesis with severe/variable anemia; confirm by analysis of *GATA1*
Autosomal dominant disorders		
Mediterranean thrombocytopenia/Bernard Soulier syndrome carrier	GPIba (17p12)	Mild thrombocytopenia; large platelets; common in Mediterranean region
MYH9-related thrombocytopenia:	*MYH9* (22q11)	Large platelets; mild-moderate thrombocytopenia; myosin heavy-chain IIA immunocytochemistry in neutrophils
May–Hegglin anomaly		Neutrophil inclusions
Sebastian syndrome		Neutrophil inclusions (distinct on TEM)
Fechtner syndrome		Neutrophil inclusions; hearing loss; nephritis; cataracts
Epstein syndrome		Platelet dysfunction; hearing loss; nephritis
Familial platelet disorder with associated myeloid leukemia	AML1/CBFA2/RUNX1 (21q22.2)	Predisposition for acute myeloid leukemia
Thrombocytopenia with radio-ulnar synostosis	*HOXA11* (7p15-p14.2)	Reduced/absent megakaryocytes; radio-ulnar synostosis; ± other malformations
Velocardiofacial (VCF) and DiGeorge syndrome	GPIbb (22q11)	Large platelets; cardiac abnormalities; parathyroid/thymus insufficiency; learning disabilities; facial dysmorphology
Platelet-type (pseudo) von Willebrand disease	GPIba (17p13)	Increased platelet aggregation with low-dose ristocetin due to gain of function mutation in platelet GPIba (ligand for VWF)
Type 2B von Willebrand disease	*VWF* (12p13)	Increased platelet aggregation with low-dose ristocetin due to gain of function mutation in VWF platelet receptor
Paris–Trousseau thrombocytopenia and Jacobsen syndrome	*FLI1* (11q23)	Cardiac and facial abnormalities; cognitive disabilities; giant platelet granules (fused α-granules)
Autosomal dominant thrombocytopenia with linkage to chromosome 10	*FLJ14813* (10p12-11.2)	Small megakaryocytes with hypolobulated nuclei; putative kinase mutation
Quebec platelet disorder	*Unknown*	Delayed-onset bleeding unresponsive to platelet transfusions; urokinase in platelets detected (Western blot)
Macrothrombocytopenia with platelet expression of glycophorin A	*Unknown*	Large platelets expressing glycophorin A (flow cytometry); decreased platelet aggregation with arachidonic acid
Autosomal recessive disorders		
Gray platelet syndrome (rarely autosomal dominant)	*Unknown*	Large pale appearing platelets in blood film; reduced/absent alpha granules in TEM
Bernard Soulier syndrome	GPIba (17p13)	Large platelets; absent platelet aggregation with ristocetin; homozygous defect in platelet GP complex Ib/IX/V
	GPIbb (22q11) GPIX (3q21	
Congenital amegakaryocytic thrombocytopenia	*MPL* (1p34)	Severe isolated hypomegakaryocytic thrombocytopenia severe thrombocytopenia; TPO receptor mutation evolving into aplastic anemia
Thrombocytopenia with absent radii (can be autosomal dominant)	*Unknown* (1q21)	Bilateral radial aplasia ± other skeletal or cardiac anomalies; severe thrombocytopenia at birth, improving with time

Platelet size according to mean platelet volume (MPV): small platelets (MPV <6 fL); normal platelets (MPV 7–11 fL); large platelets (MPV >11 fL). *Abbreviations:* TEM, transmission electron microscopy; VWF, von Willebrand factor.

Table 10.3 Drugs causing thrombocytopenia (adapted from George et al. [8] and Aster [9]).

Drug Immune-mediated	Mechanism
Acetaminophen	
Aminoglutethimide	
Aminosalicylic acid	
Amiodarone	
Amphotericin B	
Carbamazepine	May also induce marrow aplasia
Cimetidine	
Chlorothiazide/hydrochlorothiazide	
Danazol	
Diatrizoate meglumine (Hypaque)	
Diclofenac	
Digoxin	
Gold/gold salts	May also induce marrow aplasia
IFN-a	May also inhibit megakaryocyte proliferation
Levamisole	
Meclofenamate	
Methyldopa	
Nalidixic acid	
Oxprenolol	
Procainamide	
Quinidine and quinine	May also produce a TTP-like picture
Ranitidine	
Rifampin	
Simvastatin	
Sulfasalazine	
Sulfisoxazole	
Trimethoprim-sulfamethoxazole	
Vancomycin	
Unique antibody-mediated process	
Heparin	PF4-heparin-antibody causes HIT by platelet activation
Abciximab, eptifibatide and tirofiban	GPIIb/IIIa (αIIbβ3 integrin) antagonist; or peptide derivative
Suppression of platelet production	
Anagrelide	Inhibits megakaryocyte maturation
Imatinib	
Thiazide diuretics	
Valproic acid	Inhibits megakaryocyte maturation; dose-related; may also induce marrow aplasia
Suppression of all hematopoietic cells	
Chemotherapeutic agents	Some also cause immune-mediated destruction
Thrombotic thrombocytopenic purpura	
Ticlopidine	May also induce marrow aplasia
Clopidogrel	
Cyclosporine and FK506 (tacrolimus)	
Mitomcyin C	Dose-related
Unknown mechanism	
Monoclonal antibodies	

associated coagulopathy (see below). It should also be highlighted that numerous infections may be associated with petechiae and/or purpura in the absence of thrombocytopenia.

Systemic diseases

Systemic diseases involving the bone marrow, such as aplastic anemia, myelofibrosis, leukemia, lymphoma, or metastatic cancers infiltrating the bone marrow, often result in thrombocytopenia, but this is often manifested as a pancytopenia involving all three cell types: platelets, erythrocytes, and leukocytes.

Other systemic illnesses, such as renal and liver disease, not only affect platelet function but also are often accompanied by mild to moderate thrombocytopenia.

Other causes

Poor nutritional intake, such as can occur in the elderly or alcoholics, may result in decreased intake of folate, resulting in megaloblastic anemia and thrombocytopenia. In addition, excessive alcohol intake has direct inhibitory effects on platelet production.

Pregnancy is commonly associated with thrombocytopenia (in approximately 5–10% of pregnant women), usually appearing during the third trimester; however, in this situation, alternative etiologies need to be considered (see below).

Transfusion history

Previous transfusions may place an individual at risk of developing post-transfusion purpura, in which severe thrombocytopenia can appear 7–14 days after the transfusion of a blood product. Transfusion-associated infection, such as HIV, HCV, CMV, West Nile virus, or malaria, may also be complicated by thrombocytopenia.

Physical examination

The clinical appearance of the patient is of paramount importance in the assessment of the thrombocytopenic patient and provides the first clue as to the likely etiology. A sick patient in the intensive care unit may have a number of possible contributing factors, including severe sepsis, DIC, drug-induced post-transfusion purpura, massive blood transfusion, and systemic illness. In contrast, a well patient with newly diag-

nosed isolated thrombocytopenia may have an inherited thrombocytopenia, ITP, or, in a neonate, auto- or alloimmune thrombocytopenia.

Certain hereditary thrombocytopenias are accompanied by typical physical findings, such as skeletal abnormalities, facial dysmorphologies, hearing deficiencies, and cataracts, as described in Table 10.2. Evidence of an enlarged spleen or other systemic findings (e.g. fever, jaundice, adenopathy, cachexia) can be helpful in deciding whether an underlying illness is the likely cause for the thrombocytopenia.

Petechiae consisting of small (<2 mm), red, flat, discrete lesions, occurring most frequently in the dependent areas on the ankles and feet, represent extravasated red cells from capillaries and are the hallmark of a primary hemostatic disorder. They are nontender and do not blanch under pressure. Purpura (<1 cm) and ecchymoses (>1 cm) represent larger areas of bleeding, and when observed in mucous membranes, such as the oropharynx, are described as "wet purpura." These findings are in contrast to delayed bleeding into joints or muscle, which suggest a coagulation disorder rather than a platelet or von Willebrand factor (VWF) problem.

Laboratory evaluation

Blood film

The importance of examining a blood film in a patient with newly diagnosed thrombocytopenia cannot be overemphasized. For example:

- Visualization of schistocytes (RBC fragments) could be indicative of thrombotic thrombocytopenic purpura/hemolytic uremic syndrome (TTP/HUS) or DIC.
- Evidence of platelet clumps would suggest pseudothrombocytopenia.
- Megathrombocytes with Döhle-like inclusions in neutrophils could be indicative of MYH9-related diseases (Figure 10.2 & Plate 10.1 top, arrow and arrowhead, respectively).
- Pale agranular-appearing platelets could represent gray platelet syndrome.
- Blasts suggest the diagnosis of leukemia or a myeloproliferative disorder.
- Macrocytes with hypersegmented neutrophils suggest megaloblastic anemia.
- Toxic granulation suggests infection.

• Spherocytes and polychromasia may be observed in Evan's syndrome (coexisting autoimmune hemolytic anemia and ITP).

Pseudothrombocytopenia resulting from EDTA-induced platelet clumping may be overcome by obtaining a film from a drop of blood smeared directly onto a slide or by collection of blood into citrate or heparin anticoagulants.

Mean platelet volume and reticulated platelets

For inherited causes of thrombocytopenia, a useful diagnostic algorithm is based on the platelet size or mean platelet volume [6]. One caveat of this approach is that not all automated counters are able to detect very small platelets (e.g. as in Wiskott–Aldrich syndrome) or very large platelets (e.g. as in Bernard Soulier syndrome), resulting in underestimation of the platelet count. This emphasizes the importance of examining the blood film.

Platelets with a higher RNA content are believed to represent younger ("immature") cells, and it has been postulated that an increase in the relative proportion of young platelets is indicative of increased platelet turnover, akin to the reticulocytosis that occurs during marrow recovery or hemolytic anemia. Many modern hematology analyzers use a flow cytometer in combination with a dye that binds to RNA within cells to provide a direct estimate of the immature platelet fraction ("reticulated platelets"). The use of this technology has not yet been clearly defined; however, the parameter may be useful in predicting platelet recovery following chemotherapy, and also in the initial diagnostic evaluation of the thrombocytopenic patient [10].

Bone marrow examination

For a typical presentation of ITP, a bone marrow examination is not required in patients under the age of 60 years. However, a bone marrow aspirate and biopsy is recommended in:
• patients before undertaking therapeutic splenectomy;
• those with additional cytopenias;
• patients with lassitude, protracted fever, or bone or joint pain;
• patients with lymphadenopathy and/or organomegaly;

• those with unexplained macrocytosis or dysplastic features on blood film; and
• patients with suboptimal response to treatment.

Specialized platelet function tests (see Chapter 5)

Specialized tests that may be indicated in the evaluation of specific hereditary thrombocytopenias include:
• platelet aggregation;
• flow cytometry using antibodies labeling GPIb (for Bernard Soulier syndrome);
• platelet electron microscopy (for gray platelet syndrome);
• specialized immunocytochemistry (for MYH9-related diseases, Figure 10.2 & Plate 10.1);
• Western blot for protein analyses (for Quebec platelet disorder); and
• DNA analysis (for confirmatory testing when genetic basis is known).

Specific conditions

Immune thrombocytopenic pupura

ITP is probably the most common immune destructive thrombocytopenia in children and adults, occurring in approximately 1 in 20,000 persons/year [11]. ITP is an autoimmune disorder in which autoantibodies are produced against platelet surface glycoproteins, resulting in increased clearance of platelets from the circulation. In children, the condition is typically acute, and spontaneous resolution is common. Conversely, in adults, it is frequently a chronic disorder with an insidious onset, often diagnosed incidentally when a blood count is performed for other reasons [12]. There is a modest female predominance in adults, whereas young boys and girls are affected equally. Although the etiology of ITP is poorly understood, infections appear to play a role because, in the case of childhood ITP, the onset is often preceded by a viral infection. Cases in which an underlying disease cannot be identified are classified as primary ITP. However 5–10% of adult patients who initially present with ITP will subsequently be diagnosed with an underlying systemic autoimmune disease. Secondary causes of ITP are observed in patients with:
• systemic lupus erythematosus (SLE);
• antiphospholipid antibody syndrome;

- immune deficiency syndromes;
- chronic infections (e.g. HIV, HCV, *Helicobacter pylori*);
- lymphoproliferative disorders; and
- neoplasia-associated immune thrombocytopenia.

Diagnosis

The diagnosis of primary ITP is predominantly one of exclusion and is suggested by the presence of isolated thrombocytopenia in an otherwise well patient in the absence of other causes. The patient may present with evidence of mucocutaneous bleeding or after a routine complete blood count (CBC) in an asymptomatic individual. A thorough history and physical examination combined with careful review of a CBC and blood film is sufficient for diagnosis in most cases. Underlying systemic diseases, drug-induced thrombocytopenias, as well as hereditary thrombocytopenias (e.g. positive family history, abnormal blood film) should be ruled out. Bone marrow aspirate and biopsy are indicated if the clinical features are atypical, or if additional abnormalities are noted on the CBC or film. In older individuals, isolated thrombocytopenia may be the initial presenting feature of myelodysplasia or malignancy, and bone marrow biopsy is recommended in adults over 60 years of age even when the findings appear typical of ITP. Platelet autoantibody assays are not sensitive nor specific enough to be clinically useful, and should not be relied on for diagnosis. Interestingly, plasma TPO levels are usually normal or mildly elevated in ITP but are greatly elevated in amegakaryocytic states (e.g. congenital amegakaryocytic thrombocytopenia, bone marrow suppression, and aplastic anemia), and therefore, may be diagnostically useful if available. However, measurement of TPO is currently limited to the research setting.

Principles of management

In adults, treatment is generally indicated if the platelet count is below 20×10^9/L or below 50×10^9/L in the presence of significant bleeding or additional risk factors for bleeding. Those with higher counts can be merely observed, as the bleeding risk is low and early treatment does not modify the course of the disease. Platelet-inhibiting drugs, such as ASA and other NSAIDs, should be avoided. Initial treatment of ITP consists of glucocorticoids (prednisone 1 mg/kg/day p.o.), IV immunoglobulin (IVIG 1 g/kg),

or IV anti-D ($50–75$ μg/kg)in Rh(D)-positive patients with intact spleens. With major bleeding episodes, or if the platelet count is less than 10×10^9/L, glucocorticoids can be given together with either IVIG or IV anti-D. In the presence of ICH, platelet transfusions are also indicated.

The natural course of acute ITP in children is that most will recover completely within a few weeks without any treatment. The major concern is ICH, which can occur when platelets fall below 20×10^9/L but usually only when they fall below 10×10^9/L. The incidence of ICH in ITP is estimated to be between 0.2% and 1%. If the child presents with wet purpura (extensive mucocutaneous bleeding) or evidence of major bleeding and/or platelet counts below 20×10^9/L, then oral prednisone ($3–4$ mg/kg/day for $3–4$ days), IV methylprednisolone ($5–30$ mg/kg/day),IVIG ($0.8–1$ g/kg), or IV anti-D ($50–75$ μg/kg) in Rh(D)-positive children are all efficacious regimens, although the response to IVIG is generally more rapid. In adults, platelet transfusions are reserved for life-threatening bleeding and ICH.

Relapsed and chronic ITP

Around 70% of patients will respond to initial therapy with corticosteroids or immunoglobulin, although in adults, the effect is most often transient or requires repeated doses to maintain response. In contrast, only 25% of children will relapse, and late spontaneous remission is well-recognized even in this subgroup. Chronic ITP is generally defined as persistence of thrombocytopenia severe enough to warrant therapy more than 6 months after initial diagnosis. Splenectomy is the currently accepted second-line approach for adults who fail to respond to first-line therapy or experience unacceptable side effects from repeated steroid exposure, and 60–70% will have a durable response to this procedure. In children, splenectomy is generally deferred as long as possible, due to the higher life-long risk of post-splenectomy sepsis and the greater chance of remission compared with adults. Numerous therapeutic regimens have been described for those patients who fail to respond or relapse after splenectomy, although evidence for efficacy is mostly limited to case series. Examples include pulsed corticosteroids, danazol, dapsone, azathioprine, cyclosporine, mycophenolate, vincristine, and cyclophosphamide.

Recent attention has focused on novel therapeutic approaches to chronic ITP, either as salvage following failed splenectomy or to avoid splenectomy altogether. Rituximab, a monoclonal anti-CD20 chimeric antibody, has shown promise in this context, with sustained responses and minimal reported toxicity in 40–60% of patients receiving a lymphoma-based regimen of 375 mg/m^2 weekly for 4 doses [13]. It should be highlighted that rituximab has not been licensed for use in this setting, and patients must be counseled accordingly. Furthermore the potent B cell suppression that follows rituximab may increase the risk of viral infection or reactivation, and this must be balanced against the risk of bacterial infection after splenectomy.

Other research has focused on the potential role of TPO-R agonists. Although ITP is predominantly a condition of increased platelet destruction, TPO levels in ITP are not elevated in proportion to the severity of thrombocytopenia, possibly due to faster TPO clearance resulting from rapid platelet turnover. First-generation TPO-R agonists, recombinant forms of human TPO, were withdrawn from development in 1998 after thrombocytopenia due to anti-TPO antibodies was observed in some healthy volunteers receiving such agents. There are numerous second-generation TPO-R agonists currently in development, and these appear to be nonimmunogenic, well-tolerated, and effective at increasing platelet count. However, at this stage, only two agents have undergone phase 3 trials, both in chronic ITP, namely romiplostim (AMG-531) and eltrombopag (SB-497115). The reader is referred to a recent review by Kuter for an overview of these new agents [3].

Evan's syndrome

The combination of ITP with autoimmune hemolytic anemia in the absence of an underlying cause is referred to as Evan's syndrome, and has a pathogenesis and clinical course distinct from that of classic ITP [14]. More than half of these patients also have autoimmune neutropenia. Response to standard therapy is often poorly sustained, and multiple relapses with significant long-term morbidity is typical. Specific disorders that mimic Evan's syndrome must be excluded, as the management of these conditions is different. These include autoimmune lymphoproliferative syndrome (ALPS), chronic variable immunodeficiency (CVID), and systemic autoimmune disease (e.g. SLE).

Drug-induced thrombocytopenia

Drug-induced thrombocytopenia is common and probably under-recognized, either because a platelet count is not measured or because thrombocytopenia is attributed to other factors. There are a large number of agents known to cause thrombocytopenia, and most of these can be broadly divided into the following categories:

• drugs that cause predictable dose-dependent marrow suppression;
• drugs that cause idiosyncratic marrow aplasia;
• drugs that specifically inhibit megakaryopoiesis;
• drugs that trigger immune destruction of platelets;
• drugs that cause a TTP-like condition; and
• drugs that induce platelet aggregation.

Chemotherapeutic agents used for malignancy or potent immunosuppression often cause dose-dependent thrombocytopenia as a result of generalized bone marrow suppression, although some of these agents can also induce immune-mediated platelet destruction. Although the mechanisms are poorly understood, a number of drugs have been implicated in aplastic anemia, including anticonvulsants, NSAIDs, sulfonamides, and gold salts. Some drugs known to specifically inhibit megakaryopoiesis are listed in Table 10.3. Anagrelide, used in the treatment of thrombocythemia in patients with myeloproliferative diseases, can cause severe thrombocytopenia. Valproic acid, commonly used in seizure disorders and for psychiatric patients, has been associated with dose-dependent thrombocytopenia resulting from direct megakaryocyte suppression. Thiazide diuretics also have a mild inhibitory effect on megakaryocytes.

Many drugs have been implicated in producing a TTP-like condition, with thrombocytopenia, hemolysis, and varying degrees of neurological or renal dysfunction, although for most agents, this appears to be an exceedingly rare event [15]. The pathogenesis is poorly understood, although direct or immune-mediated endothelial injury may be an important trigger. Drugs for which a causal association seems likely include mitomycin C (dose-related), calcienurin inhibitors, such as cyclosporine and tacrolimus (1–3% incidence), and the thienopyridine derivitives ticlopidine (<0.1% incidence) and clopidogrel (rare).

Interestingly, quinine can also cause TTP, although it is better known for inducing antibody-mediated platelet destruction.

Drug-induced antibody-mediated platelet destruction is the most common mechanism of iatrogenic thrombocytopenia [9]. There are several mechanisms of drug-induced ITP, although the "quinine-type" accounts for the majority:

• Drugs that bind to platelet glycoproteins forming a "compound epitope" include penicillin, quinidine, quinine, and sulfonamide. The antibody binding to such platelets is dependent on the presence of the offending drug.

• Gold salts and procainamide, on the other hand, can induce true autoantibodies, which subsequently can bind to platelets in the absence of the original offending drug.

• Antiplatelet agents such as tirofiban, eptifibatide, and abciximab, which specifically target the GPIIb/IIIa (αIIbβ3 integrin) receptor on platelets, cause thrombocytopenia in 1–5% of cardiac patients via antibody-mediated processes.

Diagnosis of drug-induced ITP requires a high index of suspicion, as systemic illness or other coexistent factors may confuse the clinical picture. Onset of thrombocytopenia within 5–7 days of commencing a new drug is an important clue. Withdrawal of the offending agent leads to resolution of thrombocytopenia in most cases, although rarely IVIG, steroids, or more aggressive management may be indicated. Inadvertent rechallenge with the causative drug may induce rapid and severe thrombocytopenia and should be avoided.

Heparin-induced thrombocytopenia

HIT differs from other thrombocytopenias in that it is a hypercoagulable state rather than a bleeding condition, manifesting as venous and/or arterial thrombosis [16]. This iatrogenic disorder is discussed in more detail in Chapter 26.

Pregnancy-associated thrombocytopenia (see also Chapter 24)

There is a physiological decline in platelet count during the course of normal pregnancy, most pronounced in the third trimester, although only 5–10% of women will become thrombocytopenic [17]. Mild thrombocytopenia (100–149 $\times$ 10^9/L) is common and

of no clinical significance; however, lower platelet counts require further evaluation. The most common causes of pregnancy-associated thrombocytopenia include:

• *Gestational thrombocytopenia* (incidental or benign thrombocytopenia of pregnancy): accounts for approximately 75% of cases.

• *Preeclampsia $\pm$ HELLP* (hemolysis, elevated liver enzymes, low platelets): accounts for approximately 20% of cases.

• *ITP $\pm$ SLE:* accounts for approximately 4% of cases.

Gestational thrombocytopenia is a diagnosis of exclusion, but in 95% of cases, it manifests as mild thrombocytopenia in an asymptomatic pregnant patient with a previously normal platelet count. This is a benign condition that requires no treatment. Although more severe thrombocytopenia can occasionaly be seen, counts below 70 $\times$ 10^9/L should raise strong suspicion of an alternative diagnosis. Similarly, the finding of thrombocytopenia in early pregnancy is more suggestive of ITP or a preexisting condition. Thrombocytopenia develops in approximately 20% of patients with preeclampsia, and there is an inverse relationship between platelet count and severity of disease. The HELLP syndrome can be a serious complication, associated with up to 20% fetal mortality. Thrombocytopenia associated with preeclampsia and HELLP syndrome improves following delivery, whereas that observed in the primary microangiopathic hemolytic anemias, TTP and HUS, does not. These conditions may sometimes be difficult to discern from preeclampsia or HELLP syndrome in a pregnant woman, and plasma exchange may be required despite an uncertain diagnosis (see below). DIC complicates a small proportion of cases, and a coagulation screen is an important component of the diagnostic work-up. ITP occurs in 1–2 per 1000 pregnancies and represents approximately 3–5% of the causes of thrombocytopenia during pregnancy. A pregnant patient with ITP can be treated with IVIG (1 g/kg prepregnant weight) and/or prednisone (1 mg/kg prepregnant weight) in the acute setting to raise the platelet count to above 10 $\times$ 10^9/L. Measurement of platelet count in the newborn is important, as 5–10% of infants born to mothers with ITP will have significant thrombocytopenia (<50 $\times$ 10^9/L). The management of ITP during pregnancy is discussed in more detail in a recent review [18].

Post-transfusion purpura

Post-transfusion purpura (PTP) is a rare disorder, which usually manisfests as severe thrombocytopenia 7–14 days following transfusion of a blood product. It is caused by the formation of high-titre alloantibodies against platelet glycoproteins and represents an anamnestic immune response in a patient previously sensitized through antigen exposure in pregnancy and/or transfusion. The antibodies are most commonly directed against the platelet alloantigen HPA-1a epitope (also known as PL^{A1} or Zw^a), where the platelet GPIIIa contains a leucine at position 33. Polymorphisms of GPIIIa result in alloantigen HPA-1a and alloantigen HPA-1b (PL^{A2} or Zw^b; proline at position 33 of GPIIIa), which occur at a frequency of approximately 86% and 14% in caucasians, respectively. Classically, the affected patient is a homozygous HPA-1b middle-aged multiparous woman; however, the condition also occurs in men and nulliparous women. The alloantibodies paradoxically cause destruction of autologous as well as transfused platelets through poorly understood mechanisms. PTP has been estimated to occur following 1/50–100,000 transfusions, although this may represent an underestimate as the diagnosis may be overshadowed by coexisting factors, such as heparin exposure or sepsis. Interestingly, in countries in which universal leukodepletion is practiced, a striking reduction in the incidence of PTP has been noted, presumably due to the fact that the process removes platelets from red cell concentrates [19]. Diagnosis of PTP requires a strong index of suspicion, followed by demonstration of high-titre HPA alloantibodies in the transfusion recipient. The observation of a decline in platelet count *below* baseline *following* a platelet transfusion can be an important clue to differentiate this condition from platelet refractoriness, which is multifactorial and far more common. Treatment of PTP consists of IVIG, corticosteroids, or plasmapheresis. Platelet transfusions are contraindicated except in rare circumstances, when HPA-1a-negative platelets may be used for life-threatening bleeding complications.

HIV-associated thrombocytopenia

There are multiple factors that contribute to the thrombocytopenia frequently associated with HIV, including immune mechanisms and defective platelet production [20]. The immune-mediated platelet destruction in HIV is indistinguishable from ITP with respect to increased destruction of antibody-coated platelets and the response to prednisone, IVIG, and splenectomy. It differs from classic ITP with respect to:
• male predominance;
• markedly elevated platelet-associated IgG, IgM, and complement C$_3$, C$_4$;
• presence of circulating immune complexes; and
• antibody-mediated peroxide lysis of platelets.

Treatment with antiretroviral therapy tends to improve the defective thrombopoiesis in HIV-infected patients. TTP is also found more frequently in HIV-infected patients.

HCV-associated thrombocytopenia

Thrombocytopenia is frequently associated with chronic liver disease, and the severity correlates with the extent of hepatocellular damage and fibrosis [21]. There are numerous contributing factors, including the underlying cause of liver disease itself (e.g. alcohol is directly toxic to megakaryocytes), associated portal hypertension with splenic sequestration of platelets, and reduction in TPO synthesis. Liver disease is discussed in greater detail in Chapter 21. However, HCV-associated thrombocytopenia warrants particular mention for several reasons:
• Thrombocytopenia in HCV frequently occurs in the absence of clinical or radiological features to suggest portal hypertension;
• There is an approximately 20-fold increase in the incidence of ITP in patients with HCV, and treatment of ITP with steroids may promote viremia;
• The presence of thrombocytopenia in HCV is an adverse prognostic factor and may limit options for therapy, as antiviral agents such as interferon-α can further reduce platelet count; and
• Results from a recent phase 2 study using eltrombopag in HCV-associated thrombocytopenia suggest that TPO-R agonists may provide sufficient increase in platelet count to permit initiation of antiviral therapy in this condition [3].

Microangiopathies

Nonimmune destructive thrombocytopenias include DIC, Kasabach–Merritt syndrome, TTP, HUS, and other conditions listed in Table 10.1. These disorders share the common pathophysiological endpoint of platelet trapping and thrombus formation in the microvasculature, with subsequent fragmentation of red cells due to direct mechanical damage. They are discussed in greater detail in Chapter 12 and Chapter 26.

Disseminated intravascular coagulation

The diagnosis of DIC is usually made in association with an overt underlying systemic disorder [22]. The most common causes in adults and older children are sepsis, acute trauma (especially involving brain), snake envenomation, and malignancy. Obstetrical causes include placental abruption, fetal demise, amniotic fluid embolism, and preeclampsia. Some neonatal causes of DIC include infection, birth asphyxia, abruptio placentae, major vessel thrombosis, necrotizing enterocolitis, brain injury, and purpura fulminans (protein C, protein S deficiency). The pathophysiology of DIC is characterized by the consumption of platelets and coagulation factors within the microvasculature. Laboratory indicators of DIC, as well as therapeutic approaches, are discussed in further detail in Chapter 12.

Kasabach–Merritt syndrome

Kasabach–Merritt syndrome (Fig. 10.3) describes the combination of thrombocytopenia, noted most commonly in a newborn infant, with a hemangioma of infancy of the histopathologic subtype kaposiform hemangioendothelioma or tufted hemangioma. Although poorly understood, the pathogenesis is thought to be caused by platelet trapping and activation within the abnormal endothelium of the heman-

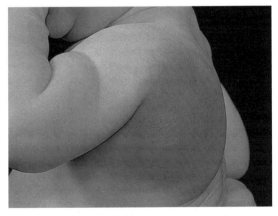

Figure 10.3 Kasabach–Merrit syndrome. Reprinted from *Blood in Systemic Disease* 1e, Greaves and Makris, 1997, with permission from Elsevier.

gioma, resulting in thrombocytopenia and laboratory evidence of DIC, including hypofibrinogenemia and increased D-dimers. It is important to highlight that the hemangioma may not be clinically obvious, and investigation of any newborn with microangiopathic hemolysis should include appropriate imaging studies, such as cranial and abdominal ultrasound, to exclude the presence of a concealed vascular lesion. Kasabach–Merritt hemangiomas tend to grow rapidly for several months followed by spontaneous regression in the first few years of life. However, individualized treatment using vascular ligation,embolization, corticosteroids, α-interferon (IFN-α), or vincristine may be required in some cases of life-threatening thrombocytopenia and coagulopathy.

TTP and HUS

These conditions are described in greater detail in Chapter 12. Briefly, however, TTP is a heterogeneous syndrome characterized by platelet aggregation in the microcirculation. Patients classically manifest with thrombocytopenia, microangiopathic hemolytic anemia, fever, renal dysfunction, and neurologic deficits; however, frequently, not all features are present at diagnosis. It is now recognized that the majority of cases result from inherited or acquired deficiency of ADAMTS13, a plasma protease important in cleaving ultra-large VWF multimers capable of causing enhanced platelet aggregation [23]. Management of TTP requires replacement of ADAMTS13 in inherited forms and plasma exchange in acquired forms.

HUS is more frequently seen in infants and young children, occurring in approximately 1 in 100,000 annually, but may be seen in patients at any age. HUS most often follows an acute diarrheal illness resulting from enterohemorrhagic *Escherichia coli* O157:H7, or *Shigella*, *Salmonella*, or *Campylobacter jejuni*. Diarrhea-associated HUS accounts for more than 90% of cases, whereas 50% of the diarrhea-negative HUS is caused by dysregulation of the complement system. Mutations have been identified in complement factor H, membrane cofactor protein, factor I, and factor B, and autoantibodies have been demonstrated against complement factor H [23]. HUS is frequently accompanied by renal failure and may be the leading cause of acute renal failure in infants and young children. The clinical presentation is sometimes difficult to distinguish from TTP, and some experts classify TTP and HUS as one disease entity, TTP/HUS. However children with HUS resulting from *E. coli* O157:H7 infection, as well as HUS caused by defects in the complement system, tend to have normal plasma levels of ADAMTS13, suggesting distinct microangiopathic mechanisms. Most importantly, the treatment of diarrhoea-associated HUS in children is distinct from adults in that supportive care is the mainstay in children. In addition, once identified, complement-deficient children can be treated with plasma transfusions. Transfusion may also be required for symptomatic anemia as well as dialysis when necessary. Antimotility agents may worsen the clinical manifestations of infectious HUS, whereas the role of antibiotics is unresolved. Because of the potentially high morbidity and mortality in TTP/HUS and the often difficult clinical distinction between TTP and HUS, children with atypical HUS, familial HUS, and all adults with HUS should be treated with plasma exchange.

Hypersplenism

When splenomegaly results in cytopenias and compensatory bone marrow hyperplasia, the term "hypersplenism" is appropriate, although bone marrow biopsy in this context is most often performed to exclude hematologic malignancy (e.g. leukemia, lymphoma, myeloproliferative disease) rather than to confirm hypersplenism per se. Numerous conditions are associated with splenomegaly and hypersplenism, including portal hypertension secondary to liver disease or portal vein thrombosis, hematological malignancies, chronic hemolytic anemias, storage disorders, leishmaniasis, and malaria. The clinical picture is usually dominated by the underlying disease rather than symptomatic pancytopenia, although in the presence of massive splenomegaly, thrombocytopenia can be severe, and increments following platelet transfusion are poor. Intervention is rarely indicated for management of thrombocytopenia alone, although improvement in counts usually follows splenectomy or splenic embolization. In the setting of portal hypertension, surgical procedures that redirect or bypass the portal circulation can reduce the risk of bleeding associated with thrombocytopenia and esophageal varices.

Thrombocytopenia in the newborn infant

Thrombocytopenia is the most common hematological abnormality observed during the noenatal period,

with an estimated incidence of 1–2% in healthy term infants. However only 1 in 10 of these cases will have a platelet count below 50×10^9/L. In contrast, thrombocytopenia affects up to 30% of infants admitted to NICU, and 1 in 5 of these will be severe. The differential diagnosis is broad. However, relatively few conditions account for the majority of cases, and many of the rare disorders can be readily identified on the basis of associated clinical and/or laboratory features [24]. A useful approach in determining the etiology of thrombocytopenia in a newborn is to differentiate based on the timing of onset and clinical condition of the infant (Table 10.4). Early-onset thrombocytopenia (<72 hours of age) is most often mild to moderate in severity, and frequently relates to placental insufficiency (e.g. preeclampsia, IUGR). In the absence of an identifiable precipitant, NAIT should always be considered when early-onset thrombocytopenia is detected in a well neonate (see below). Severe early-onset thrombocytopenia (<50×10^9/L) in a sick newborn commonly results from perinatal infection (e.g. group B *Streptococcus*) or asphyxia (e.g. meconium aspiration syndrome). Late-onset thrombocytopenia (>72 hours of age) is most often due to bacterial or fungal sepsis and/or necrotizing enterocolitis and is frequently severe in this setting.

Most thrombocytopenia in the neonatal period is self-limited or resolves with treatment of the underlying condition. Treatment of severe nonimmune-mediated thrombocytopenia in neonates consists of platelet transfusion according to transfusion threshold guidelines reviewed by Roberts and colleagues [24].

Neonatal alloimmune thrombocytopenia

NAIT is the most likely cause of thrombocytopenia in the well-appearing full-term infant. The overall incidence of NAIT is estimated to be 1 in 1000–2000 live births, although severe NAIT is somewhat less frequent (around 1 in 5000 births). NAIT also occurs in preterm infants, although the diagnosis may frequently be overshadowed by other contributing factors often present in this group. The importance of recognition and accurate diagnosis lies not only in the immediate management of the affected infant, but also in the approach to future pregnancies of the affected mother.

In NAIT, the destruction of fetal or neonatal platelets results from transplacental passage of

Table 10.4 Causes of thrombocytopenia in newborns.

Early onset, well infant
Placental insufficiency (e.g. preeclampsia, IUGR)*
Alloimmune (NAIT)*
Autoimmune (e.g. maternal ITP, SLE)
Artefactual (clumping ex vivo)
Renal vein thrombosis
Hereditary thrombocytopenia (see Table 10.2)

Early onset, sick infant
Perinatal asphyxia*
Perinatal infection (maternal flora, e.g. GBS, *E.coli*)*
DIC (± evidence of infection or asphyxia)*
Exchange/massive transfusion
Congenital infection (e.g. rubella, CMV, toxoplasmosis)
Severe Rh(D) hemolytic disease
Nonimmune hydrops fetalis
Kasabach–Merritt syndrome
Inborn errors of metabolism (e.g. organic acidurias)
Congenital leukemia
Osteopetrosis (severe form)

Early onset, associated congenital anomalies
Aneuploidy (trisomy 21, 13, 18; Turner syndrome)
Hereditary thrombocytopenia (see Table 10.2)
Bone marrow failure syndromes (e.g. Fanconi anemia)
Congenital infection (e.g. rubella)

Late onset, well infant
Late detection of an early onset condition*
Drug-induced (antimicrobials, heparin)
Infection (pre-sepsis)

Late onset, sick infant
Infection (skin/gut flora, e.g. *Pseudomonas sp., Candida sp.*)*
Necrotizing enterocolilitis*
Extensive thrombosis
Exchange/massive transfusion
Familial TTP

Early onset, <72 hours of age or present at birth; late onset, >72 hours of age; IUGR, intrauterine growth restriction; GBS, group B *Streptococcus*.
*Most common.

maternal platelet-specific alloantibodies. This is similar to the pathogenesis of Rh(D) hemolytic disease; however, in contrast to this condition, NAIT frequently affects the first pregnancy. In contrast to neonatal ITP, where the platelet count is low in both the mother and the neonate or fetus, NAIT is not associated with maternal thrombocytopenia, making it a useful labo-ratory distinction. The most frequent platelet antigen polymorphism in caucasian populations causing NAIT is the HPA-1a epitope (also known as PL^A1 or Zw^a), where the platelet GPIIIa contains a leucine at position 33. Alloantibodies (anti-HPA-1a) can form if the mother is homozygous for HPA-1b (PL^A2 or Zw^b; proline at position 33 of GPIIIa) with a significantly increased risk of developing NAIT if the mother also has HLA class-II DRB3*0101. Alloimmunization to HPA-5b (Br^a; lysine at position 505 of the α2 chain of the α2β1 or GPIa/IIa collagen receptor) may also be relatively common, although the severity is usually milder. HPA-4a alloantibodies (Pen^a; arginine at position 143 of GPIIIa) are the most common cause of severe NAIT in Asian populations.

Because ICH frequently occurs antenatally, and as NAIT can present during the first pregnancy, it is often difficult to alter the clinical course of these patients. However, a history of a previously affected infant can be predictive for NAIT in a subsequent fetus, with the potential of antenatal intervention. With few exceptions, untreated at-risk fetuses (antigen-positive) have more severe disease than their previously affected siblings. Antenatal intervention can effectively ameliorate the disease course, although the ideal approach to management remains unresolved. Such intervention may involve either weekly infusions of IVIG with or without corticosteroids given to the mother or repeated in utero fetal platelet transfusions. The risk of fetal blood sampling must be balanced against the risk of exsanguinating hemorrhage after cordocentesis.

A definitive diagnosis of NAIT requires the demonstration of fetomaternal incompatibility for a platelet antigen and presence in the maternal serum of a platelet antibody reactive with platelets from the infant and/or biologic father, but non-reactive with maternal platelets. However, these serologic tests may not be readily available, and neonates with suspected NAIT and severe thrombocytopenia should be managed as emergency cases. The treatment of choice is antigen-negative platelets harvested from the mother (washed and irradiated) or a donor known to be compatible through prior HPA-typing. If such a product is not available, random donor (unmatched) platelets may be used. Recent studies have demonstrated efficacy with this approach, and it may not be appropriate to delay transfusion in a severely thrombocytopenic neonate while waiting for serological confirmation and/or antigen-matched units. If the platelet increment following transfusion is subopti-mal, a trial of high-dose IVIG (1 g/kg for 2 days) is warranted. In extreme situations, plasma exchange should be considered, although in practice this is rarely necessary. Corticosteriods are not beneficial in this clinical setting, in contrast to neonatal autoimmune thrombocytopenia (secondary to maternal ITP), where first-line therapy for severely thrombocytopenic ba-bies consists of high-dose IVIG with or without added corticosteriods.

Inherited thrombocytopenia

Although inherited thrombocytopenias are rare, re-cent progress has been made in determining the molecular defects, thus improving our understand-ing of normal megakaryopoesis and platelet function, as well as providing new diagnostic avenues. Several conditions are highlighted in this chapter (see also Table 10.2); however, a detailed overview of inher-ited thrombocytopenia is beyond the scope of this text, and the reader is referred to some recent reviews for additional information [25–27]. Treatment modal-ities depend on the severity of the bleeding diathe-sis, and include desmopressin (DDAVP), tranexamic acid, platelet transfusion, and, during life-threatening bleeding episodes, recombinant factor VIIa.

Congenital thrombocytopenia with megakaryocytic hypoplasia

These disorders typically present in the newborn pe-riod with isolated severe thrombocytopenia, often in association with significant bleeding. Examination of the bone marrow demonstrates marked reduc-tion or complete absence of megakaryocytes. Con-genital amegakaryocytic thrombocytopenia (CAMT) is an autosomal recessive disorder due to muta-tions in the *c-mpl* gene (TPO-R), and ultimately pro-gresses to complete bone marrow failure in later life. Thrombocytopenia-absent radius syndrome (TAR) is the combination of bilateral radial aplasia with con-genital thrombocytopenia, frequently associated with other skeletal or cardiac defects. The inheritance is variable, and the condition is often sporadic; how-ever, a microdeletion in the region of chromosome 1q21 appears to be contributory. The thrombocytope-nia improves with age, and TAR should be differen-tiated from Fanconi anemia, in which the thumbs

are hypoplastic, and thrombocytopenia with radio-ulnar synostosis, in which the bones of the forearm are fused. Multiple congenital anomalies in associa-tion with thrombocytopenia should also raise suspi-cion of aneuploidy (particularly trisomy 13, 18, or 21) and congenital infection (e.g. CMV or rubella).

Autosomal dominant macrothrombocytopenia

Several disorders are characterized by autosomal dom-inant inheritance of large platelets in association with mild to moderate thrombocytopenia and a variable de-gree of platelet dysfunction. The molecular basis has been determined for many of these, and abnormali-ties in the MYH9 gene (encoding a non-muscle myosin heavy chain IIA) comprise the majority. MHY9-related disease incorporates several overlapping syndromes that were previously separated on the basis of pres-ence or absence of Döhle-like inclusions in neu-trophils (May-Grünwald-Giemsa stained blood films, Figure 10.2 & Plate 10.1, top) and non-hematological abnormalities. The recognition that these inclusions consist of misfolded (aggregated) non-muscle myosin heavy chain IIA has allowed sensitive immunofloures-cent visualization of aggregates in blood films, sup-porting the diagnosis (Figure 10.2 & Plate 10.1, bot-tom). Significant bleeding is rare in MYH9-related thrombocytopenia; however, long-term follow-up of these patients is important, as a significant propor-tion may develop sensorineural hearing loss, nephri-tis, and/or cataracts in later childhood or early adult life. Bernard Soulier syndrome (BSS) is an autoso-mal recessive disorder in which giant platelets are found in association with moderate thrombocytope-nia and severe platelet dysfunction. This condition is discussed in Chapter 11. However, it should be high-lighted that heterozygous carriers of BSS mutations may have macrothrombocytopenia, and this accounts for many of the cases previously included under the term "benign Mediterranean macrothrombocytope-nia." Similarly, macrothrombocytopenia observed in some patients with DiGeorge syndrome results from a hemizygous 22q11 microdeletion that incorporates one of the BSS genes. Autosomal dominant thrombo-cytopenia is also observed in type 2B and "platelet-type" VWD, discussed further in Chapter 8 and Chap-ter 11, respectively.

Sex-linked thrombocytopenia

Familial thrombocytopenia affecting only the male members of a pedigree should raise suspicion of an X-linked disorder. Despite presentation with thrombocytopenia in early infancy and failure to respond to standard therapy, these boys are frequently misdiagnosed with ITP, highlighting the importance of a thorough family history. Wiskott-Aldrich syndrome (WAS) is characterized by small platelets, eczema, and a variable degree of immune deficiency depending on the nature of the underlying gene defect. Isolated microthrombocytopenia due to point mutations in the WAS gene has previously been referred to as "X-linked thrombocytopenia" (XLT). Interestingly, the thrombocytopenia may improve following splenectomy in WAS/XLT, although the only curative option for the immune deficiency is hemopoietic stem cell transplantation. Mutations in the GATA-1 gene underlie a number of primary hematologic disorders, including XLT with dyserythropoiesis. However, the platelets in this disorder are large, thereby differentiating it from WAS/XLT.

Thrombocytosis

Thrombocytosis is defined as a platelet count of greater than 400×10^9/L. Reactive thrombocytosis (RT; secondary thrombocytosis) is much more frequent (90% of cases) than primary thrombocytosis (PT) in both children and adults [28]. A variety of clinical conditions can lead to RT, including:

- infection,
- malignancy,
- blood loss,
- inflammation,
- rebound thrombocytosis,
- tissue damage, and
- splenectomy.

PT may be a result of rare cases of familial thrombocytosis caused by an autosomal dominant gain-of-function mutation in the TPO gene, resulting in overproduction of TPO. More commonly, PT is caused by clonal proliferation of megakaryocyte precursors seen in essential thrombocythemia, polycythemia vera, chronic myelogenous leukemia, myelofibrosis, and myelodysplastic syndrome (observed least frequently). The evaluation and treatment approach to myeloproliferative disorders, as well as their differentiation from reactive disorders, are discussed in detail in Chapter 14.

Acknowledgment

Jeremy Robertson was the 2007/2008 recipient of the Baxter BioScience Fellowship in Hemostasis at The Hospital for Sick Children, Toronto, Canada.

References

1 Slichter SJ. Relationship between platelet count and bleeding risk in thrombocytopenic patients. *Trans Med Rev* 2004;18(3):153–67.

2 Kaushansky K. Thrombopoietin: the primary regulator of platelet production. *Blood* 1995;86:419–31.

3 Kuter DJ. New thrombopoietic growth factors. *Blood* 2007;109:4607–16.

4 Junt T, Schulze H, Chen Z, et al. Dynamic visualization of thrombopoiesis within bone marrow. *Science* 2007;317:1767–70.

5 Chong BH, Ho S-J. Autoimmune thrombocytopenia. *J Thromb Haemost* 2005;3:1763–72.

6 Balduini CL, Cattaneo M, Fabris F, et al. Inherited thrombocytopenias: a proposed diagnostic algorithm from the Italian Gruppo di Studio delle Piastrine. *Haematologica* 2003;88:582–92.

7 Drachman JG. Inherited thrombocytopenia: when a low platelet count does not mean ITP. *Blood* 2004;103:390–8.

8 George JN, Raskob GE, Shah SR, et al. Drug-induced thrombocytopenia: a systematic review of published case reports. *Ann Intern Med* 1998;129:886–90.

9 Aster RH, Bougie DW. Drug-induced immune thrombocytopenia. *N Engl J Med* 2007;357:580–7.

10 Salvagno GL, Montagnana M, Degan M, et al. Evaluation of platelet turnover by flow cytometry. *Platelets* 2006;17(3):170–7.

11 Gernsheimer T. Epidemiology and pathophysiology of immune thrombocytopenic purpura. *Eur J Haematol* 2008;80(Suppl 69):3–8.

12 Cines DB, Blanchette VS. Immune thrombocytopenic purpura. *N Engl J Med* 2002;346:995–1008.

13 Garvey B. Rituximab in the treatment of autoimmune haematological disorders. *Br J Haematol* 2008;141:149–69.

14 Norton A, Roberts I. Management of Evans syndrome. *Br J Haematol* 2005;132:125–37.

15 Dlott JS, Danielson CFM, Blue-Hnidy, et al. Drug-induced thrombotic thrombocytopenic purpura/hemolytic uremic syndrome: a concise review. *Ther Apher Dial* 2004;8(2):102–11.

16 Chong BH. Heparin-induced thrombocytopenia. *J Thromb Haemost* 2003;1:1471–8.

17 McCrae KR. Thrombocytopenia in pregnancy: differential diagnosis, pathogenesis, and management. *Blood Rev* 2003;17:7–14.

18 Gernsheimer T, McCrae KR. Immune thrombocytopenic purpura in pregnancy. *Curr Opin Hematol* 2007;14:574–80.

19 Williamson LM, Stainsby D, Jones H, et al. The impact of universal leukodepletion of the blood supply on hemovigilance reports of posttransfusion purpura and transfusion-associated graft-versus-host disease. *Transfusion* 2007;47:1455–67.

20 Liebman HA, Stasi R. Secondary immune thrombocytopenic purpura. *Curr Opin Hematol* 2007;14:557–73.

21 Weksler BB. The pathophysiology of thrombocytopenia in hepatitis C virus infection and chronic liver disease. *Aliment Pharmacol Ther* 2007;26(Suppl 1):13–19.

22 Levi M. Disseminated intravascular coagulation. *Crit Care Med* 2007;35:2191–5.

23 Zheng XL, Sadler JE. Pathogenesis of thrombotic microangiopathies. *Annu Rev Pathol* 2008;3:249–57.

24 Roberts I, Stanworth S, Murray NA. Thrombocytopenia in the neonate. *Blood Rev* 2008;22:173–86.

25 Geddis AE, Kaushansky K. Inherited thrombocytopenias: toward a molecular understanding of disorders of platelet production. *Curr Opin Pediatr* 2004;16:15–22.

26 Nurden AT, Nurden P. Inherited disorders of platelets: an update. *Curr Opin Hematol* 2006;13:157–62.

27 Nurden P, Nurden AT. Congenital disorders associated with platelet dysfunctions. *Thromb Haemost* 2008;99:253–63.

28 Vannucchi AM, Barbui T. Thrombocytosis and thrombosis. *Hematology (Am Soc Hematol Educ Program)* 2007;363–70.

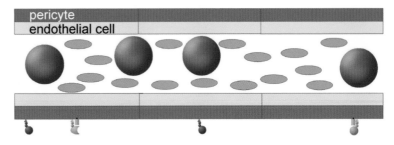

Plate 1.1 *Intact vessel.* An intact blood vessel is pictured with the endothelial cells (tan) and surrounding pericytes (dark brown). Within the vessel are red blood cells and platelets (blue). Associated with the pericytes, tissue factor complexed with factor VII(a) is shown in green. Factor IX, shown in blue, is associated with collagen IV in the extravascular space.

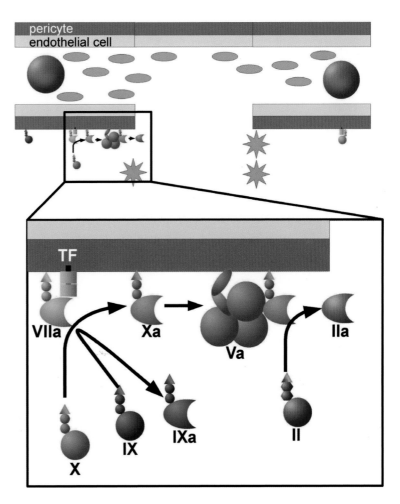

Plate 1.2 *Initiation.* A break in the vasculature brings plasma coagulation factors and platelets into contact with the extravascular space. Unactivated platelets within the vessel are shown as blue disks. Platelets adhering to collagen in the extravascular space are activated and are represented as blue star shapes to indicate cytoskeletal-induced shape change. The expanded view shows the protein reactions in the initiation phase. Factor VIIa/tissue factor activates both factor IX and factor X. Factor Xa, in complex with factor Va released from platelets, can activate a small amount of thrombin (IIa).

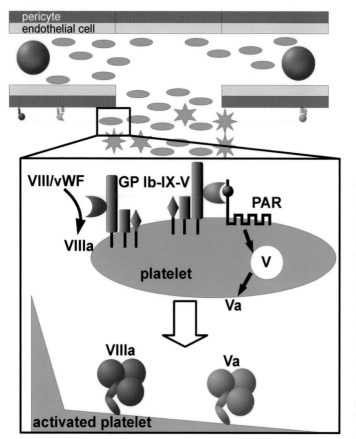

Plate 1.3 *Amplification.* Platelets, shown as blue discs, aggregate to stop blood loss from the break in the vasculature. Activated platelets are shown as star shapes. The expanded view shows thrombin (red) generated during the initiation phase binding to the glycoprotein Ib-IX-V complex (GP Ib-IX-V) on platelets. When bound, thrombin is somewhat protected from inhibition and can cleave protease activated receptor (PAR) 1 at the recognition site (black sphere). When the new amino-terminal folds back on the seven transmembrane domain, a signaling cascade is initiated leading to surface exposure of phosphatidylserine as well as degranulation of alpha (white circle) or dense (not shown) granules. Factor Va is released from alpha granules and further activated by thrombin. Also, factor VIII is activated by cleavage and release from von Willebrand factor (vWF).

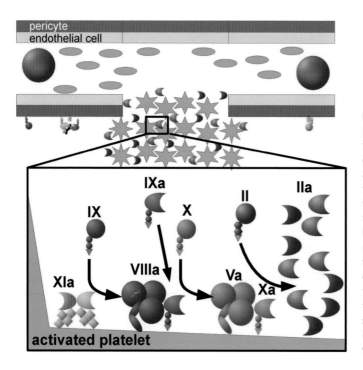

Plate 1.4 *Propagation.* The expanded view shows platelet surface thrombin generation. Factor IXa, formed during the initiation phase, can move into a complex with factor VIIIa formed during the amplification phase. This IXa/VIIIa complex cleaves factor X. Factor Xa, in complex with platelet surface factor Va, generates a burst of thrombin (IIa). This thrombin can feedback and activate platelet surface bound factor XI, the resulting factor XIa can feed more factor IXa into the reaction. This additional factor IXa enhances factor Xa and thrombin generation. As shown in the overview, the burst of thrombin stabilizes the initial platelet plug as all of the platelets are now activated (represented as blue star shapes as opposed to the disc shaped platelets in circulation). The factor VIIa/tissue factor complex with associated factor Xa is inhibited by TFPI.

Plate 1.5 *Localization.* Thrombin generated during the propagation phase cleaves fibrinopeptides A and B leading to fibrin assembly (shown as brown distributed among and associated with the blue star shapes that represent activated platelets). The result is a stable platelet plug with fibrin and bound thrombin distributed throughout the plug. The expanded view shows the interface between the platelet plug (blue) and healthy endothelium. Thrombin released into the circulation is inhibited by antithrombin (AT) to form a thrombin-antithrombin complex (TAT). Also, thrombin (IIa) that reaches the endothelial cell surface binds tightly to thrombomodulin (TM). The thrombin-thrombomodulin complex actives protein C (PC) in a reaction enhanced by the endothelial cell protein C receptor (EPCR). Activated protein C (APC) in a reaction enhanced by protein S (PS) can cleave factor Va to inactivated factor Va (iVa). So thrombin on healthy endothelium participates in a negative feedback process that prevents thrombin generation away from the platelet plug that seals an injury.

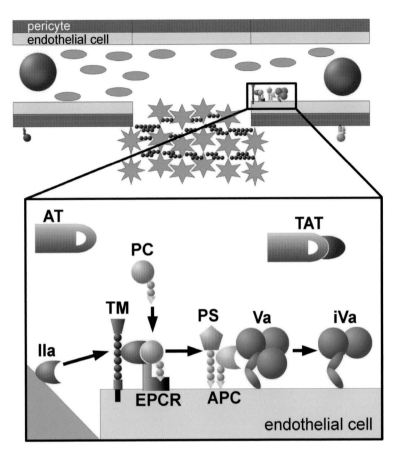

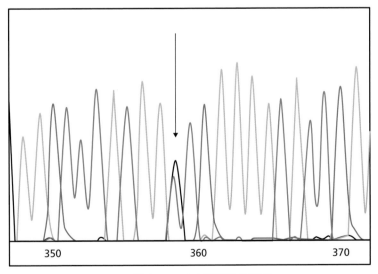

Plate 4.1 DNA sequence derived from a carrier of hemophilia A. The sequence shows a double peak (G + A) shown by the arrow in the sequencing chromatogram. This woman is heterozygous for a glutamine to premature stop codon mutation in exon 9 of the factor VIII gene.

Heterozygous FVIII Sequence

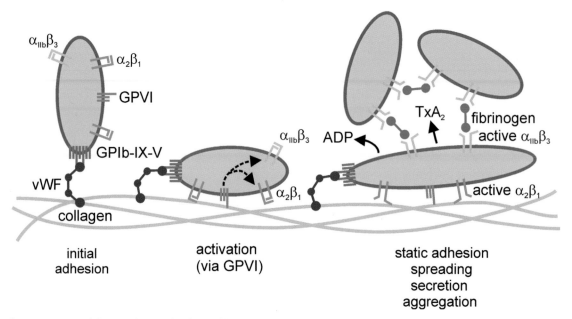

initial
adhesion

activation
(via GPVI)

static adhesion
spreading
secretion
aggregation

Plate 5.1 A general diagram showing the phases of hemostatic plug/thrombus formation at medium and high rates of shear. Platelets are initially captured (tethered) by von Willebrand factor (VWF) bound to immobilized collagen. Collagen activates platelets via Gp VI leading to an increase in affinity of the integrins $\alpha_{IIb}\beta_3$ and $\alpha_2\beta_1$ for VWF/fibrinogen and collagen, respectively. This activated state mediates stable platelet adhesion and potentiates activation through further activation of Gp VI and also release of ADP and TxA_2. The formation of a procoagulant surface also supports formation of thrombin. VWF and fibrinogen, in combination with ADP, TxA_2 and thrombin, mediate thrombus formation (aggregation), spreading and stabilization (clot retraction).

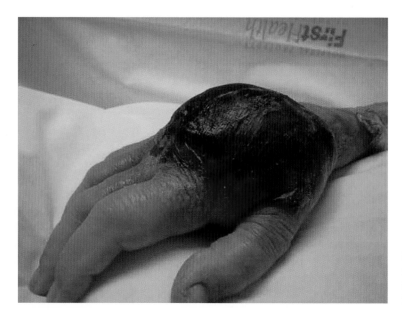

Plate 7.1 Iatrogenic hematoma from a needle stick on the dorsum of the hand of a patient with acquired hemophilia A. (Courtesy of Dr Stephan Moll).

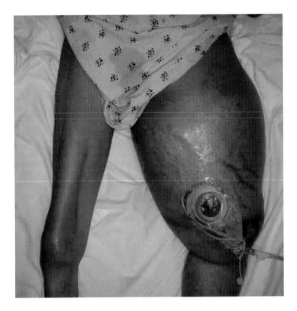

Plate 7.2 Large pseudotumor involving the entire left thigh in a patient with congenital hemophilia A and a high titer inhibitor to factor VIII. Note the draining fistula. The patient eventually underwent surgical limb disarticulation following induction of immune tolerance. (Courtesy of Dr Stephan Moll).

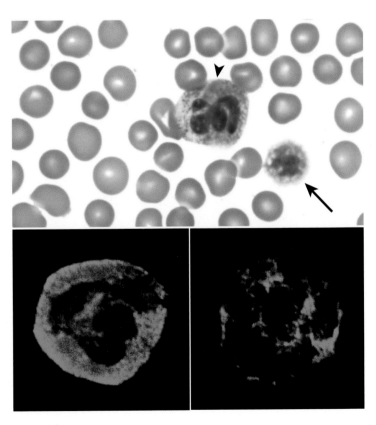

Plate 10.1 May-Grünwald-Giemsa stained blood film (top) demonstrating giant platelet (arrow) and neutrophil inclusion (arrowhead). Immunofluorescent visualization of non-muscle myosin heavy chain IIA aggregates (bottom): normal homogenous cytoplasmic staining (lower left), abnormal variable speckled cytoplasmic staining (lower right).

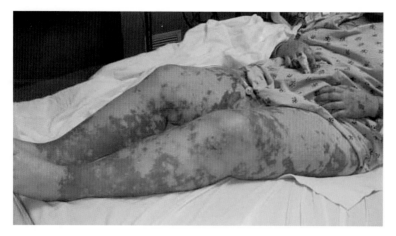

Plate 12.1 Purpura fulminans in a patient with meningococcemia. Purpura fulminans is associated with underlying DIC and is characterized by widespread ecchymosis and ischemic infarction of the skin. (Courtesy of Dr Stephan Moll).

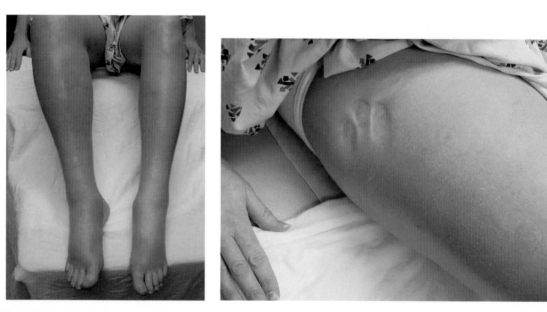

Plate 13.1 Acute right lower extremity deep vein thrombosis. Note the swelling, erythema, and pitting edema. (Courtesy of Dr Stephan Moll).

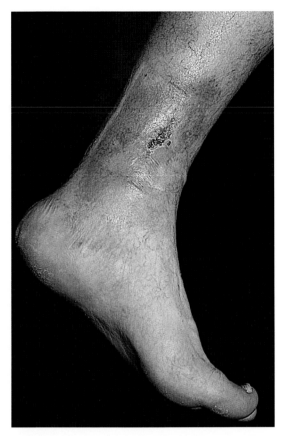

Plate 13.2 Post-thrombotic syndrome. Although usually the symptoms are confined to itching, mild swelling and pain, when severe there is pigmentation and ulceration over the medial malleolus. Reprinted from Blood in Systemic Disease 1e, Greaves and Makris, 1997, with permission from Elsevier.

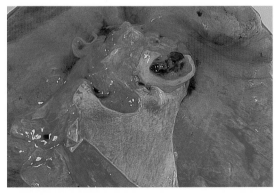

Plate 13.3 Pulmonary embolus in the pulmonary artery causing sudden death in a young woman who was using the combined contraceptive pill. Reprinted from Blood in Systemic Disease 1e, Greaves and Makris, 1997, with permission from Elsevier.

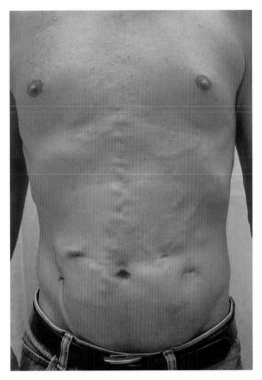

Plate 13.4 Prominent superficial venous collaterals in a patient with inferior vena caval (IVC) thrombotic occlusion, occurring as a late complication of an IVC filter. (Courtesy of Dr Stephan Moll).

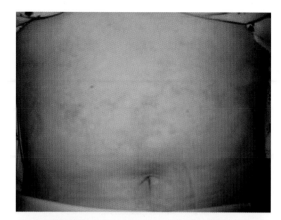

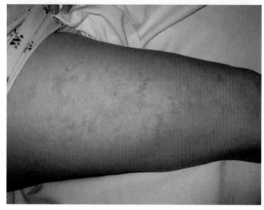

Plate 17.1 Livedo reticularis in a patient with catastrophic anti-phospholipid syndrome. This lacy reticular purplish rash is a manifestation of venular occlusion in the skin. Livedo reticularis may occur as an isolated benign idiopathic condition, or as a secondary condition in a variety of conditions including anti-phospholipid syndrome (as a manifestation of small vessel thrombosis). (Courtesy of Dr Stephan Moll).

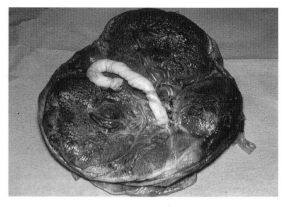

Plate 17.2 Unusually massive, macroscopic, late pregnancy placental infarction in primary antiphospholipid syndrome. Reprinted from Blood in Systemic Disease 1e, Greaves and Makris, 1997, with permission from Elsevier.

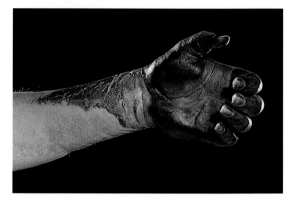

Plate 23.1 Arterial thrombosis in a patient with malignancy. Reprinted from Blood in Systemic Disease 1e, Greaves and Makris, 1997, with permission from Elsevier.

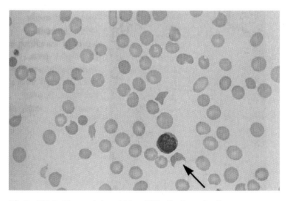

Plate 26.1 The peripheral blood film in thrombotic thrombocytopenic purpura (TTP) showing schistocytes (arrowed) and thrombocytopenia. Reprinted from Blood in Systemic Disease 1e, Greaves and Makris, 1997, with permission from Elsevier.

11 Qualitative platelet disorders

Marco Cattaneo

Introduction

Abnormalities of platelet function are associated with a heightened risk for bleeding, proving that platelets have an important role in hemostasis. Typically, patients with platelet disorders have mucocutaneous bleeding of variable severity and excessive hemorrhage after surgery or trauma.

In this chapter, the main inherited and acquired qualitative platelet defects are reviewed. Abnormalities of platelet function resulting from defects of plasma proteins (e.g. von Willebrand disease, afibrinogenemia) will not be considered here, as they are discussed in Chapters 8 and 9.

Inherited qualitative platelet defects

Inherited disorders of platelet function are generally classified according to the functions or responses that are abnormal. However, because platelet functions are intimately related, a clear distinction between disorders of platelet adhesion, aggregation, activation, secretion, and procoagulant activity is, in many instances, problematic. For this reason, a classification of the inherited disorders of platelet function is proposed based on abnormalities of platelet components that share common characteristics (Table 11.1):

- platelet receptors for adhesive proteins;
- platelet receptors for soluble agonists;
- platelet granules;
- signal-transduction pathways;
- procoagulant phospholipids; and
- miscellaneous disorders (less well characterized).

Abnormalities of the platelet receptors for adhesive proteins

Gp Ib/V/IX complex (VWF binding site)

The Bernard–Soulier syndrome (BSS) is characterized by:

- autosomal recessive inheritance (with one exception of autosomal dominant inheritance);
- prolonged bleeding time;
- thrombocytopenia;
- giant platelets (often not detected on automatic counters);
- decreased platelet survival; and
- lack of platelet agglutination with ristocetin.

The lack of ristocetin-induced agglutination is not corrected by the addition of normal plasma. The platelet responses to physiologic agonists are normal, with the exception of low concentrations of thrombin, because Gp Ibα (one of the two components of Gp Ib) has a critical role in the platelet aggregatory, secretory, and procoagulant responses to thrombin.

Bleeding events, which may be very severe in homozygous BSS, can be controlled by platelet transfusion. Most heterozygotes do not have a bleeding diathesis but are the most common cause of macrothrombocytopenia in some parts of the world [1].

BSS is caused by defects in the genes for Gp Ibα, Ibβ, or IX, but not Gp V. The molecular defects that are responsible for BSS (frameshifts, deletions, point mutations) are summarized at the following Web site: http://www.bernard-soulier.org/mutations.

Platelet-type, or pseudo, von Willebrand disease (VWD) is not caused by defects of VWF, but by a gain-of-function phenotype of the platelet Gp Ibα [2].

Table 11.1 Inherited platelet defects.

Abnormalities of the platelet receptors for adhesive proteins:
Gp Ib/V/IX complex (BSS, platelet-type VWD, Bolin–Jamieson syndrome)
Gp IIb/IIIa (α_{IIb}/β_3) (GT)
Gp Ia/IIa (α_2/β_1)
Gp VI
Gp IV

Abnormalities of the platelet receptors for soluble agonists:
Thromboxane A_2 receptor
α_2-Adrenergic receptor
$P2Y_{12}$ receptor

Abnormalities of the platelet granules:
δ-Granules (δ-SPD, HPS, CHS, TAR syndrome, Wiskott–Aldrich syndrome)
α-Granules (gray platelet syndrome, Quebec platelet disorder, Paris–Trousseau syndrome, Jacobsen syndrome)
α- and δ-Granules (α,δ-SPD)

Abnormalities of the signal-transduction pathways:
Abnormalities of the arachidonate–thromboxane A_2 pathway, Gaq deficiency, partial selective PLC-β_2 isoenzyme deficiency, defects
  in pleckstrin phosphorylation, defective Ca^{2+} mobilization, hyper-responsiveness of platelet Gsa

Abnormalities of membrane phospholipids:
Scott syndrome
Stormorken syndrome

Miscellaneous abnormalities of platelet function:
Primary secretion defects
Other platelet abnormalities (Montreal platelet syndrome, osteogenesis imperfecta, Ehlers–Danlos syndrome, Marfan syndrome,
  hexokinase deficiency, glucose-6-phosphate deficiency)

This abnormal receptor has an increased avidity for VWF, leading to the binding of the largest VWF multimers to resting platelets and their clearance from the circulation. Because the high-molecular-weight VWF multimers are the most hemostatically active, their loss is associated with an increased bleeding risk, as in type 2B VWD (which is caused by a gain-of-function abnormality of the VWF molecule; see Chapter 8). Platelet-type VWD is an autosomal dominant disease caused by gain-of-function missense mutations of Gp Ibα and associated with amino acid substitutions occurring within the disulfide-bonded double loop region of Gp Ibα (G233V, G233S, and M239V).

Bolin–Jamieson syndrome is a rare, autosomal-dominant, mild bleeding disorder associated with a larger form of Gp Ibα in one allele. It has been pro-posed that it is associated with a large multimer form of the size polymorphism occurring in the mucin-like domain.

Abnormalities of Gp IIb/IIIa (αIIb/β3)

Glanzmann thrombasthenia (GT) is an autosomal re-cessive disease caused by lack of expression or quali-tative defects of one of the two glycoproteins forming the integrin α_{IIb}/β_3 (in activated platelets, these ad-hesive glycoproteins bridge adjacent platelets, secur-ing platelet aggregation). The diagnostic hallmark is the lack, or severe impairment, of platelet aggregation induced by all agonists. Platelet clot retraction is defec-tive and GT platelets bind to the subendothelium but they fail to spread.

The disease is associated with bleeding manifesta-tions that are similar to those of patients with BSS, although of less severity [3]. GT patients are grouped into three types, according to the severity of α_{IIb}/β_3 deficiency on their platelet membranes:

- *Type I patients:* $\alpha 5\%$ (characterized by lack of fibrinogen in platelet α-granules);
- *Type II patients:* 10–20%; and
- *Type III (variant) patients:* 50–100%.

The GT defect is caused by mutations or deletions in the genes encoding one of the two glycoproteins forming the α_{IIb}/β_3 integrin. In GT caused by mutations in the α_3 integrin, the levels of the platelet vitronectin receptor (α_v/β_3) are also decreased, but the phenotype of these patients is no different from that of the other GT patients.

Abnormalities of Gp Ia/IIa ($\alpha 2/\beta 1$)

Two patients with mild bleeding disorders associated with deficient expression of the platelet receptor for collagen Gp Ia/IIa (α_2/β_1) and selective impairment of platelet responses to collagen have been described [4]. Their platelet defect spontaneously recovered after the menopause, suggesting that α_2/β_1 expression is under hormonal control.

Abnormalities of Gp VI

A selective defect of collagen-induced platelet aggregation was also described in another mild bleeding disorder, characterized by the deficiency of the platelet Gp VI, a member of the immunoglobulin superfamily of receptors, which mediates platelet activation by collagen. The molecular defects that are responsible for the platelet abnormality have not been characterized in the patients described so far [5]. The possibility should be explored that the molecular abnormality lies in the gene encoding for the Fcα receptor, which is the signaling subunit of Gp VI.

Abnormalities of Gp IV

Gp IV binds collagen, thrombospondin and probably other proteins. Its physiological role is unclear, because its deficiency, common in healthy individuals from Japan and other East Asian populations, is not associated with an abnormal phenotype.

Abnormalities of the platelet receptors for soluble agonists

Thromboxane A2 receptor

In 1993, a patient with a mild bleeding disorder was described whose platelets had a defective response to the TxA$_2$ analog U46619, albeit having a normal number of TxA$_2$ binding sites and normal equilibrium dissociation rate constants. Despite the normal number of TxA$_2$ receptors, the TxA$_2$-induced IP3 formation, Ca^2 mobilization and GTPase activity were abnormal, suggesting that the abnormality in these platelets was impaired coupling between the TxA$_2$ receptor, G protein, and PLC [6]. This patient was subsequently found to have an Arg 60 to Leu mutation in the first cytoplasmic loop of the TxA$_2$ receptor, affecting both isoforms of the receptor.

$\alpha 2$-Adrenergic receptors

Subjects with a selective impairment of platelet response to epinephrine, a decreased number of the platelet α_2-adrenergic receptors, and mildly prolonged bleeding times have been described. However, the relationship between this defect and bleeding manifestations still needs to be defined.

P2Y12 receptor for ADP

Human platelets express three distinct P2 receptors stimulated by adenosine nucleotides:

- P2X$_1$;
- P2Y$_1$ receptor for ADP with a role in the initiation of platelet activation; and
- P2Y$_{12}$ receptor for ADP essential for a sustained, full aggregation response to ADP.

The concurrent activation of both P2Y receptors is necessary for full platelet aggregation induced by ADP. P2Y$_{12}$ also mediates the potentiation of platelet secretion by ADP and the stabilization of thrombin-induced platelet aggregates.

Only patients with congenital defects of the platelet P2Y$_{12}$ receptors have been described. The first patient (V.R. described in 1992 by Cattaneo et al. [7]) had a life-long history of excessive bleeding, a prolonged bleeding time, and abnormalities of platelet aggregation similar to those observed in patients with defects of platelet secretion (reversible aggregation in response to weak agonists and impaired aggregation in response to low concentrations of collagen or thrombin), except that the aggregation response to ADP was severely impaired.

Other measures of platelet function found in this patient were:
• No inhibition by ADP of PGE_1-stimulated platelet adenylyl cyclase;
• Normal shape change and normal (or mildly reduced) mobilization of cytoplasmic ionized calcium induced by ADP; and
• Presence of approximately 30% of the normal number of platelet binding sites for $[^{33}P]2MeSADP$ or $[]^3H[]ADP$;

Three additional patients with very similar characteristics were later described. All of these patients displayed base pair deletions in the $P2Y_{12}$ gene, shifting the reading frame for several residues before introducing a premature stop codon, causing an early truncation of the protein.

A fifth patient (A.C.) with a congenital bleeding disorder associated with abnormal $P2Y_{12}$-mediated platelet responses to ADP has more recently been characterized. The platelet phenotype is very similar to that of patients with $P2Y_{12}$ deficiency, except that the number and affinity of $[]^{33}P[]$-2MeSADP binding sites was normal [8]. Analysis of the patient's $P2Y_{12}$ gene revealed, in one allele, a G-to-A transition changing the codon for Arg 256 in the sixth transmembrane domain to Gln, and, in the other allele, a C-to-T transition changing the codon for Arg 265 in the third extracellular loop to Trp. Neither mutation interfered with receptor surface expression, but both altered function, suggesting that the structural integrity of these regions corresponding to the extracytoplasmic end of TM 6 and EL 3 is necessary for the normal function of this G protein-coupled receptor.

The study of the children of patient M.G. and patient A.C. allowed the characterization of patients with a heterozygous $P2Y_{12}$ defect whose platelets do not secrete normal amounts of ATP after stimulation with different agonists. This secretion defect was not caused by impaired production of thromboxane A_2 or low concentrations of platelet granule contents, and is therefore very similar to that described in patients with an ill-defined group of congenital defects of platelet secretion, sometimes referred to by the general term "primary secretion defect" (PSD; see below), which

is the most common congenital disorder of platelet function.

$P2Y_{12}$ deficiency is probably much more common than currently recognized; it is therefore important to emphasize that this condition should be suspected when ADP, even at relatively high concentrations (10 μM or higher), induces a slight and rapidly reversible aggregation that is preceded by normal shape change. The confirmatory diagnostic test is based on the ability of ADP to inhibit the platelet adenylyl cyclase after its stimulation by prostaglandins or forskolin.

Abnormalities of the platelet granules

Abnormalities of the δ-granules (δ-storage pool deficiency)

The term δ-storage pool deficiency (δ-SPD) defines a congenital abnormality of platelets characterized by deficiency of dense granules in megakaryocytes and platelets [9]. It may present as an isolated platelet function defect or associate with a variety of congenital disorders. Between 10% and 18% of patients with congenital abnormalities of platelet function have SPD. The inheritance is autosomal recessive in some families but autosomal dominant in others.

δ-SPD is characterized by:
• a bleeding diathesis of variable degree;
• mildly to moderately prolonged skin bleeding time, inversely related to the amount of ADP or serotonin contained in the granules;
• abnormal platelet secretion induced by several platelet agonists;
• impaired platelet aggregation in 75% of cases (only 33% have aggregation tracings typical for a platelet secretion defect); and
• decreased levels of δ-granule constituents: ATP and ADP, serotonin, calcium, and pyrophosphate.

Lumiaggregometry, which measures platelet aggregation and secretion simultaneously, may prove a more accurate technique than platelet aggregometry for diagnosing patients with δ-SPD and, more generally, with platelet secretion defects.

Hermansky–Pudlak syndrome (HPS) and Chédiak–Higashi syndrome (CHS) are rare syndromic forms of δ-SPD. HPS is an autosomal recessive disease of subcellular organelles of many tissues involving abnormalities of melanosomes, platelet δ-granules, and lysosomes. It is characterized by tyrosinase-positive oculocutaneous albinism, a bleeding diathesis resulting from δ-SPD, and ceroid-lipofuscin lysosomal storage disease. HPS can arise from mutations in different genetic loci [9].

CHS is a lethal disorder (death usually in the first decade of life) with:
• autosomal recessive inheritance;
• variable degrees of oculocutaneous albinism;
• very large peroxidase-positive cytoplasmic granules in a variety of hematopoietic (neutrophils) and non-hematopoietic cells;
• easy bruisability as a result of δ-SPD;
• recurrent infections, associated with neutropenia, impaired chemotaxis, and bactericidal activity; and
• abnormal natural killer (NK) cell function.

Two types of hereditary thrombocytopenia may be associated with δ-SPD:
1 Thrombocytopenia and absent radii syndrome (TAR); and
2 Wiskott–Aldrich syndrome.

Abnormalities of the α-granules
Gray platelet syndrome (GPS) derives its name from the gray appearance of the patient's platelets in peripheral blood smears as a consequence of the rarity of platelet granules. The inheritance pattern seems to be autosomal recessive, although in a single family, it seemed to be autosomal dominant.

Affected patients have a lifelong history of mucocutaneous bleeding, which may vary from mild to moderate in severity, and prolonged bleeding time [10]. They have mild thrombocytopenia with abnormally large platelets and isolated reduction of the platelet α-granule content. Mild to moderate myelofibrosis has been described in some (hypothetically ascribed to the action of cytokines released by the hypogranular platelets and megakaryocytes in the bone marrow). The basic defect in GPS is probably defective targeting and packaging of endogenously synthesized proteins in α-granules.

The Quebec platelet disorder is an autosomal dominant qualitative platelet abnormality, characterized by:
• severe posttraumatic bleeding complications unresponsive to platelet transfusion;
• abnormal proteolysis of α-granule proteins;
• severe deficiency of platelet factor V;

• deficiency of multimerin;
• reduced to normal platelet counts; and
• markedly decreased platelet aggregation induced by epinephrine.

Multimerin, one of the largest proteins found in the human body, is present in platelet α-granules and in endothelial cell Weibel–Palade bodies. It binds factor V and its activated form, factor Va. Its deficiency in patients with the Quebec platelet disorder is probably responsible for the defect in platelet factor V, which is likely to be degraded by abnormally regulated platelet proteases, notably urokinase plasminogen activator [11].

Jacobsen or Paris–Trousseau syndrome is a rare syndrome that is associated with:
• a mild hemorrhagic diathesis;
• congenital thrombocytopenia with normal platelet life span;
• increased number of marrow megakaryocytes (many presenting with signs of abnormal maturation and intramedullary lysis); and
• a deletion of the distal part of one chromosome 11 [del(11)q23.3→qter] has been found in affected patients.

Abnormalities of the α- and δ-granules
α,δ-SPD is characterized by deficiencies of both α- and δ-granules. The clinical picture and the platelet aggregation abnormalities are similar to those of patients with GPS or δ-SPD.

Abnormalities of the signal-transduction pathways

Congenital abnormalities of the arachidonate–thromboxane A_2 pathway, involving the liberation of arachidonic acid from membrane phospholipids, defects of cyclo-oxygenase, or thromboxane synthetase, are associated with platelet function defects and mild bleeding [12]. Other congenital abnormalities of the platelet signal-transduction pathways have been described involving:
• G-proteins (Gαq deficiency);
• phosphatidylinositol metabolism (partial selective PLC-β2 isozyme deficiency); or
• defects in pleckstrin phosphorylation and hyper-responsiveness of platelet Gsα.

Abnormalities of membrane phospholipids

Scott syndrome is a rare bleeding disorder associated with the maintenance of the asymmetry of the lipid bilayer in the membranes of blood cells, including platelets leading to reduced thrombin generation and defective wound healing. The cause of the defect is still unclear.

In Stormorken syndrome, resting, unstimulated platelets from patients with this syndrome display a full procoagulant activity. Therefore, this condition represents the exact opposite in terms of platelet membrane function to the Scott syndrome; yet, surprisingly, it is also associated with a bleeding tendency. Platelets from patients with this condition respond normally to all agonists, with the exception of collagen.

Miscellaneous abnormalities of platelet function

Primary secretion defects

The term primary secretion defect was probably used for the first time by Weiss, to indicate all those ill-defined abnormalities of platelet secretion not associated with platelet granule deficiencies. The term was later used to indicate the platelet secretion defects not associated with platelet granule deficiencies and abnormalities of the arachidonate pathway, or all the abnormalities of platelet function associated with defects of signal transduction [13].

With the progression of our knowledge of platelet pathophysiology, this heterogeneous group, which brings together the majority of patients with congenital disorders of platelet function, will become progressively smaller, losing those patients with better defined biochemical abnormalities responsible for their platelet secretion defect. An example is heterozygous $P2Y_{12}$ deficiency state, which was included in this group of disorders until its biochemical abnormality was identified.

Other platelet abnormalities

Spontaneous platelet aggregation and decreased responses to thrombin are observed in patients with the Montreal platelet syndrome, a rare and poorly characterized congenital thrombocytopenia with large platelets [14].

Platelet function abnormalities have also been reported in osteogenesis imperfecta, Ehlers–Danlos syndrome, Marfan syndrome, hexokinase deficiency, and glucose-6-phosphate deficiency [15].

Acquired platelet defects

Platelet function can be impaired in several hematologic and non-hematologic conditions and by medications (Table 11.2) [16].

Uremia

The bleeding time (BT) may be severely prolonged in patients with uremia, but it can be corrected by increasing the hematocrit with RBC transfusions or with erythropoietin, suggesting that, in many instances, the defective primary hemostasis in uremia is a consequence of anemia. (It is known that RBCs normally facilitate the platelet interaction with the vessel wall.)

However, correction of the hematocrit fails to correct the BT in some patients, suggesting that other factors impair platelet–vessel wall interaction in this condition. Abnormalities of interaction of adhesive glycoproteins with their platelet receptors,

Table 11.2 Acquired platelet defects.

Medications affecting platelet function
Uremia
Dysproteinemias
Acute leukemias and myelodysplastic syndromes
Cardiopulmonary bypass
Liver disease
Antiplatelet antibodies
Myeloproliferative disorders
    Essential thrombocythemia
    Polycythemia vera
    Chronic myelogenous leukemia
    Agnogenic myeloid metaplasia

defective platelet activation, and platelet procoagulant activity have been described. Both dialyzable and non-dialyzable substances may be responsible.

Myeloproliferative disorders

Functional and biochemical abnormalities of platelets from patients with myeloproliferative disorders include:

- decreased release of arachidonic acid from membrane phospholipids;
- reduced conversion of arachidonic acid to its active metabolites;
- reduced responsiveness to TxA_2;
- deficiency of platelet granules;
- deficiency of the α_2/β_1 integrin; and
- decreased number of α_2-adrenergic receptors.

Other factors, in addition to platelet functional defects, contribute to the bleeding diathesis of these patients, including increased whole blood viscosity and thrombocytosis [17].

Cardiopulmonary bypass

Cardiopulmonary bypass causes transient thrombocytopenia and platelet function defects, which contribute to the increased bleeding risk of these patients. Platelet function defects associated with extracorporeal circulation include:

- defective aggregation,
- platelet granule deficiencies,
- abnormal interaction with VWF, and
- generation of platelet-derived microparticles.

These abnormalities result from platelet activation and fragmentation, hypothermia, contact with the blood–air interface, and exposure to traces of platelet agonists such as thrombin, ADP, and plasmin.

Table 11.3 Drugs affecting platelet function.

NSAIDs:
Aspirin, indomethacin, ibuprofen, sulindac, naproxen, phenylbutazone

Thienopyridines:
Ticlopidine, clopidogrel, thromboxane A2 receptor

Gp IIb/IIIa antagonists:
Abciximab, eptifibatide, tirofiban

Drugs that increase the platelet cAMP or cGMP levels:
Prostacyclin, iloprost, dipyridamole, theophylline, nitric oxide, nitric oxide donors

Anticoagulants and fibrinolytic agents:
Heparin, streptokinase, tPA, urokinase

Cardiovascular drugs:
Nitroglycerin, isosorbide dinitrate, propranolol, frusemide, calcium-channel blockers, quinidine, ACE inhibitors, verapamil, diltiazem

Volume expanders:
Dextran, hydroxyethyl starch

Psychotropic drugs, anesthetics:
Imipramine, amitriptyline, nortriptyline, chlorpromazine, promethazine, fluphenazine, trifluoperazine, haloperidol, halothane, dibucaine, tetracaine, butacaine, nepercaine, procaine plaquenil

Chemotherapeutic agents:
Mitomycin, daunorubicin, BCNU

Miscellaneous drugs:
Antihistamines, radiographic contrast agents, clofibrate

Abbreviations: ACE, angiotensin-converting enzyme; cGMP, cyclic guanosine 3′,5′-monophosphate; CAMP, cyclic adenosine 3′,5′-monophosphate.

Medications

Many drugs affect platelet function (Table 11.3), sometimes causing a prolongation of the BT. In some instances, the inhibition of platelet function is the target of the drug, as in the case of antiplatelet agents that are given to reduce the risk of cardiovascular or cerebrovascular accidents. In other cases, the induced abnormalities of platelet function are to be considered side effects of the drug, which are in most instances without obvious clinical consequences.

Liver disease

Chronic liver disease is associated with a prolongation of the BT disproportionate to the degree of thrombocytopenia that usually complicates this condition. Whether the described defects are caused by intrinsic or extrinsic abnormalities of the platelets is unclear.

Therapy

Platelet transfusions should be used only in severe bleeding episodes, which are usually seen in patients with BSS or, less frequently, GT. Recombinant factor VIIa is a good, albeit expensive, alternative to platelet transfusions [18]. Antifibrinolytic agents, such as aprotinin and tranexamic acid, or the vasopressin analog desmopressin (DDAVP) should be used in all other circumstances, because they are relatively cheap, do not cause platelet refractoriness, and are not associated with the risk of transmitting blood-borne viral diseases [19].

References

1 Pham A, Wang J. Bernard-Soulier syndrome: an inherited platelet disorder. *Arch Pathol Lab Med* 2007;131(12):1834–6.

2 Budde U. Diagnosis of von Willebrand disease subtypes: implications for treatment. *Haemophilia* 2008;14(Suppl 5):27–38.

3 Nair S, Ghosh K, Kulkarni B, Shetty S, Mohanty D. Glanzmann's thrombasthenia: updated. *Platelets* 2002;13(7):387–93.

4 Moroi M, Jung SM. Platelet receptors for collagen. *Thromb Haemost* 1997;78(1):439–44.

5 Arthur JF, Dunkley S, Andrews RK. Platelet glycoprotein VI-related clinical defects. *Br J Haematol* 2007;139(3):363–72.

6 Higuchi W, Fuse I, Hattori A, Aizawa Y. Mutations of the platelet thromboxane A2 (TXA2) receptor in patients characterized by the absence of TXA2-induced platelet aggregation despite normal TXA2 binding activity. *Thromb Haemost* 1999;82(5):1528–31.

7 Cattaneo M, Lecchi A, Randi AM, McGregor JL, Mannucci PM. Identification of a new congenital defect of platelet function characterized by severe impairment of platelet responses to adenosine diphosphate. *Blood* 1992;80(11):2787–96.

8 Cattaneo M, Gachet C. ADP receptors and clinical bleeding disorders. *Arterioscler Thromb Vasc Biol* 1999;19(10):2281–5.

9 Nurden P, Nurden AT. Congenital disorders associated with platelet dysfunctions. *Thromb Haemost* 2008;99(2):253–63.

10 Nurden AT, Nurden P. The gray platelet syndrome: clinical spectrum of the disease. *Blood Rev* 2007;21(1):21–36.

11 Diamandis M, Veljkovic DK, Maurer-Spurej E, Rivard GE, Hayward CP. Quebec platelet disorder: features, pathogenesis and treatment. *Blood Coagul Fibrinolysis* 2008;19(2):109–19.

12 Rao AK. *Congenital Platelet Signal Transduction Defects.* Cambridge: Cambridge University Press, 2002.

13 Cattaneo M. *Congenital Disorders of Platelet Secretion.* Cambridge: Cambridge University Press, 2002.

14 Balduini CL, Cattaneo M, Fabris F, et al. Inherited thrombocytopenias: a proposed diagnostic algorithm from the Italian Gruppo di Studio delle Piastrine. *Haematologica* 2003;88(5):582–92.

15 Cattaneo M. Inherited platelet-based bleeding disorders. *J Thromb Haemost* 2003;1(7):1628–36.

16 Bennett J. *Acquired Platelet Function Defects.* Cambridge: Cambridge University Press, 2002.

17 Elliott MA, Tefferi A. Thrombosis and haemorrhage in polycythaemia vera and essential thrombocythaemia. *Br J Haematol* 2005;128(3):275–90.

18 Poon M-C. *Factor VIIa.* Orlando, FL: Academic Press, 2003.

19 Mannucci PM, Levi M. Prevention and treatment of major blood loss. *N Engl J Med* 2007;356(22):2301–11.

12 Disseminated intravascular coagulation and other microangiopathies

Raj S. Kasthuri and Nigel S. Key

Disseminated intravascular coagulation

Disseminated intravascular coagulation (DIC) is an acquired clinicopathologic syndrome characterized by chaotic activation of the coagulation system, resulting in widespread intravascular deposition of fibrin-rich thrombi. DIC is not itself a disease state, but rather is a secondary manifestation of some other underlying disorder. Depending on the underlying cause and rapidity of the process, the clinical spectrum may range from subclinical laboratory abnormalities (compensated DIC or non-overt DIC) to multiorgan failure, metabolic derangement, hemodynamic instability, widespread bleeding, and death.

The following definition of DIC has been proposed by the DIC Scientific and Standardization Committee of the International Society on Thrombosis and Hemostasis (ISTH): "DIC is an acquired syndrome characterized by the intravascular activation of coagulation with loss of localization arising from different causes. It can originate from and cause damage to the microvasculature, which if sufficiently severe, can produce organ dysfunction" [1].

Synonyms for DIC in the medical literature include the defibrination syndrome, consumption coagulopathy, generalized intravascular coagulation, thrombohemorrhagic phenomenon, and disseminated intravascular fibrin formation.

Etiology

A broad range of pathological conditions (the most important of which are listed in Table 12.1) may trigger DIC. Sepsis syndromes are among the most frequently encountered causes. Although the highest risk is seen with Gram-negative bacterial infections, Gram-positive infections as well as nonbacterial infections can also be associated with DIC. Complications of pregnancy and malignancy are other common causes of DIC in clinical practice.

Pathogenesis

The pathogenesis of DIC involves simultaneous dysregulation of several homeostatic mechanisms (Fig. 12.1). These can be broadly divided into:

1 excessive activation of coagulation;
2 downregulation of physiologic anticoagulant pathways; and
3 inhibition of fibrinolysis.

Dysfunction of the vascular endothelium, a vast and pervasive organ, is prominent as both a cause and a consequence of these processes. The net result is widespread generation of thrombin and conversion of circulating fibrinogen to insoluble fibrin thrombi, aggravated by the relative inability of the fibrinolytic mechanism to remove intravascular fibrin.

Obstruction of small and medium-sized vessels caused by intravascular fibrin deposition may lead to (multiple) organ dysfunction, especially affecting the kidneys, brain, lung, liver, and heart. The widespread activation of coagulation leads to consumption of clotting factors and platelets, a process that is aggravated by simultaneous impaired hepatic production of these factors. Thus, abnormal prolongation of coagulation screening tests, thrombocytopenia, and a seemingly paradoxical bleeding tendency may occur in some patients with more advanced forms of DIC.

The passage of erythrocytes through the fibrin meshwork in the microvascular circulation may lead to red cell fragmentation. This microangiopathic

Table 12.1 Conditions associated with disseminated intravascular coagulation (DIC).

Infection:
- Sepsis syndromes (Gram-positive and Gram-negative bacteria)
- Viral infections (e.g. dengue, Ebola)
- Other (e.g. ricketsial, malarial infections)

Trauma/tissue damage:
- Head injury
- Pancreatitis
- Fat embolism
- Any other serious tissue damage (crush or penetrating injury)

Malignancy:
- Solid tumors
- Acute leukemias (especially AML-M3)
- Chronic leukemias (CMML)

Obstetric complications:
- Abruptio placentae
- Amniotic fluid embolism
- Eclampsia and preeclampsia
- Retained dead fetus

Vascular disorders:
- Giant hemangiomas (Kasabach–Merritt syndrome)
- Other vascular malformations
- Large aortic aneurysm

Severe allergic/toxic reactions:
- Toxic shock syndrome
- Snake, spider venoms

Severe immunologic reactions:
- Acute hemolytic transfusion reactions
- Heparin-induced thrombocytopenia, type II

hemolytic anemia (MAHA) is much less common in DIC than in the group of disorders known as the "thrombotic microangiopathies," where it is, in fact, a *sine qua non*.

Excessive activation of coagulation

Although coagulation may be initiated in vitro by both the intrinsic (contact) and extrinsic (tissue factor) pathways, the tissue factor pathway is the primary initiator of coagulation in vivo [2]. Unlike most other soluble clotting factors circulating in plasma, tissue factor (TF) is a cell-bound transmembrane protein. By virtue of its predominant extravascular location, TF is nor-

mally present on cells that are relatively inaccessible to blood clotting factors in the absence of vessel injury, such as smooth muscle cells and fibroblasts. However, the systemic response to infection and injury results in the synthesis and release of pro-inflammatory cytokines, such as tumor necrosis factor TNF-α, interleukin 1 (IL-1), and IL-6, which trigger TF synthesis by monocytes and endothelial cells (Fig. 12.1) [2]. With other forms of DIC, it is likely that additional stimuli capable of activating and/or propagating coagulation (such as fat, brain lipids, cancer procoagulant protein, or amniotic fluid) are released into the circulation.

Downregulation of physiological anticoagulant pathways

DIC is associated with an acquired deficiency of naturally occurring anticoagulants, particularly antithrombin (III) and protein C. Plasma levels are decreased secondary to consumption and increased enzymatic degradation by activated neutrophils [3]. Endothelial dysfunction adversely affects the protein C/protein S/thrombomodulin pathway in other ways also. The same proinflammatory cytokines that up-regulate TF synthesis simultaneously down-regulate endothelial synthesis of the cofactors thrombomodulin and endothelial cell protein C receptor [4]. The end result is decreased conversion of protein C to activated protein C on the endothelial cell surface.

Inhibition of fibrinolysis

The role of the fibrinolytic system is to generate plasmin on fibrin surfaces, in an effort to restore vascular patency via enzymatic digestion of fibrin strands. In many forms of DIC, fibrinolysis is actively suppressed because of elevated levels of plasminogen activator inhibitor type 1 (PAI-1) [5]. PAI-1 inhibits the plasminogen activators tissue plasminogen activator and urokinase, preventing the generation of plasmin from plasminogen. Thus, by failing to clear intravascular fibrin thrombi, the inhibition of fibrinolysis by PAI-1 also contributes to the net procoagulant state and end-organ hypoperfusion in DIC.

Clinical manifestations

As predicted from the complex underlying pathophysiological derangements, patients with DIC may

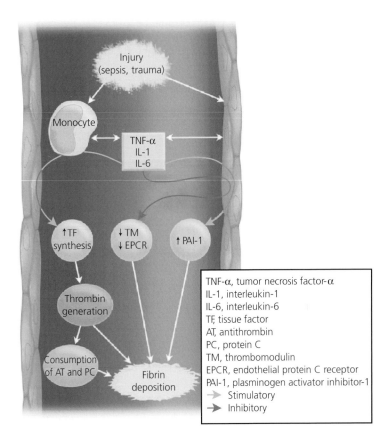

Figure 12.1 Pathogenesis of DIC.

suffer simultaneous bleeding and thrombotic manifestations. Clinical features are determined to some extent by the underlying etiology. Thus, whereas vaso-occlusive manifestations are significantly more prevalent overall, certain subtypes of DIC may be associated with bleeding, usually in the form of microvascular oozing from mucocutaneous surfaces. In obstetric disorders, this may be explained by the hyperacuity of the process leading to rapid consumption of clotting factors and platelets, whereas in acute promyelocytic leukemia (AML-M3), production of plasminogen activators by leukemic cells may lead to hyperfibrinolytic bleeding [6].

The most common result of microvascular occlusion is end-organ dysfunction, as in sepsis syndromes. This process may lead to renal, cardiac, and/or pulmonary failure. Vaso-occlusion may occasionally lead to more clinically overt thrombotic manifestations, such as purpura fulminans in meningococcal or pneumococcal sepsis, which is a clinical syndrome present-

ing as skin necrosis (Plate 12.1) and digital gangrene (Fig. 12.2). The systemic prothrombotic state may also lead to the development of a localized large-vessel arterial or venous thromboembolic event.

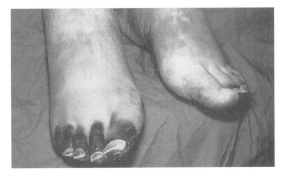

Figure 12.2 Gangrenous feet resulting from pneumococcal infection and DIC. Splenectomy had been performed 11 years earlier. Reprinted with permission from Blood in Systemic Disease 1e, Greaves and Makris, 1997, published by Elsevier.

It is important to realize that a substantial subset of patients with DIC may suffer only subclinical laboratory abnormalities, with insidious or even absent clinical features. This condition has been referred to as compensated DIC or non-overt DIC (discussed below).

Diagnosis

The diagnosis of DIC should take into account both the clinical presentation as well as laboratory findings. It is important to appreciate that DIC is a syndrome that is *always secondary* to another underlying pathological condition and that there is no single diagnostic laboratory test for DIC. A diagnostic scoring algorithm using widely available coagulation tests has been proposed by the DIC Scientific and Standardization Committee of the ISTH [1]. The design of this scoring system has a pathophysiologic basis, incorporating the concept of "overt" (decompensated, Table 12.2) and "non-overt" (compensated, Table 12.3) DIC as distinct entities. To some extent, these subsets reflect differ-

ent points in the continuum, although non-overt DIC may be associated with adverse outcomes in critically ill patients independently of progression to overt DIC. Under this scoring system, a score of 5 or more meets the definition of "overt" DIC. It should be noted that the term "fibrin-related products" in the scoring system includes:
• direct assays for the presence of fibrin (e.g. soluble fibrin monomers); and
• indirect assays of fibrin generation [e.g. D-dimer, fibrin degradation products (FDPs)].

Importantly, the proposed scoring algorithm should be applied only if an underlying disorder known to be associated with DIC (e.g. sepsis, severe trauma) exists. This scoring system has been validated prospectively in the diagnosis of DIC, and it has been shown that DIC is an independent predictor of mortality in sepsis patients. Additionally, the severity of DIC based on the DIC score also correlates with poor outcomes in these patients [7]. Despite these recent data, the DIC scoring system has not yet been widely adopted in clinical practice.

Table 12.2 Diagnostic scoring system for overt DIC [Do not use this algorithm unless the patient has an underlying disorder that is associated with DIC].

Global coagulation test results	Score (0, 1, or 2 points)
Platelet count	$>100 \times 10^9/L = 0$ $50–100 \times 10^9/L = 1$ $<50 \times 10^9/L = 2$
Elevated fibrin-related markers (soluble fibrin monomers, D-dimers, fibrin degradation products)	No increase = 0 Moderate increase = 1 Strong increase = 2
Prolonged prothrombin time (in seconds above upper limit of normal)	<3 s = 0 3–6 s = 1 >6 s = 2
Fibrinogen level	>1.0 g/L = 0 <1.0 g/L = 1

Total score =
If score ≥5, compatible with overt DIC, recommend repeating score daily.
If score <5, suggestive (not affirmative) for non-overt DIC, repeat scoring in 1–2 days.

Adapted from Taylor FB Jr, Toh CH, Hoots WK, Wada H, Levi M. Towards definition, clinical and laboratory criteria, and a scoring system for disseminated intravascular coagulation. *Thromb Haemost* 2001;86:1327–30.

Table 12.3 Diagnostic scoring system for non-overt DIC.*

Criteria	Score (0, 1, or 2 points)	
1. Risk assessment		
Is there an underlying disorder that is associated with DIC?	Yes = 2 No = 0	
2. Major criteria		
Platelet count	$>100 \times 10^9$/L = 0	+ Rising = −1
	$<100 \times 10^9$/L = 1	Stable = 0
		Falling = 1
Prothrombin time (in seconds above upper limit of normal)	<3 s = 0	+ Falling = −1
	>3 s = 1	Stable = 0
		Rising = 1
Soluble fibrin or FDPs	Normal = 0	+ Falling = −1
	Raised = 1	Stable = 0
		Rising = 1
3. Specific criteria		
Antithrombin	Normal = −1	
	Low = 1	
Protein C	Normal = −1	
	Low = 1	
TAT complexes	Normal = −1	
	High = 1	
Total score =		

*At the present time, although this scoring system has been proposed, interpretations with regards to cut-off scores for diagnosis of non-overt DIC are unclear. In general, trends over time will be more useful than individual single point scores.

Abbreviations: FDP, fibrin degradation product; TAT, thrombin–antithrombin complex.

Adapted from Taylor FB Jr, Toh CH, Hoots WK, Wada H, Levi M. Towards definition, clinical and laboratory criteria, and a scoring system for disseminated intravascular coagulation. *Thromb Haemost* 2001;86:1327–30.

Overt DIC

This is defined as a state in which the vascular endothelium, and blood and its components, have lost the ability to compensate and restore homeostasis in response to injury. The result is a progressively decompensating state that is manifest as thrombotic multiorgan dysfunction and/or bleeding.

Non-overt DIC

This is defined as a clinical vascular injury state that results in great stress to the hemostatic system, the response to which, for the moment, is sufficient to forestall further rampant inflammatory and hemostatic activation.

The scoring system for the diagnosis of non-overt DIC (Table 12.3) includes, in addition to global studies of coagulation [protrombin time (PT), FDPs], more specific (but less widely available) tests that are surrogate markers of intravascular thrombin generation [thrombin–antithrombin (TAT) complexes] and ongoing consumption of coagulation inhibitors [such as antithrombin (AT) and protein C (PC) levels]. However, in a recent summary reviewing the evidence to date on the DIC scoring system, the ISTH Scientific Committee on DIC questioned the value of including AT and PC levels in the "non-overt DIC" scoring system [8]. Therefore, the definition of non-overt DIC continues to undergo additional refinement.

Although perceived as a classic finding, a low plasma fibrinogen level is not a sensitive marker of DIC [9]. In fact, high plasma fibrinogen levels are much more frequently encountered. Fibrinogen levels are probably influenced more by the degree of activation of secondary fibrino(geno)lysis than the degree of consumption during thrombus formation.

Treatment

The development of DIC in patients with sepsis or trauma has been shown to be independently associated with increased morbidity and mortality. Thus, prompt and at times preemptive therapy becomes important in these patients.

Managing the underlying disease

The mainstay of treatment in patients with DIC is management of the underlying disease. The reversibility of DIC depends to a large degree on the underlying cause. Delivery of the fetus and placenta may promptly restore homeostasis in patients with obstetric DIC. Eradication of infection with antibiotics and/or surgery may not necessarily have the same rapid effect in sepsis syndromes, possibly because of established widespread endothelial injury.

Supportive care and blood products

Good supportive care in the management of patients with DIC includes adequate hemodynamic support to maintain perfusion and appropriate supportive transfusion of blood products. Given the mechanisms involved in the development of DIC, there is always the theoretical fear of "fueling the fire" with transfused blood cells and plasma products, although the evidence that this occurs in practice is underwhelming. To complicate matters further, there are no consensus guidelines for optimal transfusion management of these patients.

Treatment of patients with DIC who are actively bleeding or at high risk for bleeding should include platelet transfusions, fresh frozen plasma, cryoprecipitate, and packed red cells as needed. Patients requiring invasive procedures should be covered peri-procedure with plasma and platelet transfusions as needed. Reasonable transfusion goals in these circumstances are platelet counts $\leq 50 \times 10^9$/L, fibrinogen ≤ 1.0 g/L, and

maintenance of PT and activated partial thromboplastin time (APTT) as close to the normal range as possible. There is no role for the prophylactic administration of blood products in patients with DIC. The approach to these patients should be individualized based on their clinical and laboratory manifestations.

Systemic anticoagulation

On the basis of the pathophysiology of DIC, an argument may be made for the use of systemic heparin anticoagulation. Although the literature remains divided about this approach, the few available controlled trials have failed to demonstrate a clear benefit [10]. The routine use of heparin in DIC not associated with a clinical thrombotic event is generally discouraged given the demonstrated risk of bleeding complications in these patients. There is some consensus that treatment is indicated for those with a documented thromboembolic event or extensive deposition of fibrin leading to acral ischemia or purpura fulminans. In the case of large-vessel thromboembolic events, full therapeutic doses of unfractionated heparin are indicated, whereas in microvascular occlusive syndromes, lower doses (e.g. 500–800 U/hour) may be preferable. Low-molecular-weight heparin has been successfully used as an alternative to unfractionated heparin in some studies. The role of direct thrombin inhibitors (such as hirudin or argatroban) in DIC also remains to be established in controlled trials. Although these agents might theoretically be more effective than heparins, they also carry a higher risk of bleeding.

Antifibrinolytic therapy

Because fibrinolysis is generally down-regulated concomitant with excessive fibrin formation in DIC, treatment with antifibrinolytic agents (such as ε-aminocaproic acid or tranexamic acid) is generally contraindicated. There may be exceptions to the rule, such as patients with acute promyelocytic leukemia who may develop a form of DIC characterized by hyperfibrinolytic bleeding that may result in intracranial hemorrhage. In this instance, judicious use of antifibrinolytics has proven effective [11].

Specific inhibitors of coagulation

In view of the depletion of natural anticoagulants during DIC, it is logical to suppose that replacement therapy using one or more of the missing natural anticoagulants is warranted.

Several preliminary trials with antithrombin, mainly in patients with sepsis, demonstrated some improvement in the duration of DIC and resolution of laboratory abnormalities. However, a significant benefit in mortality could not be demonstrated in a large, randomized controlled study of sepsis (the KyberSept Trial) [12]. Although a post hoc subgroup analysis in this trial suggested a benefit with the use of AT without concomitant heparin in a subset of patients with DIC [13], the role of AT therapy in patients with DIC remains unclear at this time.

On the other hand, a large, randomized, controlled trial (the PROWESS Study) using recombinant activated PC (Drotrecogin alfa,activated) to treat patients with sepsis did demonstrate improved survival compared with placebo [14]. This effect was probably mediated not only by an antithrombotic effect, but also by anti-inflammatory and profibrinolytic effects of this agent. However, excess bleeding was seen in patients treated with activated PC, which inactivates factors Va and VIIIa. Therefore, caution is required in patients with severe thrombocytopenia ($\leq 30 \times 10^9/L$) or otherwise at high risk of bleeding. This pivotal phase III study has been further dissected using extensive subgroup analyses, which have suggested a greater benefit for rhAPC in patients with severe sepsis (≥ 2 organs affected, APACHE II score >25) and those patients with sepsis with coexisting DIC [15]. Additionally, patients that received concomitant therapy with rhAPC and heparin tended to have higher mortality rates. These issues have been specifically addressed in subsequent clinical trials evaluating the role of rhAPC in less severe sepsis (APACHE II score <25, the ADDRESS study), which showed no benefit to the use of rhAPC; and the concomitant use of heparin and rhAPC in patients with severe sepsis (the XPRESS study), which failed to demonstrate significant differences with use of heparin [16,17]. The role of activated PC in the treatment of other forms of DIC has not been adequately evaluated.

Thrombotic microangiopathies

The thrombotic microangiopathies are a group of related disorders characterized by widespread microvas-

Table 12.4 Underlying etiologies of thrombotic microangiopathies.

Thrombotic thrombocytopenic purpura:
- Familial (ADAMTS-13 deficiency)
- Acquired
  - o Idiopathic
  - o Drug-related (quinine, ticlopidine)

Hemolytic uremic syndrome:
- Familial (including factor H deficiency)
- Acquired

Secondary thrombotic microangiopathies:
- Malignancy
- Malignant hypertension
- Transplantation
  - o Stem cell transplantation
  - o Solid organ transplantation
- Pregnancy-related
  - o Preeclampsia
  - o HELLP syndrome
- Collagen vascular disease
  - o Scleroderma renal crisis
  - o Systemic lupus erythematosus
  - o Antiphospholipid antibody syndrome

cular occlusion by platelet-rich aggregates. The accelerated consumption of platelets results in thrombocytopenia. Red cell fragmentation occurs secondary to turbulent blood flow in areas of the microcirculation obstructed by platelet-rich thrombi. Peripheral blood smear examination reveals the presence of fragmented red cells (schistocytes or helmet cells) associated with elevated serum lactate dehydrogenase levels, a condition known as microangiopathic hemolytic anemia (MAHA) [18].

A number of syndromes are included under the rubric of thrombotic microangiopathies (Table 12.4), and a clear distinction between them at the time of presentation may be difficult or impossible. This is especially true of thrombotic thrombocytopenic purpura (TTP) and the hemolytic uremic syndrome (HUS).

The classic clinical pentad in TTP includes:
- thrombocytopenia,
- MAHA,
- renal failure,
- neurologic abnormalities, and
- fever,

but frequently not all features are present.

"Classic" HUS is characterized by:
- MAHA,
- thrombocytopenia, and
- prominent renal failure, following an acute diarrheal illness.

The clinical presentation of many of the secondary thrombotic microangiopathies may also be indistinguishable on initial evaluation. The diagnostic dilemma is further compounded by the urgent requirement for plasma exchange in a subset of these patients (discussed below). Therefore, it is appropriate to use the generic diagnosis of "TTP/HUS" in patients presenting with thrombocytopenia and MAHA in the absence of a clinically apparent cause or DIC. Plasma exchange should then be initiated while further evaluation to rule out an alternative diagnosis continues [19].

Pathophysiology

Although the clinical manifestations of these syndromes show considerable overlap, pathogeneses (where understood) of some of the individual entities may differ considerably.

Thrombotic thrombocytopenic purpura

Unlike the case with DIC, microvascular thrombi are relatively fibrin-poor, but are enriched in von Willebrand factor (VWF) and platelets. Microvascular platelet deposition in TTP is secondary to endothelial secretion of unusually large VWF multimers. Under normal conditions, these unusually large multimers (which are particularly "sticky" for platelets) are prevented from entering the circulation by an enzyme that cleaves VWF. Predominantly synthesized in the liver, this metalloprotease enzyme is known as ADAMTS-13 (*a d*isintegrin-like *a*nd *m*etalloprotease with *t*hrombo*s*pondin repeats) [20]. A qualitative or quantitative defect of ADAMTS-13 allows the unusually large multimers of VWF to remain anchored to endothelial cells, resulting in widespread platelet adherence, microvascular obstruction, and end-organ dysfunction.

Studies have demonstrated that many (but apparently not all) patients with definite TTP have ≤5% activity of ADAMTS-13 in their plasma. In the familial form of TTP, affected individuals are usually homozygous or doubly heterozygous for mutations in the gene for ADAMTS-13, located on chromosome 9. In the idiopathic acquired form of TTP, immunoglobulin G (IgG) antibodies against the enzyme have been detected, suggesting an autoimmune etiology [21]. More modest reductions in ADAMTS-13 enzyme activity in plasma (5–50%) may be found in liver disease, malignancy, inflammation, pregnancy, and in the neonatal period.

Hemolytic uremic syndrome

Microvascular platelet thrombus formation in the classic form of HUS is believed to be toxin-induced. Specifically, prodromal infection of the gastrointestinal tract by verotoxin-producing *Escherichia coli* O157:H7, or certain other serotypes of *E. coli* or *Shigella dysenteriae*, is characteristic of this disorder. These toxins, which gain access to blood via the colonic circulation, ultimately target cerebral and glomerular epithelium, mesangial cells and tubular epithelium in the kidneys, and vascular endothelium. In these locations, verotoxins mediate cytokine release, endothelial activation and injury, and direct activation of platelets. The release of platelet adhesogens from damaged endothelium results in microvascular platelet thrombi formation and renal injury.

The small subset of individuals with familial HUS tend to have more severe disease and a greater risk of recurrence. Some of these patients are deficient in complement factor H, which inactivates C3b, a product of the alternate complement pathway. The absence of this regulatory mechanism can lead to autoantibody or immune complex-mediated glomerular injury, with platelet activation, increase in local endothelial procoagulant properties, and ultimately microvascular thrombus formation.

Other thrombotic microangiopathies

Ticlopidine, clopidogrel, and (particularly) quinine appear to cause thrombotic microangiopathy through an antibody-mediated mechanism. The pathogenesis of many of the other secondary thrombotic microangiopathies listed in Table 12.4 remains poorly understood.

Differential diagnosis

Faced with a thrombocytopenic patient with MAHA, DIC should be ruled out by review of the history (to rule out an underlying disorder associated with DIC) and by confirmation that screening studies of coagulation, such as the PT, APTT, and fibrinogen level, are normal. The direct antiglobulin (Coombs) test should be obtained to screen for immune-mediated hemolysis. Stool cultures are indicated if there has been a preceding diarrheal illness. A careful review of drug exposures, particularly for drugs such as quinine, is essential.

In a pregnant patient—particularly one in the latter stages or in the immediate postpartum period—it may be very difficult to distinguish TTP/HUS (which requires urgent plasma exchange) from preeclampsia with or without the associated HELLP (**h**emolysis, **e**levated **l**iver enzymes and **l**ow-**p**latelets) syndrome. In general, these syndromes resolve promptly with delivery, whereas TTP/HUS may persist.

The utility of a low-plasma ADAMTS-13 activity remains uncertain. The presence of a very low level (<5%) is probably diagnostic but not necessarily exclusive to TTP, and laboratory demonstration of an inhibitory antibody to the enzyme helps to identify an autoimmune etiology. However, measuring enzyme levels is unlikely to be useful in making the diagnosis in the acute setting for the following reasons. First, most centers do not have the capability for real-time ADAMTS-13 testing, and there is a significant lag time before test results are available. Second, roughly a quarter of patients with idiopathic TTP do not have ADAMTS-13 deficiency. Finally, and most important, patients with TTP respond well to plasma exchange regardless of underlying ADAMTS-13 deficiency [22]. However, measurement of ADAMTS-13 activity may provide valuable information in aiding long-term management of these patients as discussed below.

Clinical manifestations

The distinction between TTP and HUS, when possible, is based on the presence of significant renal failure and preceding history. Thus, in the classic (endemic) form of acquired HUS, which is most common in children less than 5 years of age, a bloody diarrhea resulting from *E. coli* or *S. dysenteriae* is a prodromal hallmark. In the epidemic form of HUS, which may occur after eating infected meat or dairy products, approximately 10–30% of infected individuals develop the full-blown syndrome. The use of antimotility agents after an *E. coli* infection may increase the risk of HUS. Recurrence of this type of HUS is uncommon. Patients with familial forms of HUS (the Upshaw–Schulman syndrome) tend to present early in childhood and frequently have a relapsing clinical course that may progress to end-stage renal disease.

Classic TTP occurs much more frequently in adulthood and is frequently associated with neurologic dysfunction, which characteristically manifests as transient focal (e.g. dysphasia) or non-focal (e.g. confusion, seizure) symptoms. Neurologic symptoms may be the first sign of relapse in a patient with a previous history of TTP. The risk of recurrence in the idiopathic acquired form of TTP is in the range of 10–30%, with most (but not all) events occurring within the first year. Patients with familial forms of TTP may present later in life than those with familial HUS.

The thrombotic microangiopathy related to chemotherapy, cyclosporine, transplantation, or total body irradiation tends to occur weeks to months following exposure to these agents. The diagnostic criteria for thrombotic microangiopathy associated with hematopoietic stem cell transplantation have recently been addressed by a consensus conference, which opted for stringent criteria to avoid misdiagnosis [23]. It was proposed that *all* of the following criteria should be met: (1) >4% schistocytes on peripheral blood smear; (2) de novo, prolonged, or progressive thrombocytopenia (platelet count <50 × 10^9/L or 50% or greater reduction from previous counts); (3) sudden and persistent increase in lactate dehydrogenase (LDH); (4) decrease in hemoglobin concentration or increased transfusion requirement; and (5) decrease in serum haptoglobin. In this disorder, the outcome is frequently very poor, renal manifestations are prominent, and plasma exchange does not appear to be efficacious.

Treatment

In the era prior to plasma exchange, the mortality rate of TTP approached 100%. Since the institution of plasma exchange, TTP has become a curable disease. Thus, prompt diagnosis is essential. The diagnostic criteria have therefore become less stringent, and, as already described, all patients with thrombocytopenia and MAHA who do not have another explanation for these findings—whether or not they have renal manifestations, fever, or neurological dysfunction—should be suspected of having TTP/HUS and treated as such.

Plasma exchange

The most important treatment modality in these patients is plasma exchange, which is superior to plasma infusion [24]. A single plasma volume exchange replacing with fresh frozen or cryosupernatant plasma should be performed daily along with monitoring of platelet counts, serum LDH, and periodic review of the peripheral smear.

Neurologic symptoms generally resolve rapidly following institution of plasma exchange. Measures of ongoing hemolysis, such as the LDH, may also improve promptly with therapy, although the anemia may persist and occasionally may require supportive transfusions. The recovery from renal failure may be unpredictable and often slow and incomplete, such that some patients may need prolonged dialysis. The platelet count is the most reliable marker of disease activity on which to base treatment decisions. An improvement reflects resolution, whereas worsening of thrombocytopenia at any point in the course of the disease may reflect an exacerbation and the need for more aggressive therapy. In those patients who fail to demonstrate an initial response, more intense therapy, such as greater volumes of plasma exchanged once or even twice daily, is indicated [19].

Plasma exchange is most beneficial in patients with TTP/HUS who fall into the "idiopathic acquired," "pregnancy-related," and "drug-related" categories. Its benefit is unclear in other forms of thrombotic microangiopathy, such as that associated with stem cell transplantation (which may be more related to the use of cyclosporine A as well as graft-versus-host disease), total body irradiation, and cytomegalovirus infection.

In responsive patients, there are no set criteria to guide the optimal duration of treatment. Once the platelet count normalizes, a decision can be made to discontinue plasma exchange. A fall in the platelet count may occur within the first 1–2 weeks, reflecting disease exacerbation, and plasma exchange then needs to be reinstituted. One approach has been to decrease the frequency of plasma exchanges rather than to abruptly discontinue. Ultimately, however, discontinuing plasma exchange is the only way to evaluate whether hematological remission has been achieved.

There is still debate as to whether plasma exchange is indicated in patients with postinfectious HUS. The vast majority of disease in young children will resolve with supportive care alone, but plasmapheresis is probably indicated and useful in affected adults.

Immunosuppression

In many centers, glucocorticoids are used as an adjunct to initial plasma exchange, but there are few data to support this practice. Certainly, it is reasonable to consider glucocorticoids in patients who are refractory to plasma exchange. Other immunosuppressive modalities, such as vincristine, have also been reported to be of value in refractory cases. Particular reference must be made here to the use of rituximab, the monoclonal antibody against CD20. Rituximab has been used in patients with relapsing or refractory TTP with encouraging results in small series of patients with recovery of ADAMTS-13 levels and achievement of durable remissions [25]. The benefit of combining rituximab and plasma exchange in the treatment of patients with TTP will be evaluated in a phase III randomized trial in the United States in the near future.

Role of ADAMTS-13 activity

Measurement of ADAMTS-13 activity and search for an autoantibody to the enzyme is often performed at the time that TTP/HUS is suspected. Because there is no consensus as to the most robust assay methodology, no specific recommendation can be made. However, at the time of writing, our understanding of the role of ADAMTS deficiency in the diagnosis and management of TTP/HUS can be briefly summarized as follows:

• A severe deficiency of ADAMTS13 activity (<5% of pooled normal plasma) is relatively specific for TTP;

• Only about 70% of patients with a firm diagnosis of acute idiopathic TTP have a severe deficiency in ADAMTS13;

• The response to plasma exchange appears to be similar in patients with or without severe ADAMTS13 deficiency;

• Secondary forms of thrombotic microangiopathy (such as that associated with hematopoietic stem cell therapy) are associated with normal levels of ADAMTS13 activity; and

• Patients with TTP associated with deficiency of ADAMTS-13 are at a greater risk for relapse compared to those without.

The major implication of these observations is that ADAMTS13 activity should not be used to decide which patients with clinically diagnosed acute idiopathic TTP/HUS are (or rather, are not) candidates for plasma exchange. On the other hand, those individuals who are subsequently proven to have severe ADAMTS13 activity caused by an autoantibody to the enzyme should be more carefully observed when in remission because of their higher risk of relapse; indeed, in this situation, a falling plasma level of ADAMTS13 may herald the onset of a relapse. It remains to be demonstrated whether these patients are more suitable candidates for more aggressive immunosuppression, as might reasonably be expected.

Other treatments

In patients with multiple relapses, splenectomy during hematologic remission may favorably alter the disease course.

In the context of ADAMTS-13 deficiency, episodes of familial TTP have been reversed or prevented by the infusion of fresh frozen or cryosupernatant plasma. These products contain the metalloprotease enzyme, and in this subset of congenitally deficient patients, plasmapheresis can therefore be avoided.

Patients with TTP/HUS rarely experience bleeding, despite sometimes very significant thrombocytopenia. Routine prophylactic platelet transfusion is contraindicated, because of fear that it may precipitate further vaso-occlusive phenomena. However, it is occasionally necessary to administer platelets to a patient with one of these syndromes who is actively bleeding.

The use of antimicrobial agents in HUS increases the release of Shiga toxin from the organism and could paradoxically increase the risk of HUS. They are therefore not recommended.

The sequence of the ADAMTS-13 metalloprotease has now been determined, and gene therapy for treatment of patients with familial forms of the disease may become a reality in the relatively near future.

References

1 Taylor FB Jr, Toh CH, Hoots WK, Wada H, Levi M. Towards definition, clinical and laboratory criteria, and a scoring system for disseminated intravascular coagulation. *Thromb Haemost* 2001;86(5):1327–30.

2 Mackman N, Tilley RE, Key NS. Role of the extrinsic pathway of blood coagulation in hemostasis and thrombosis. *Arterioscler Thromb Vasc Biol* 2007;27(8):1687–93.

3 Levi M, de Jonge E, van der Poll T. Rationale for restoration of physiological anticoagulant pathways in patients with sepsis and disseminated intravascular coagulation. *Crit Care Med* 2001;29(7 Suppl):S90–4.

4 Levi M. Disseminated intravascular coagulation. *Crit Care Med* 2007;35(9):2191–5.

5 Biemond BJ, Levi M, Ten Cate H, et al. Plasminogen activator and plasminogen activator inhibitor I release during experimental endotoxaemia in chimpanzees: effect of interventions in the cytokine and coagulation cascades. *Clin Sci (Lond)* 1995;88(5):587–94.

6 Falanga A. Mechanisms of hypercoagulation in malignancy and during chemotherapy. *Haemostasis* 1998;28(Suppl 3):50–60.

7 Angstwurm MW, Dempfle CE, Spannagl M. New disseminated intravascular coagulation score: A useful tool to predict mortality in comparison with Acute Physiology and Chronic Health Evaluation II and Logistic Organ Dysfunction scores. *Crit Care Med* 2006;34(2):314–20.

8 Toh CH, Hoots WK. The scoring system of the Scientific and Standardisation Committee on Disseminated Intravascular Coagulation of the International Society on Thrombosis and Haemostasis: a 5-year overview. *J Thromb Haemost* 2007;5(3):604–6.

9 Levi M, de Jonge E, van der Poll T, ten Cate H. Disseminated intravascular coagulation. *Thromb Haemost* 1999;82(2):695–705.

10 Feinstein DI. Diagnosis and management of disseminated intravascular coagulation: the role of heparin therapy. *Blood* 1982;60(2):284–7.

11 Schwartz BS, Williams EC, Conlan MG, Mosher DF. Epsilon-aminocaproic acid in the treatment of patients with acute promyelocytic leukemia and acquired

alpha-2-plasmin inhibitor deficiency. *Ann Intern Med* 1986;105(6):873–7.

12 Warren BL, Eid A, Singer P, et al. Caring for the critically ill patient. High-dose antithrombin III in severe sepsis: a randomized controlled trial. *JAMA* 2001;286(15):1869–78.

13 Kienast J, Juers M, Wiedermann CJ, et al. Treatment effects of high-dose antithrombin without concomitant heparin in patients with severe sepsis with or without disseminated intravascular coagulation. *J Thromb Haemost* 2006;4(1):90–7.

14 Bernard GR, Vincent JL, Laterre PF, et al. Efficacy and safety of recombinant human activated protein C for severe sepsis. *N Engl J Med* 2001;344(10):699–709.

15 Ely EW, Laterre PF, Angus DC, et al. Drotrecogin alfa (activated) administration across clinically important subgroups of patients with severe sepsis. *Crit Care Med* 2003;31(1):12–19.

16 Abraham E, Laterre PF, Garg R, et al. Drotrecogin alfa (activated) for adults with severe sepsis and a low risk of death. *N Engl J Med* 2005;353(13):1332–41.

17 Levi M, Levy M, Williams MD, et al. Prophylactic heparin in patients with severe sepsis treated with drotrecogin alfa (activated). *Am J Respir Crit Care Med* 2007;176(5):483–90.

18 Moake JL. Thrombotic microangiopathies. *N Engl J Med* 2002;347(8):589–600.

19 George JN. How I treat patients with thrombotic thrombocytopenic purpura-hemolytic uremic syndrome. *Blood* 2000;96(4):1223–9.

20 Tsai HM. Physiologic cleavage of von Willebrand factor by a plasma protease is dependent on its conformation and requires calcium ion. *Blood* 1996;87(10):4235–44.

21 Furlan M, Robles R, Galbusera M, et al. von Willebrand factor-cleaving protease in thrombotic thrombocytopenic purpura and the hemolytic-uremic syndrome. *N Engl J Med* 1998;339(22):1578–84.

22 Sadler JE, Moake JL, Miyata T, George JN. Recent advances in thrombotic thrombocytopenic purpura. *Hematology Am Soc Hematol Educ Program* 2004:407–23.

23 Ruutu T, Barosi G, Benjamin RJ, et al. Diagnostic criteria for hematopoietic stem cell transplant-associated microangiopathy: results of a consensus process by an International Working Group. *Haematologica* 2007;92(1):95–100.

24 Rock GA, Shumak KH, Buskard NA, et al. Comparison of plasma exchange with plasma infusion in the treatment of thrombotic thrombocytopenic purpura. Canadian Apheresis Study Group. *N Engl J Med* 1991;325(6):393–7.

25 Garvey B. Rituximab in the treatment of autoimmune haematological disorders. *Br J Haematol* 2008;141(2):149–69.

13 Venous thromboembolism

Lori-Ann Linkins and Clive Kearon

Pathogenesis of venous thromboembolism

Virchow was the first to identify stasis, vessel wall injury, and hypercoagulability as the pathogenic triad responsible for thrombosis. This classification of risk factors for venous thromboembolism (VTE) remains valuable. A summary of risk factors for VTE is given in Table 13.1.

Venous stasis

The importance of venous stasis as a risk factor for VTE is demonstrated by the fact that most deep vein thrombi (DVTs) associated with stroke affect the paralyzed leg and most DVT associated with pregnancy affect the left leg, the iliac veins of which are prone to extrinsic compression by the pregnant uterus and the right common iliac artery.

Vessel damage

Venous endothelial damage, as a consequence of accidental injury, manipulation during surgery (e.g. hip replacement), or iatrogenic injury, is an important risk factor for VTE. Hence, three-quarters of proximal DVTs that complicate hip surgery occur in the operated leg, and thrombosis is common with indwelling venous catheters.

Hypercoagulability

A complex balance of naturally occurring coagulation and fibrinolytic factors, and their inhibitors, serve to maintain blood fluidity and hemostasis. Inherited or acquired changes in this balance predispose to thrombosis.

Inherited predisposition to VTE

The most important inherited biochemical disorders that are associated with VTE result from:

- defects in the naturally occurring inhibitors of coagulation: deficiencies of antithrombin, protein C, or protein S; and
- resistance to activated protein C, which is caused by the factor V Leiden mutation in the majority of cases.

The first three of these disorders are rare in the general population (combined prevalence of <1%), have a combined prevalence of approximately 5% in patients with a first episode of VTE, and are associated with a 10- to 40-fold increase in the risk of VTE [1]. The factor V Leiden mutation is common, occurring in approximately 5% of Caucasions and approximately 20% of patients with a first episode of VTE (i.e. an approximate 4-fold increase in VTE risk).

A mutation in the 3′ untranslated region of the prothrombin gene (G20210A), which is associated with an approximately 25% increase in prothrombin levels, occurs in about 2% of Caucasians and approximately 5% of those with a first episode of VTE (i.e. an approximate 2.5-fold increase in risk).

Elevated levels of a number of coagulation factors (I, II, VIII, IX, XI) are associated with thrombosis in a "dose-dependent" manner. It is probable that such elevations are often inherited, with strong evidence for this in the case of factor VIII. Abnormalities of the fibrinolytic system have questionable importance as risk factors for VTE.

Acquired predisposition to VTE

Acquired hypercoagulable states include estrogen therapy, antiphospholipid antibodies (anticardiolipin antibodies and/or lupus anticoagulants), systemic lupus erythematosus, malignancy, combination chemotherapy, and surgery [2]. Patients who develop heparin-induced thrombocytopenia (HIT) also have a very high risk of developing arterial and venous thromboembolism [3]. Finally,

Table 13.1 Risk factors for VTE.

Patient factors:
Previous VTE*
Age over 40
Pregnancy, purpureum
Obesity
Inherited hypercoagulable state

Underlying condition and acquired factors:
Malignancy*
Estrogen therapy
Cancer chemotherapy
Paralysis*
Prolonged immobility
Major trauma*
Lower limb injuries*
Heparin-induced thrombocytopenia
Antiphospholipid antibodies
Lower limb orthopedic surgery*
Surgery requiring general anesthesia >30 minutes

Combinations of factors have at least an additive effect on the risk of VTE.

*Common major risk factors for VTE.

Table 13.2 Natural history of VTE.

- VTE usually starts in the calf veins.
- About 80% of symptomatic DVTs are proximal.
- Two-thirds of asymptomatic DVT detected postoperatively by screening venography are confined to the distal (calf) veins.
- About 20% of symptomatic isolated calf DVTs subsequently extend to the proximal veins, usually within a week of presentation.
- PE usually arises from proximal DVT.
- 70% of patients with symptomatic proximal DVT have asymptomatic PE (high probability lung scans in 40%), and vice versa.
- Only one-quarter of patients with symptomatic PE have symptoms or signs of DVT.
- 50% of untreated symptomatic proximal DVTs are expected to cause symptomatic PE.
- 10% of symptomatic PE are rapidly fatal.
- 30% of untreated symptomatic non-fatal PE will have a fatal recurrence.

hyperhomocysteinemia, whether due to hereditary or acquired causes, is also a risk factor for VTE.

Prevalence and natural history of VTE

VTE is rare before the age of 16 years, likely because the immature coagulation system is resistant to thrombosis. However, the risk of VTE increases exponentially with advancing age (i.e. 1.9-fold per decade), rising from an annual incidence of approximately 30 in 100,000 at 40 years, to 90 in 100,000 at 60 years, and 260 in 100,000 at 80 years. Clinically important components of the natural history of VTE are summarized in Table 13.2.

Management of VTE

Diagnosis of VTE

Objective testing for DVT and pulmonary embolism (PE) is essential because clinical assessment alone is unreliable. Failure to diagnose VTE is associated with a high mortality, whereas inappropriate anticoagula-

tion can lead to serious complications, including fatal hemorrhage.

Diagnosis of DVT

The clinical features of DVT include localized swelling, erythema, tenderness, and distal edema (Plate 13.1). However, these features are nonspecific, and approximately 85% of ambulatory patients with suspected DVT will have another cause for their symptoms. The differential diagnosis for DVT includes:

- cellulitis;
- ruptured Baker cyst;
- muscle tear, muscle cramps, muscle hematoma;
- external venous compression;
- superficial thrombophlebitis; and
- post-thrombotic syndrome (see Plate 13.2).

Venography

Venography is the reference standard test for the diagnosis of DVT. It has advantages over other tests in that it is capable of detecting both proximal vein thrombosis and isolated calf vein thrombosis. However, the disadvantages are that it:

- is invasive, expensive, and requires technical expertise; and
- exposes patients to the risks associated with contrast media, including the potential for an allergic reaction or renal impairment.

Table 13.3 Test results that confirm or exclude DVT.

Diagnostic for first DVT

Venography: Intraluminal filling defect

Venous ultrasound: Noncompressible proximal veins at two or more of the common femoral, popliteal, and calf trifurcation sites

Excludes first DVT

Venography: All deep veins seen, and no intraluminal filling defects

D-dimer: Normal test which has a very high sensitivity (i.e. ≥98%) and at least a moderate specificity (i.e. ≥40%)

Venous ultrasound: Fully compressible proximal veins and (a) low clinical suspicion for DVT at presentation; (b) normal D-dimer test which has a moderately high sensitivity (i.e. ≥85%) and specificity (i.e. ≥70%) at presentation; or (c) normal serial testing (at 7 days)

Low clinical suspicion for DVT at presentation *and* a normal D-dimer test which has moderately high sensitivity (i.e. ≥85%) and specificity (i.e. ≥70%) at presentation

Diagnostic for recurrent DVT

Venography: Intraluminal filling defect

Venous ultrasound: (a) A new noncompressible common femoral or popliteal vein segment or (b) 4.0 mm increase in diameter of the common femoral or popliteal vein during compression compared to a previous recent test

Excludes Recurrent DVT

Venogram: All deep veins seen and no intraluminal filling defects

Venous ultrasound: Normal or ≤1mm increase in diameter of the common femoral or popliteal veins on venous ultrasound compared to a previous test, *and* remains normal (no progression of venous ultrasound) at 2 and 7 days

D-dimer: Normal test which has a very high sensitivity (i.e. ≥98%) and at least a moderate specificity (i.e. ≥40%)

For these reasons, noninvasive tests such as venous ultrasonography and D-dimer testing, alone or in combination with clinical assessment, have largely replaced venography [4]. A summary of the test results that effectively confirm or exclude DVT is given in Table 13.3.

Clinical assessment

Although clinical assessment cannot unequivocally confirm or exclude DVT, clinical evaluation using empiric assessment or a structured clinical model (Table 13.4) can stratify patients as having:

- Low probability of DVT (prevalence of DVT approximately 5%);
- Moderate probability of DVT (prevalence of DVT approximately 25%); or
- High probability of DVT (prevalence of DVT approximately 60%) [5].

Such categorization is useful in guiding the performance and interpretation of objective testing [6].

Compression venous ultrasonography

This is the noninvasive method of choice for diagnosing DVT. The common femoral vein, superficial femoral vein, popliteal vein, and proximal deep calf veins are imaged in real time and compressed with the transducer probe. Inability to compress the vein fully is diagnostic of venous thrombosis.

Venous ultrasonography is highly accurate for the detection of proximal vein thrombosis with a sensitivity of approximately 97%, specificity of approximately 94%, and negative predictive value of approximately 98% in symptomatic patients. If DVT cannot be excluded by a normal proximal venous ultrasound in combination with other results (e.g. low clinical probability or normal D-dimer), a follow-up ultrasound is performed after 1 week to check for extending calf vein thrombosis (present in approximately 2% of patients). If the second ultrasound is normal, the risk of symptomatic VTE during the next 6 months is less than 2%.

The accuracy of venous ultrasonography is substantially lower if its findings are discordant with the clinical assessment [7] and/or if abnormalities are confined to short segments of the deep veins. Ideally, these patients should have a venogram because the result of the venogram will differ from the venous ultrasound in approximately 25% of these cases. If venography is not available, additional testing (e.g. D-dimer, serial venous ultrasonography) may help to clarify the diagnosis and avoid inappropriate anticoagulant therapy.

Venous ultrasonography of the calf veins is more difficult to perform (e.g. sensitivity 70%), and its value is controversial. Some investigators have proposed that a single complete compression ultrasound that includes examination of the calf veins should be used to exclude DVT. Studies using this method have reported an incidence of VTE of 0.5% during 3 months follow-up after a negative examination, establishing that a negative venous ultrasound that includes the

Table 13.4 Wells' Model for determining clinical suspicion of DVT (adapted from Wells et al., *N Engl J Med* 2003;349:1227–35).

Variables	Points
Active cancer (treatment ongoing or within previous 6 months or palliative)	1
Paralysis, paresis or recent plaster immobilization of the lower extremities	1
Bedridden >3 days or major surgery within 4 weeks	1
Localized tenderness along the distribution of the deep venous system	1
Entire leg swollen	1
Calf swelling 3 cm > asymptomatic side (measured 10 cm below tibial tuberosity)	1
Pitting edema confined to the symptomatic leg	1
Collateral dilated superficial veins (non-varicose)	1
Previously documented DVT	1
Alternative diagnosis as likely or more likely than DVT	−2

Pretest probability calculated as follows:

	Total Points
DVT likely	≥2
DVT unlikely	0 or 1

Note: In patients with symptoms in both legs, the more symptomatic leg is used.

calf veins excludes VTE [8]. However, this method has the potential to diagnose calf DVT that would have spontaneously lysed without treatment and to yield false-positive results, thereby exposing patients to the risk of bleeding due to anticoagulant therapy without clear benefit.

D-dimer blood testing

D-dimer is formed when cross-linked fibrin is broken down by plasmin, and levels are usually elevated with DVT and/or PE. Normal levels can help to exclude VTE, but elevated D-dimer levels are nonspecific and have low positive predictive value [9,10].

D-dimer assays differ markedly in their diagnostic properties for VTE. A normal result with a very sensitive D-dimer assay (i.e. sensitivity of approximately 98%) excludes VTE on its own [i.e. it has a high negative predictive value (NPV)]. However, very sensitive D-dimer tests have low specificity (approximately 40%), which limits their use because of high false-positive rates. In order to exclude DVT and/or PE, a normal result with a less sensitive D-dimer assay (i.e. approximately 85%) needs to be *combined* with either a low clinical probability or another objective test that has a high NPV, but is nondiagnostic on its own (e.g., negative venous ultrasound of the proximal veins; Table 13.3) [11]. As less sensitive D-dimer assays are

more specific (approximately 70%), they yield fewer false-positive results.

Specificity of D-dimer decreases with aging and with comorbid illness, such as cancer. Consequently, D-dimer testing may have limited value as a diagnostic test for VTE in hospitalized patients (more false-positive results) and is unhelpful in the early postoperative period.

Computed tomographic (CT) venography and magnetic resonance (MR) venography

CT venography and MR venography have the potential to diagnose DVT in settings where the accuracy of compression ultrasonography is limited (e.g. isolated pelvic DVT, asymptomatic patients). The sensitivity and specificity of CT venography compared with compression ultrasonography for detecting all DVT has been reported between 89% and 100%, and 94% and 100%, respectively [12]. However, given the cost, exposure to radiation, and limited availability of CT venography, this modality currently plays a limited role in the diagnosis of DVT. A meta-analysis of studies comparing MR venography with conventional venography reported a pooled sensitivity of 92% and specificity of 95% of MR venography for proximal DVT [13]. As with CT venography, cost and availability will inhibit the widespread use of MR for diagnosis of acute DVT.

Diagnosis of recurrent DVT

Persistent abnormalities of the deep veins on ultrasound examination are common following DVT. Therefore, diagnosis of recurrent DVT requires evidence of new clot formation. Tests that can diagnose or exclude recurrent DVT are noted in Table 13.3.

Diagnosis of DVT in pregnancy

Pregnant patients with suspected DVT can generally be managed in the same way as nonpregnant patients; although, with the exception of serial impedance plethysmography (now rarely used), diagnostic approaches have not been well evaluated in this population. Pregnant patients with normal noninvasive tests who still have a high clinical suspicion of isolated iliac DVT should be considered for venography or an MRI.

Diagnosis of PE (Plate 13.3)

The clinical features of PE may include:
- pleuritic chest pain,
- shortness of breath,
- syncope,
- hemoptysis, and
- palpitations.

As with DVT, these features are nonspecific, and objective testing must be performed to confirm or exclude the diagnosis of PE.

Pulmonary angiography

This is the reference standard test for the diagnosis of PE (Fig. 13.1). However, it has many of the same limitations as venography. A summary of tests that confirm or exclude PE is given in Table 13.5.

Computed tomographic pulmonary angiography (CTPA)

Spiral CT (also know as helical CT) with peripheral injection of radiographic contrast (CTPA) is the current standard diagnostic test for PE [14,15]. In comparison with ventilation-perfusion lung scanning, CTPA is less likely to be "nondiagnostic" (i.e. approximately 10% vs. 60%) and has the potential to identify an alternative etiology for the patient's symptoms. This technique has a sensitivity of 83%, specificity of 96%, NPV of 95%, and positive predictive value of 86% for PE.

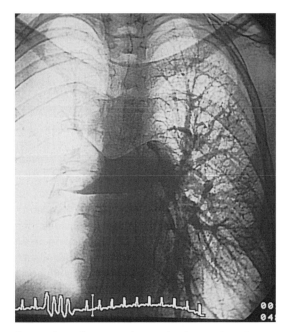

Figure 13.1 Pulmonary angiogram showing massive pulmonary embolism in the right pulmonary artery. Reprinted from Blood in Systemic Disease 1e, Greaves and Makris, 1997, with permission from Elsevier.

Accuracy of CTPA varies according to the size of the largest pulmonary artery involved and according to clinical pretest probability. For example, the positive predictive value of CTPA is 97% for pulmonary emboli in the main or lobar artery, but drops to 68% for segmental arteries, and is lower still for PE in the subsegmental arteries (25%). In patients with a high clinical pretest probability of PE, the positive predictive value of CTPA is 96%, but this value falls to 92% in patients with an intermediate clinical pretest probability of PE, and to 58% in patients with a low clinical pretest probability of PE.

In management studies that used CTPA to diagnose PE, less than 2% of patients who had anticoagulant therapy withheld based on a negative CTPA went on to have symptomatic VTE during follow-up. Taken together, these observations suggest the following:
- A good-quality, normal CTPA excludes PE if clinical suspicion is low or moderate.
- Lobar or larger pulmonary artery intraluminal defects are generally diagnostic for PE.
- Segmental pulmonary artery intraluminal defects are generally diagnostic for PE if clinical suspicion is

Table 13.5 Test results that confirm or exclude PE.

Diagnostic for PE

Pulmonary angiography: Intraluminal filling defect
CTPA: Lobar or main pulmonary artery intraluminal filling
  defect. Segmental intraluminal filling defect and moderate
  or high clinical suspicion
Ventilation-perfusion scan: High probability scan and moderate/
  high clinical suspicion
Diagnostic test positive for DVT: With non-diagnostic
  ventilation-perfusion scan or CTPA

Excludes PE

Pulmonary angiography: Normal
Ventilation-perfusion scan: Normal
D-dimer: Normal test which has a very high sensitivity
  (approximately 98%) and at least a moderate specificity
  (approximately 40%)
CTPA: Negative good quality study *and*
(a) Low or moderate clinical suspicion, *or*
(b) High clinical suspicion and negative bilateral leg ultrasounds
Non-diagnostic CTPA *and* negative bilateral leg ultrasounds *and*
(a) Low clinical suspicion, *or*
(b) Normal D-dimer with sensitivity ≥85%, *or*
(c) Negative bilateral leg ultrasounds at day 7 and day 14
Non-diagnostic ventilation-perfusion scan *and* normal
  proximal venous ultrasound *and*
(a) Low clinical suspicion for PE, *or*
(b) Normal D-dimer test which has at least a moderately
  high sensitivity (i.e. ≥85%) and specificity (i.e. ≥70%)
Low clinical suspicion for PE *and* normal D-dimer which has
  at least a moderately high sensitivity (i.e. ≥85%) and
  specificity (i.e. ≥70%)

CTPA, computed tomographic pulmonary angiography.

Ventilation–perfusion lung scanning

In the past, ventilation–perfusion lung scanning was the initial investigation in patients with suspected PE, and it is still useful in patients with contraindications to x-ray contrast dye (e.g. renal failure) and patients at higher risk for developing breast cancer from radiation exposure (e.g. young women). A normal perfusion scan excludes PE, but is only found in a minority of patients (10–40%). Perfusion defects are nonspecific; only approximately one-third of patients with perfusion defects have PE. The probability that a perfusion defect is caused by PE increases with size and number and the presence of a normal ventilation scan ("mismatched" defect). A lung scan with mismatched segmental or larger perfusion defects is termed "high-probability." A single mismatched defect is associated with a prevalence of PE of approximately 80%. Three or more mismatched defects are associated with a prevalence of PE of approximately 90%. Lung scan findings are highly age-dependent, with a relatively high proportion of normal scans and a low proportion of nondiagnostic scans in younger patients. A high frequency of normal lung scans are also seen in pregnant patients who are investigated for PE.

Clinical assessment:

As with suspected DVT, clinical assessment is useful for categorizing probability of PE (Table 13.6) [16].

D-dimer testing:

As previously discussed when considering the diagnosis of DVT, a normal D-dimer result, alone or in combination with another negative test, can be used to exclude PE (Table 13.5).

Patients with nondiagnostic combinations of noninvasive tests for PE

Patients with nondiagnostic test results for PE at presentation have a prevalence of PE of approximately 20%; therefore, further investigations to exclude PE are required. The first step is to perform venous ultrasonography to look for DVT. If DVT is confirmed, it can be concluded that the patient's symptoms are due to PE. Negative tests for DVT do not rule out PE, but they do reduce the probability of PE and suggest that the short-term risk of recurrent PE is low.

moderate or high, but should be considered nondiagnostic if suspicion is low or there are discordant findings (e.g. negative D-dimer).

• Subsegmental pulmonary artery intraluminal defects are nondiagnostic, and patients with such findings require further testing.

A note of caution: If possible, CTPA should be avoided in younger women (e.g. younger than 40 years) because it delivers a substantial dose of radiation to the chest, which increases the risk of breast cancer.

Table 13.6 Wells' model for determining clinical suspicion of PE (adapted from Wells et al., *Thromb Haemost* 2000;83:416–20).

Variables	Points
Clinical signs and symptoms of deep vein thrombosis (minimum leg swelling and pain with palpation of the deep veins)	3.0
Pulmonary embolism is the most likely diagnosis.	3.0
Heart rate >100 bpm	1.5
Immobilization or surgery in the previous 4 weeks	1.5
Previous DVT/PE	1.5
Hemoptysis	1.0
Malignancy (treatment ongoing or within previous 6 months or palliative)	1.0

Pretest probability calculated as follows:.

	Total Points		Total Points
High	>6	PE likely	≥ 4
Moderate	2–6	PE unlikely	<4
Low	<2		

If imaging studies are negative for DVT, we recommend one of the following management strategies:
• Withhold anticoagulants and perform serial venous ultrasounds to check for evolving proximal DVT (after 1 and 2 weeks). The subsequent risk of recurrent VTE during the next 3 months if serial ultrasounds are negative is <1%, which is similar to that after a normal pulmonary angiogram.
• Perform CTPA or lung scanning if either of these tests has not been performed.
• Repeat CTPA after 24 hours (to reduce the risk of contrast-induced nephrotoxicity).

As an additional precaution, patients who have had PE and/or DVT excluded should routinely be asked to return for reevaluation if symptoms of PE and/or DVT persist or recur. A diagnostic algorithm for PE is given in Fig. 13.2.

Diagnosis of PE in pregnancy

Pregnant patients with suspected PE can be managed similarly to nonpregnant patients, with the following modifications:
• Venous ultrasound of the legs should be performed first followed by ventilation–perfusion lung scanning if there is no DVT.

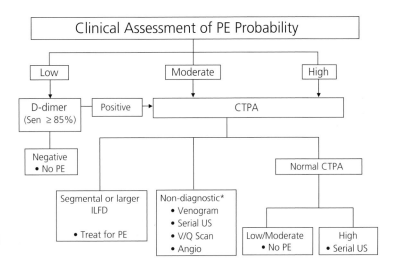

Figure 13.2 Diagnostic algorithm for PE. *Choice of additional diagnostic testing depends on clinical presentation and local expertise. CTPA, computerized tomographic pulmonary angiography (multidetector); US, ultrasound; V/Q, ventilation–perfusion; angio, angiography; ILFD, intraluminal filling defect.

• The amount of radioisotope used for the perfusion scan should be reduced and the duration of scanning extended.

• If pulmonary angiography is performed, the brachial approach with abdominal screening is preferred.

• The use of CTPA in pregnancy is discouraged, primarily because of radiation exposure to the mother.

Treatment of VTE

Initiation of anticoagulant therapy with heparin

Heparin is a highly sulfated glycosoaminoglycan that produces its anticoagulant effect by binding to antithrombin, markedly accelerating the ability of this naturally occurring anticoagulant to inactivate thrombin, activated factor X (factor Xa), and activated factor IX (factor IXa). At therapeutic concentrations, heparin has a half-life of approximately 60 minutes. Heparin binds to a number of plasma proteins, a phenomenon that reduces its anticoagulant effect by limiting its accessibility to antithrombin. The concentration of heparin-binding proteins increases during illness, which contributes to the variability in anticoagulant response in patients with thromboembolism. Because of this variability, response to intravenous heparin should be monitored with the activated partial thromboplastin time (APTT) [17].

Many trials have established that weight-adjusted low-molecular-weight heparin (LMWH) is as safe and effective as adjusted-dose heparin for the treatment of acute VTE. LMWHs are derived from standard, commercial-grade heparin by chemical depolymerization to yield fragments approximately one-third the size of heparin. Depolymerization of heparin results in less binding to heparin-binding proteins and, consequently, improved bioavailability. LMWH therefore has a more predictable anticoagulant response than heparin, which reduces the need for laboratory monitoring. Additional advantages of LMWH are that it can be used to treat patients without hospital admission and need only be injected subcutaneously once daily.

Other potential side effects include HIT and osteoporosis. These complications occur less frequently in patients receiving LMWH. Patients with HIT, with or without associated thrombosis, can be treated with danaparoid, hirudin, or argatroban.

Current clinical practice is to treat patients with acute VTE for a minimum of 5 days with: (1) intravenous heparin in a regimen of at least 30,000 IU/day or 18 IU/kg/hour adjusted to achieve an APTT ratio of 1.5 to 2.5; (2) LMWH at a weight-adjusted dose of either approximately 100 IU/kg every 12 hours or approximately 150–200 IU/kg once daily; (3) subcutaneous heparin administered twice daily, either monitored (initial dose of 17,500 U twice daily or a weight-adjusted dose of 250 U/kg twice daily, with dose adjustment to achieve an APTT ratio of 1.5 to 2.5 six hours after injection) or unmonitored (initial dose of 333 U/kg followed by a twice daily dose of 250 U/kg); or (4) fondaparinux 5.0 mg (2.5 mg if <50 kg; 7.5 mg if >100 kg) once daily by subcutaneous injection [18]. This initial treatment is usually overlapped with a course of oral anticoagulants.

Long-term therapy with oral anticoagulants

Vitamin K antagonists (e.g. warfarin) are coumarin compounds that produce their anticoagulant effect through the production of hemostatically defective, vitamin K-dependent coagulant proteins (prothrombin, factor VII, factor IX, and factor X). The dose of warfarin must be monitored closely because the anticoagulant response is influenced by interactions with other medications and changes in diet [19]. The international normalized ratio (INR) replaced the prothrombin time (PT) for monitoring oral anticoagulant therapy in the 1970s because, unlike the PT, the INR takes into account differences in the responsiveness of thromboplastins to oral anticoagulants. The target INR for treatment of acute VTE is 2.0–3.0.

Oral anticoagulants are typically started on day 1 or 2 of treatment of acute VTE and continued for a length of time determined on an individual basis (discussed below). Long-term treatment with LMWH (50–75% of acute treatment dose) has also been shown to be effective in treating VTE.

Duration of anticoagulant therapy
The optimal duration of anticoagulant therapy is determined by both patient- and disease-related factors. The most important factors are outlined below.

Major transient risk factors
These include recent surgery (within 3 months of surgery with general anesthesia), plaster cast

immobilization of a leg, and hospitalization. The risk of recurrence after stopping anticoagulant therapy is low, approximately 3% in the first year after stopping anticoagulant therapy and 10% in the first 5 years. Three months of anticoagulant therapy is considered adequate for patients with VTE secondary to these risk factors.

Minor transient risk factors

These include estrogen therapy, prolonged travel (i.e. >10 hours), pregnancy, less marked leg injuries, and immobilization. The risk of recurrence after stopping anticoagulant therapy is expected to be higher than in those patients with a major transient risk factor, but lower than those patients with an unprovoked VTE (e.g. approximately 5% in the first year). Three months of anticoagulant therapy is also considered adequate in this setting.

Unprovoked VTE

The risk of recurrent VTE, after 6 months or more of treatment, when anticoagulant therapy is stopped following an unprovoked VTE is approximately 10% in the first year and approximately 30% after 5 years. Given the persistent risk of recurrence, and the greater than 90% risk reduction with oral anticoagulants targeted at an INR of 2.5, long-term anticoagulation is the preferred option for patients who have a low risk of bleeding. The rationale for long-term anticoagulation is even stronger for patients with unprovoked PE. As patients with isolated calf DVT have half the risk of recurrence of those with proximal DVT, 3 months of anticoagulant therapy is considered adequate.

Active malignancy

Patients with cancer who have VTE are three-fold more likely to have recurrent VTE than patients who do not have cancer. The patients at highest risk of recurrence (e.g. patients with metastatic disease, poor mobility, or ongoing chemotherapy) should be considered for indefinite anticoagulant therapy. One large randomized trial has shown that extended duration LMWH (minimum of 6 months) reduces the risk of recurrent VTE in patients with malignancy by approximately 50% compared with conventional anticoagulant treatment (LMWH for 5–7 days followed by oral anticoagulant therapy) [20].

Hypercoagulable states

Patients who have an antiphospholipid antibody (e.g., anticardiolipin antibodies and/or lupus anticoagulant) have a higher risk of recurrence and should receive indefinite anticoagulant therapy. Patients heterozygous for factor V Leiden or the G20210A prothrombin gene mutation do not appear to have a clinically important increased risk for recurrence. The implications for duration of treatment of other abnormalities, such as homozygous factor V Leiden, double heterozygous for factor V Leiden and the G20210A prothrombin gene mutation, as well as elevated levels of clotting factors VIII, IX, XI, and homocysteine, and deficiencies of protein C, protein S, and antithrombin, are uncertain.

PE versus DVT

Patients who present with PE appear to have the same risk of recurrent VTE as those who present with proximal DVT. However, patients who initially present with a symptomatic PE are three times more likely to have a PE as their recurrent VTE event (approximately 60%) than patients who initially present with a symptomatic DVT (approximately 20%). Consequently, the case fatality of recurrent VTE in patients who initially presented with a PE is expected to be two-fold higher (10%) after a PE than after an initial DVT (5%).

Other potential indicators for increased risk of recurrent VTE

Patients who experience a second episode of VTE have an increased risk of recurrence (RR 1.5), and indefinite anticoagulant therapy is recommended if both episodes were unprovoked. Male gender, presence of residual DVT on ultrasound examination, and an elevated D-dimer level after stopping anticoagulant therapy may all be associated with an increased risk of recurrent VTE, but the implication of these factors for duration of anticoagulant therapy is currently uncertain.

Risk of bleeding on anticoagulant therapy

The risk of bleeding on anticoagulants differs markedly among patients, depending on the prevalence of risk factors (e.g. advanced age, previous bleeding or stroke, renal failure, anemia, antiplatelet therapy, malignancy, poor anticoagulant control) [21]. A meta-analysis in patients who were considered average risk for bleeding and received oral anticoagulant therapy for VTE for 3 months (at a target INR range of 2.0–3.0) demonstrated a case fatality of major bleeding of 9% [22]. Consequently, the case fatality with an episode of major bleeding appears to be similar to the case fatality of recurrent VTE after an initial PE, and twice that of a recurrence after an initial DVT. Based on these observations, for a patient to be considered for long-term anticoagulant therapy, the estimated risk of recurrence off anticoagulant therapy needs to be greater than the risk of major bleeding on anticoagulant therapy.

Thrombolytic therapy

Systemic thrombolytic therapy accelerates the rate of resolution of PE, which can be life-saving for patients with hemodynamic compromise (i.e. severe hypotension and/or hypoxia). However, this benefit comes at the cost of about a two- to four-fold increase in the frequency of major bleeding, and a five- to ten-fold increase in intracranial bleeding [23]. One trial conducted in patients with submassive PE demonstrated a significant reduction in the combined endpoint of in-hospital death and clinical deterioration, requiring escalation of treatment for patients who received thrombolysis in addition to heparin in comparison with patients who received heparin alone. The groups did not differ in all-cause mortality, recurrent PE, or major bleeding. Whether thrombolytic therapy decreases the incidence of pulmonary hypertension or recurrences in the long term is yet to be determined. Similarly, thrombolytic therapy may reduce the risk of the post-thrombotic syndrome following DVT, but this does not appear to justify its associated risks. Catheter-based treatments of DVT (e.g., thrombolytic therapy combined with mechanical removal of thrombus) may be more rapidly effective and associated with a lower risk of bleeding, but require further evaluation before they can be recommended.

When thrombolysis is indicated, regimens that are given within 2 hours or less, such as 100 mg rt-PA over 2 hours, appear preferable.

Major contraindications to thrombolytic therapy include:
- active internal bleeding,
- stroke within the past 3 months, and
- intracranial disease.

Relative contraindications include:
- major surgery within the past 10 days,
- recent organ biopsy,
- recent puncture of a noncompressible vessel,
- recent gastrointestinal bleeding,
- liver or renal disease,
- severe arterial hypertension, and
- severe diabetic retinopathy.

Surgical treatment

Pulmonary endarterectomy is beneficial in selected patients with thromboembolic pulmonary hypertension. Urgent pulmonary embolectomy is reserved for patients with shock whose blood pressure cannot be maintained despite administration of thrombolytic therapy or those with an absolute contraindication to thrombolytic therapy.

Inferior vena caval filters

A randomized trial demonstrated that a filter, as an adjunct to anticoagulation in patients with proximal DVT, reduced the rate of PE (asymptomatic and symptomatic) from 4.5% to 1.0% during the 12 days following insertion, with a suggestion of fewer fatal episodes (0% vs. 2%) [24]. However, after 2 years, patients with a filter had a significantly higher rate of recurrent DVT (21% vs. 12%) and only a nonstatistically significant reduction in the frequency of symptomatic PE (3% vs. 6%). After 8 years of follow up, there was a reduction in PE, an increase in DVT, and no difference in DVT and PE combined. This study supports the use of vena caval filters to prevent PE in patients with acute DVT and/or PE who cannot be anticoagulated (i.e. bleeding) but does not support more liberal use of filters. Patients should receive a course of anticoagulation if this subsequently becomes safe, which should be continued for the same duration as if the patient did not have a vena caval filter in situ. A rare late complication of IVC filters is extensive IVC thrombosis (Plate 13.4).

Treatment of VTE during pregnancy

Heparin and LMWH do not cross the placenta and are safe for the fetus, whereas oral anticoagulants cross the placenta and can cause fetal bleeding and malformations. Therefore, pregnant women with acute VTE should be treated with therapeutic doses of subcutaneous heparin or LMWH throughout pregnancy. Care should be taken to avoid delivery while the mother is therapeutically anticoagulated; one management approach involves stopping subcutaneous heparin 24 hours prior to induction of labor and switching to intravenous heparin if there is a high risk of embolism. After delivery, warfarin, which is safe for infants of nursing mothers, should be given (with initial heparin overlap) for 6 weeks and until a minimum of 3 months of treatment has been completed.

Prevention of VTE

VTE prophylaxis following surgery

Surgical patients can be stratified according to their risk factors for VTE into low-, moderate-, and high-risk categories [25].

Low risk

This category includes patients under 40 years of age who undergo uncomplicated surgery and have no additional risk factors. The rate of asymptomatic proximal DVT detected by surveillance bilateral venography is 0.4%, and the rate of symptomatic PE and fatal PE is 0.2% and <0.01%, respectively. Recommended VTE prophylaxis in this group is limited to early mobilization.

Moderate risk

This category includes patients over 40 years of age who undergo prolonged and/or complicated surgery or have additional minor risk factors. The rate of asymptomatic proximal DVT is 5%, and the rate of symptomatic PE and fatal PE is 2% and 0.5%, respectively. Recommended VTE prophylaxis in this group includes unfractionated heparin (5000 U/day preoperatively, and two to three times daily postoperatively), LMWH (approximately 3000 U/day), or graduated compression stockings alone or in combination with pharmacologic methods.

High risk

This category includes patients who undergo major surgery for malignancy, hip or knee surgery, or those who have a history of previous VTE. The rate of asymptomatic proximal DVT is 15%, and the rate of symptomatic PE and fatal PE is 5% and 1%, respectively. Recommended VTE prophylaxis in this group includes LMWH (4000 to 6000 U/day, as a single or divided dose); warfarin (usually started postoperatively and adjusted to achieve an INR of 2.0–3.0); or fondaparinux (2.5 mg once daily, usually started postoperatively) or intermittent pneumatic compression devices alone or in combination with other methods of prophylaxis. Mechanical methods of prophylaxis should be used in patients who have a moderate or high risk of VTE if anticoagulants are contraindicated (e.g. neurosurgical patients).

Pharmacologic agents for VTE prophylaxis in orthopedic surgery

Meta-analyses support the finding that LMWH is more effective than heparin following orthopedic surgery and is associated with a similar frequency of bleeding. Warfarin (target INR 2–3 for approximately 7–10 days) is less effective than LMWH at preventing DVTs that are detected by venography soon after surgery, but appears to be similarly effective at preventing symptomatic VTE over a 3-month period. An additional 3 or 4 weeks of LMWH after hospital discharge further reduces the frequency of symptomatic VTE after orthopedic surgery (from 3.3% to 1.3%). There is evidence that aspirin reduces the risk of postoperative VTE by one-third. However, as warfarin and LMWH are expected to be more effective (at least a two-thirds reduction in VTE), aspirin alone is not recommended during the initial postoperative period. Fondaparinux has been shown to be more effective than LMWH following major orthopedic surgery but may cause marginally more bleeding.

VTE prophylaxis in medical patients

Primary prophylaxis with anticoagulants and/or mechanical methods should be used in hospitalized patients who have a moderate or high risk of VTE. In recent years, three large, randomized, controlled trials have shown that LMWH (enoxaparin 40 mg or dalteparin 5000 IU subcutaneously once daily for 10 days) and fondaparinux (2.5 mg once daily) reduce the rate of VTE by about 50% (range 45–63%) compared with placebo in acutely ill medical patients.

References

1 Kearon C, Crowther M, Hirsh J. Management of patients with hereditary hypercoagulable disorders. *Annu Rev Med* 2000;51:169–85.

2 Anderson FA Jr, Spencer FA. Risk factors for venous thromboembolism. *Circulation* 2003;107:I9–16.

3 Warkentin TE, Greinacher A, Koster A, Lincoff AM. Treatment and prevention of heparin-induced thrombocytopenia: American College of Chest Physicians Evidence-Based Clinical Practice Guidelines (8th Edition). *Chest* 2008;133:340S–80S.

4 Kearon C, Julian JA, Newman TE, Ginsberg JS. Noninvasive diagnosis of deep venous thrombosis. McMaster Diagnostic Imaging Practice Guidelines Initiative. *Ann Intern Med* 1998;128:663–77.

5 Wells PS, Anderson DR, Rodger M, et al. Evaluation of D-dimer in the diagnosis of suspected deep-vein thrombosis. *N Engl J Med* 2003;349:1227–35.

6 Wells PS, Owen C, Doucette S, Fergusson D, Tran H. Does this patient have deep vein thrombosis? *JAMA* 2006;295:199–207.

7 Wheeler HB, Hirsh J, Wells P, Anderson FA Jr. Diagnostic tests for deep vein thrombosis. Clinical usefulness depends on probability of disease. *Arch Intern Med* 1994;154:1921–8.

8 Stevens SM, Elliott CG, Chan KJ, Egger MJ, Ahmed KM. Withholding anticoagulation after a negative result on duplex ultrasonography for suspected symptomatic deep venous thrombosis. *Ann Intern Med* 2004;140:985–91.

9 Kelly J, Rudd A, Lewis RR, Hunt BJ. Plasma D-dimers in the diagnosis of venous thromboembolism. *Arch Intern Med* 2002;162:747–56.

10 Stein PD, Hull RD, Patel KC, et al. D-dimer for the exclusion of acute venous thrombosis and pulmonary embolism: a systematic review. *Ann Intern Med* 2004;140:589–602.

11 Fancher TL, White RH, Kravitz RL. Combined use of rapid D-dimer testing and estimation of clinical probability in the diagnosis of deep vein thrombosis: systematic review. *Br Med J* 2004;329:821.

12 Kanne JP, Lalani TA. Role of computed tomography and magnetic resonance imaging for deep venous thrombosis and pulmonary embolism. *Circulation* 2004;109:I15–21.

13 Sampson FC, Goodacre SW, Thomas SM, van Beek EJ. The accuracy of MRI in diagnosis of suspected deep vein thrombosis: systematic review and meta-analysis. *Eur Radiol* 2007;17:175–81.

14 Stein PD, Fowler SE, Goodman LR, et al. Multidetector computed tomography for acute pulmonary embolism. *N Engl J Med* 2006;354:2317–27.

15 Roy PM, Colombet I, Durieux P, Chatellier G, Sors H, Meyer G. Systematic review and meta-analysis of strategies for the diagnosis of suspected pulmonary embolism. *Br Med J* 2005;331:259.

16 Wells PS, Anderson DR, Rodger M, et al. Excluding pulmonary embolism at the bedside without diagnostic imaging: management of patients with suspected pulmonary embolism presenting to the emergency department by using a simple clinical model and d-dimer. *Ann Intern Med* 2001;135:98–107.

17 Hirsh J, Bauer KA, Donati MB, Gould M, Samama MM, Weitz JI. Parenteral anticoagulants: American College of Chest Physicians Evidence-Based Clinical Practice Guidelines (8th Edition). *Chest* 2008;133:141S–59S.

18 Kearon C, Kahn SR, Agnelli G, Goldhaber S, Raskob GE, Comerota AJ. Antithrombotic therapy for venous thromboembolic disease: American College of Chest Physicians Evidence-Based Clinical Practice Guidelines (8th Edition). *Chest* 2008;133:454S–545S.

19 Ansell J, Hirsh J, Hylek E, Jacobson A, Crowther M, Palareti G. Pharmacology and management of the vitamin K antagonists: American College of Chest Physicians Evidence-Based Clinical Practice Guidelines (8th Edition). *Chest* 2008;133:160S–98S.

20 Lee AY, Levine MN, Baker RI, Bowden C, Kakkar AK, Prins M, et al. Low-molecular-weight heparin versus a coumarin for the prevention of recurrent venous thromboembolism in patients with cancer. *N Engl J Med* 2003;349:146–53.

21 Schulman S, Beyth RJ, Kearon C, Levine MN. Hemorrhagic complications of anticoagulant and thrombolytic treatment: American College of Chest Physicians Evidence-Based Clinical Practice Guidelines (8th Edition). *Chest* 2008;133:257S–98S.

22 Linkins LA, Choi PT, Douketis JD. Clinical impact of bleeding in patients taking oral anticoagulant therapy for venous thromboembolism: a meta-analysis. *Ann Intern Med* 2003;139:893–900.

23 Agnelli G, Becattini C, Kirschstein T. Thrombolysis vs heparin in the treatment of pulmonary embolism: a clinical outcome-based meta-analysis. *Arch Intern Med* 2002;162:2537–41.

24 Decousus H, Leizorovicz A, Parent F, et al. A clinical trial of vena caval filters in the prevention of pulmonary embolism in patients with proximal deep-vein thrombosis. Prevention du Risque d'Embolie Pulmonaire par Interruption Cave Study Group. *N Engl J Med* 1998;338:409–15.

25 Geerts WH, Bergqvist D, Pineo GF, et al. Prevention of venous thromboembolism: American College of Chest Physicians Evidence-Based Clinical Practice Guidelines (8th Edition). *Chest* 2008;133:381S–453S.

14 | Myeloproliferative neoplasms: Essential thrombocythemia, polycythemia vera, and primary myelofibrosis

Ayalew Tefferi

Introduction

Myeloproliferative neoplasms (MPN) are a category of chronic myeloid malignancies that includes chronic myelogenous leukemia (CML), polycythemia vera (PV), essential thrombocythemia (ET), primary myelofibrosis (PMF), and other less known clinico-pathologic entities [1]. From a pathogenetic standpoint, all members of the MPN arise out of an acquired oncogenic mutation that occurs at the stem cell level. Therefore, the MPN are often referred to as clonal stem cell diseases. However, at present, the disease-causing mutation is known only for CML and involves the cytoplasmic tyrosine kinase ABL (*BCR-ABL*). In early 2005, an activating Janus kinase 2 mutation (*JAK2*V617F) was discovered in PV, ET, and PMF [2]. In 2006 and 2007, additional *JAK2* (exon 12 mutations) and *MPL* (thrombopoietin receptor) mutations were described in these diseases [2]. Current estimates of *JAK2* and *MPL* mutational frequencies in PV are 100% and 0%, for ET 50% and 5%, and for PMF 70% and 10%, respectively.

Clinical presentation

Annual incidence rates for ET, PV, and PMF are estimated at 2.5, 1.0, and 0.5, respectively. Prevalence figures are much higher, especially in cases of ET and PV because of their relatively good prognosis. The median age at diagnosis for all of these three MPN is approximately 60 years. In general, clinical manifestations are similar in ET and PV but different than those in PMF.

Essential thrombocythemia and polycythemia vera

Most patients with ET or PV are asymptomatic at presentation. Approximately one-third of patients present with microvascular symptoms: headaches, lightheadedness, visual symptoms such as blurring and scotomata, palpitations, chest pain, erythromelalgia, and distal paresthesias. Erythromelalgia is the most dramatic vasomotor symptom, characterized by erythema, warmth, and pain in distal extremities. Other non-life-threatening complications in ET and PV include constitutional symptoms, pruritus that is often provoked by water contact, superficial thrombophlebitis, minor mucocutaneous bleeding, and increased propensity for first trimester miscarriage. At least two-thirds of PV patients have splenomegaly at diagnosis.

PV and ET are associated with an increased risk of thrombosis and bleeding. Table 14.1 (at diagnosis) [3–14] and Table 14.2 (during follow-up) [3–15] present incidence figures of "major" thrombotic events in a selected series of large studies in PV and ET. Major thrombosis at diagnosis ranges from 9.7% to 29.4% for ET and 34% to 38.6% for PV; the corresponding figures for major thrombosis during follow-up are 8% to 30.7% for ET and 8.1% to 19% for PV.

In general, arterial events (strokes, transient ischemic attacks, myocardial infarctions, angina pectoris, peripheral artery occlusions) are more prevalent than venous events (pulmonary embolism, deep vein thrombosis, hepatic/portal/mesenteric vein thrombosis, sagittal sinus thrombosis, retinal vein thrombosis) in ET or PV. For example, in one recent study of 470 patients with either ET or PV, who experienced first

Table 14.1 Thrombotic, hemorrhagic, and microvascular events in PV and ET reported at diagnosis

	n	Major thrombosis (%)	Major arterial thrombosis* (%)	Major venous thrombosis* (%)	MVD (%)	Total bleeds (% major)
ET						
Fenaux, 1990	147	18	83	17	34	18 (4)
Cortelazzo, 1990	100	11	91	9	30	9 (3)
Colombi, 1991	103	23.3	87.5	12.5	33	3.6 (1.9)
Besses, 1999	148	25	NA	NA	29	6.1 (NA)
Jensen, 2000	96	14	85	15	23	9 (5.2)
Chim, 2005	231	13	96.7	3.3	5.6	3 (1.7)
Wolanskyj, 2006	150	21.3	NA	NA	13.3	9.3
Campbell, 2005	776	9.7	82.7	17.3	NA	NA
Carobbio, 2006	439	29.4	68.2	31.8	NA	NA
PV						
GISP, 1995[†]	1213	34	~66[†]	~33[†]	NA	NA
Passamonti, 2000	163	34	64	36	24	3 (NA)
Marchioli, 2005	1638	38.6	~75	~25	5.3	8.1 (4.8)

With permission from Tefferi and Elliott [20].
Abbreviations: MVD, microvascular disturbances; NA, not available.
*Percent of total major thrombotic events.
[†] Estimate per Gruppo Italiano Studio Policitemia (GISP).

thrombosis, the event was arterial in 70% and venous in 30% of cases [16]. Specifically, cerebrovascular accidents (CVA) occurred in 184 cases (39%), coronary syndrome in 102 (22%), lower extremity deep vein thrombosis (DVT) in 102 (22%), and other DVT in 40 (9%) [16]. Also, thrombosis is more prevalent, as well as more relevant as a cause of death, than bleeding in these disorders.

DVT in MPN includes catastrophic abdominal vein thrombosis (AVT) [17]. The incidence of AVT in ET was recently reported at 4% (19 cases among 469 consecutive patients with ET) [17]. In another study of 501 patients with MPDs, including 23 cases of ET, 18 cases of AVT were identified, and the disease-specific rates were 10% for PV, 13% for ET, and 1% for chronic idiopathic myelofibrosis [17].

It has long been recognized that a substantial proportion of "idiopathic" AVT might represent latent MPN. This contention was recently affirmed by the demonstration of a *JAK2* mutation in such cases; in a recent study of 241 patients presenting with AVT, including Budd-Chiari syndrome and portal vein throm-

bosis, *JAK2*V617F was found in 45% of Budd-Chiari syndrome and 34% of portal vein thrombosis cases, whereas *JAK2* exon 12 and *MPL*515 mutations were not detected [18]. However, more than 90% of the cases could have been diagnosed with bone marrow examination or other diagnostic methods, although mutation screening would have made such investigations unnecessary in approximately 40% of the patients. Notably, the presence of *JAK2*V617F in AVT did not affect survival. In a large Mayo Clinic study ($n = 664$) of unexplained nonsplanchnic venous and arterial thrombosis, the incidence of JAK2V617F was too low (<1%) to warrant mutation screening as part of the hypercoagulable workup [19].

Primary myelofibrosis

Anemia, often requiring red blood cell transfusions, and marked splenomegaly are the typical clinical hallmarks of PMF. Spleen and liver enlargement in PMF is secondary to extramedullary hematopoiesis. Patients also suffer from hypercatabolic symptoms (profound fatigue, weight loss, night sweats, low-grade

Table 14.2 Thrombotic and hemorrhagic events in PV and ET reported at follow-up.

	n	Major thrombosis (%)	Major arterial thrombosis (%)*	Major venous thrombosis (%)*	Total bleeds (% major)	% of deaths from hemorrhage	% of deaths from thrombosis
ET							
Fenaux, 1990	147	13.6	86	14	NA (0.7)	0	25
Cortelazzo, 1990	100	20	71	29	NA (1)	0	100
Colombi, 1991	103	10.6	91	9	8.7 (5.8)	0	27.3
Besses, 1999	148	22.3	94	6	11.5 (4.1)	0	13.3
Jensen, 2000	96	16.6	69	31	13.6 (7.3)	3.3	16.7
Chim, 2005	231	10	91.3	8.7	6.5 (5.2)	10	10
Passamonti, 2004	435	10.6	71.7	28.3	NA	1	26
Wolanskyj, 2006	150	30.7	NA	NA	10%	NA	NA
Campbell, 2005	776	8	74.2	25.8	4.1 (3.5)		
Carobbio, 2006	439	17.8	65.4	34.6	NA	NA	NA
PV							
GISP, 1995[†]	1213	19	62.5	37.5	NA	2.6	29.6
Passamonti, 2000	163	18.4	80	15	NA (1.8)	6	19
Marchioli, 2005	1638	13.4	57.1	42.9	2.9 (0.8)	4.3	41
Passomonti, 2004	396	8.1	59.4	40.6	NA	2	20

With permission from Tefferi and Elliott [20].

*Percent of total major thrombotic events.

[†] GISP, Gruppo Italiano Studio Policitemia.

fever), peripheral edema (from venous compression), diarrhea, early satiety (from gastric compression), and portal hypertension. Splenomegaly in PMF may be complicated by splenic infarction manifested by left upper quadrant pain and referred left shoulder pain. Extramedullary hematopoiesis can also occur at other sites, including lymph nodes, skin, pleura, peritoneum, lung, and the paraspinal and epidural spaces. Acute myeloid leukemia (AML) occurs in approximately 20% of PMF patients over the first 10 years of disease.

Pathogenesis of thrombosis and bleeding in ET and PV

The pathogenesis of microvascular symptoms in ET and PV is believed to involve abnormal thromboxane A_2 (TX A_2) generation and platelet–endothelial interactions [20]. In regards to thrombosis, recent information implicates granulocytes rather than platelets as being more important, but both platelets and endothelial cells might have a subordinating role [20]. In this regard, patients with ET or PV display increased baseline/induced platelet P-selectin expression, platelet–granulocyte/platelet–monocyte complexes, granulocyte activation, and baseline/lipopolysaccharide-induced expression of tissue factor (TF) by both monocytes and neutrophils [20]. Similarly, a recent study suggested in vivo down-regulation of both neutrophil TF expression and number of neutrophil–platelet complexes by hydroxyurea therapy, in patients with either ET or PV [20].

Study after study has failed to show a definite association between platelet count per se and either thrombosis or bleeding in PV or ET [20]. On the other hand, it is now well established that approximately 50% of patients with MPN-associated extreme thrombocytosis display laboratory evidence of acquired von Willebrand syndrome (AVWS) whose origin might involve a platelet count-dependent increased proteolysis of high-molecular-weight von Willebrand protein [21]. However, the degree of the abnormality is seldom clinically relevant, (i.e. associated with bleeding or a ristocetin cofactor activity of <30%) [21].

Other qualitative platelet defects in ET are believed to play a minor role in disease-associated hemorrhage and include defects in epinephrine-, collagen-, and ADP-induced platelet aggregation, decreased ATP secretion, and acquired storage pool deficiency that results from abnormal in vivo platelet activation. Spontaneous platelet aggregation is another characteristic finding in MPN, but it has no apparent clinical relevance.

Diagnosis

Table 14.3 outlines the current WHO diagnostic criteria for PV, ET, and PMF [1]. Figures 14.1–14.3 provide WHO-based diagnostic algorithms for these diseases [1]. Virtually all patients with PV carry a *JAK2* mutation. Therefore, peripheral blood *JAK2*V617F screening is currently the preferred initial test for evaluating a patient with suspected PV (Fig. 14.1). The concomitant determination of serum erythropoietin (Epo) level is encouraged in order to minimize the consequences of false-positive or false-negative molecular test results. Mutation screening for an exon 12 *JAK2* mutation and bone marrow examination should be considered in a *JAK2*V617F-negative patient who displays subnormal serum Epo levels (Fig. 14.1). Because *JAK2*V617F also occurs in approximately 50% of patients with either ET or PMF, it is reasonable to include mutation screening in the diagnostic work-up of both thrombocytosis (Fig. 14.2) and bone marrow fibrosis (Fig. 14.3).

Prognosis

Median survival in both ET and PV exceeds 15 years, and the 10-year risk of developing either myelofibrosis (MF; <4% and <10%, respectively) or AML (;2% and <6%, respectively) is relatively low. Compared with both PV and ET, PMF has a significantly worse prognosis with a median survival of 6 years and 10-year risk of AML estimated at 20%.

Several studies have identified advanced age (>60 years) and thrombosis history as risk factors for thrombosis in both PV and ET (Table 14.4) [20]. In ET, two recent, large, single-institution studies ($n = 322$ and $n = 439$, respectively) [9,14] confirmed the prothrombotic effect of advanced age (≥60 years) and history of thrombosis, although the latter association was significant in regards to arterial but not venous events in one of the two studies [9]. In addition, both studies identified leukocytosis (≥15 × 10^9/L in one study [9] and >8.7 × 10^9/L in the other [14]), but neither thrombocytosis nor the presence of *JAK2*V617F, as an additional independent risk factor for thrombosis. Similarly, the presence of cardiovascular risk factors did not modify thrombosis risk in one of the two studies [9], as well as in another recent study [16].

In PV, a series of reports from the European Collaboration on Low-Dose Aspirin in Polycythemia Vera (ECLAP) group have addressed multiple clinical issues, including thrombotic complications. In their most recent report ($n = 1638$), Landolfi and colleagues, on behalf of ECLAP, confirmed the strong association between advanced age and thrombosis and, in addition, identified leukocytosis (>15 × 10^9/L as opposed to ≤10 × 10^9/L) as an independent predictor of myocardial infarction [20]. History of arterial or venous events predicted recurrence of a similar vascular event. In contrast, neither the platelet count nor the hematocrit level affected thrombosis risk. Similarly, controlled prospective studies are needed to clarify the prognostic relevance of hereditary and acquired causes of thrombophilia, pattern of X chromosome inactivation in granulocyte-derived DNA (i.e. monoclonal vs. polyclonal), and altered PRV-1, platelet Mpl, or EEC expression [20].

Current evidence is inconclusive regarding the prognostic relevance of *JAK2* or *MPL* mutations in MPNs. In ET, overall or leukemia-free survival does not appear to be affected by either the presence of *JAK2*V617F or its allele burden. The impact on the risk of thrombosis or fibrotic transformation is less clear [20]. Equally unclear is the prognostic relevance of *JAK2*V617F allele burden in PV where a higher mutant allele burden is implicated by some but not by others as an adverse prognostic factor for fibrotic

Table 14.3 The 2008 World Health Organization diagnostic criteria for PV, ET, and PMF [29].

		2008 WHO Diagnostic Criteria		
		PV*	ET*	PMF*
Major criteria	1	Hgb > 18.5 g/dL (men) > 16.5 g/dL (women) *or* Hgb > 17 g/dL (men), or > 15 g/dL (women) if associated with a sustained increase of ≥2 g/dL from baseline that cannot be attributed to correction of iron deficiency *or*[‡]	1 Platelet count ≥ 450 × 10⁹/L	1 Megakaryocyte proliferation and atypia[†] accompanied by either reticulin and/or collagen fibrosis. *or* In the absence of reticulin fibrosis, the megakaryocyte changes must be accompanied by increased marrow cellularity, granulocytic proliferation, and often decreased erythropoiesis (i.e. pre-fibrotic PMF).
	2	Presence of *JAK2*V617F or similar mutation	2 Megakaryocyte proliferation with large and mature morphology. No or little granulocyte or erythroid proliferation.	2 Not meeting WHO criteria for CML, PV, MDS, or other myeloid neoplasm
			3 Not meeting WHO criteria for CML, PV, PMF, MDS, or other myeloid neoplasm	3 Demonstration of *JAK2*V617F or other clonal marker *or* no evidence of reactive marrow fibrosis
			4 Demonstration of *JAK2*V617F or other clonal marker *or* no evidence of reactive thrombocytosis	
Minor criteria	1	BM trilineage myeloproliferation		1 Leukoerythroblastosis
	2	Subnormal serum Epo level		2 Increased serum LDH
	3	EEC growth		3 Anemia
				4 Palpable splenomegaly

*Diagnosis of PV requires meeting either both major criteria and one minor criterion *or* the first major criterion and two minor criteria; diagnosis of ET requires meeting all four major criteria; and diagnosis of PMF requires meeting all three major criteria and two minor criteria.

†Small to large megakaryocytes with aberrant nuclear/cytoplasmic ratio and hyperchromatic and irregularly folded nuclei and dense clustering.

‡or Hgb or Hct >99th percentile of reference range for age, sex, or altitude of residence *or* red cell mass >25% above mean normal predicted.

Abbreviations: Hgb, hemoglobin; Hct, hematocrit; Epo, erythropoietin; EEC, endogenous erythroid colony; WHO, World Health Organization; CML, chronic myelogenous leukemia; MDS, myelodysplastic syndrome; LDH, lactate dehydrogenase.

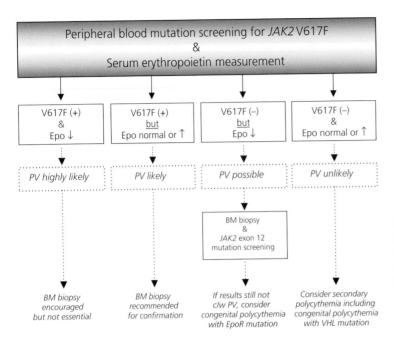

Figure 14.1 Diagnostic algorithm for suspected PV (with permission from Tefferi and Vardiman [1]). *Abbreviations*: PV, polycythemia vera; SP, secondary polycythemia; CP, congenital polycythemia; BM, bone marrow; V617F, JAK2V617F; Epo, erythropoietin; EpoR, erythropoietin receptor; VHL, von Hippel-Lindau; c/w, consistent with.

transformation, thrombosis, and need for chemotherapy [20]. In PMF, *JAK2*V617F presence was associated with inferior survival in one but not in another study [20]. Similarly divergent results were reported in terms of leukemic transformation rate and need for chemotherapy or splenectomy.

Treatment

PV and ET

Controlled studies have shown significant reductions in the incidence of thrombotic complications in

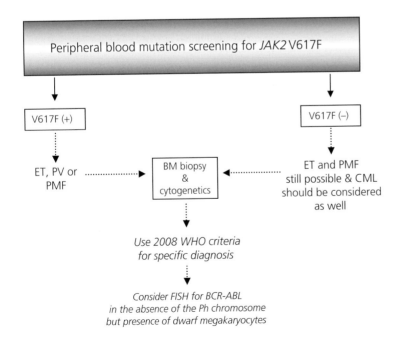

Figure 14.2 Diagnostic algorithm for suspected ET (with permission from Tefferi and Vardiman [1]). *Abbreviatioins*: PV, polycythemia vera; ET, essential thrombocythemia; PMF, primary myelofibrosis; CML, chronic myeloid leukemia; MDS, myelodysplastic syndrome; MPN, myeloproliferative neoplasm; WHO, World Health Organization; RT, reactive thrombocytosis; FISH, fluorescent in situ hybridization; Ph, Philadelphia; BM, bone marrow; V617F, JAK2V617F.

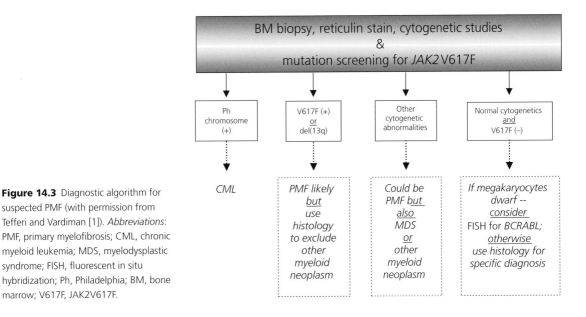

Figure 14.3 Diagnostic algorithm for suspected PMF (with permission from Tefferi and Vardiman [1]). *Abbreviations*: PMF, primary myelofibrosis; CML, chronic myeloid leukemia; MDS, myelodysplastic syndrome; FISH, fluorescent in situ hybridization; Ph, Philadelphia; BM, bone marrow; V617F, JAK2V617F.

patients with PV treated with low-dose aspirin [22] and in high-risk patients with ET treated with hydroxyurea [23]. Also, there is compelling, although not controlled, evidence to support the use of phlebotomy in all patients with PV and hydroxyurea in those with high-risk disease. Taken together, current recommendations for treatment in PV include phlebotomy and low-dose aspirin in all patients and the addition of hydroxyurea in high-risk disease (Table 14.4). In this regard, it is generally recommended but not mandated to keep the hematocrit level below 45% in men and 42% in women during phlebotomy for PV. This treatment strategy, with the exception of phlebotomy, also applies to ET (Table 14.4). Finally, new evidence suggests that aspirin therapy in PV and ET might be most effective in preventing CVA, whereas cytoreductive therapy and systemic anticoagulation might be needed for minimizing the risk of coronary event and DVT, respectively [16].

The use of aspirin in both PV and ET requires the absence of clinically relevant AVWS, which might occur in patients with extreme thrombocytosis (platelet count >1000 × 10⁹/L). On the other hand, extreme thrombocytosis neither defines high-risk disease nor warrants the use of cytoreductive therapy [24]. The frequently cited association of extreme thrombocytosis with gastrointestinal bleeding is based on anecdotal observation and may, in some instances, be attributed to occult AVWS.

Very few studies in PV or ET have directly compared the efficacy of other cytoreductive agents with that of hydroxyurea. In ET, hydroxyurea (plus aspirin) was shown to be superior to anagrelide (plus aspirin) in terms of preventing arterial thrombosis, and anagrelide performed better in terms of venous thrombosis; in addition, anagrelide therapy was less tolerated and was associated with significantly more occurrences of severe hemorrhage and fibrotic transformation [25]. Non-controlled studies have shown the efficacy of pipobroman or busulfan in both PV and ET, and these agents might be considered in patients failing hydroxyurea therapy. Single-agent activity, sometimes associated with modest reductions in JAK2V617F allele burden, has also been demonstrated for alpha interferon (α-IFN) in PV and ET. However, there is no controlled study that proves the drug's superiority over hydroxyurea.

There is an increased rate of first-trimester miscarriages (approximately 30%) in both ET and PV, and a recent study suggested that this risk might be higher in JAK2V617F-positive patients [26]. However, there is no controlled evidence to suggest that specific treatment influences outcome. Other pregnancy-associated complications in ET and PV are infrequent, and

Table 14.4 Current management and risk stratification in ET, PV, and PMF.

Risk categories	ET	PV	PMF Age <50 years	PMF Age ≥50 years
Low	Low-dose aspirin	Low-dose aspirin + Phlebotomy	Observation *or* Experimental drug therapy	Observation *or* Experimental drug therapy
Low but with extreme thrombocytosis* for ET and PV Intermediate for PMF	Low-dose aspirin[†]	Low-dose aspirin[†] + Phlebotomy	Experimental drug therapy *or* RIC[‡] transplant	Experimental drug therapy *or* Conventional drug therapy
High	Low-dose aspirin + Hydroxyurea	Low-dose aspirin + Phlebotomy + Hydroxyurea	Experimental drug therapy *or* Full transplant	Experimental drug therapy *or* RIC[‡] transplant

*Extreme thrombocytosis is defined as a platelet count of 1000×10^9/L or more.
[†]Clinically significant acquired von Willebrand syndrome (ristocetin co-factor activity <30%) should be excluded before the use of aspirin in patients with a platelet count of over 1000×10^9/L.
[‡]RIC, reduced intensity conditioning.

Risk stratification for ET and PV:
High risk: Age ≥60 years *or* previous thrombosis
Low risk: Neither of the above

Risk stratification of PMF according to the Mayo Prognostic Scoring System:[30]
(One point each for hemoglobin <10 g/dL, leukocyte count <4 or >30×10^9/L, platelet count <100×10^9/L, or monocyte count ≥1×10^9/L)
Low risk: score 0
Intermediate risk: score 1
High risk: score ≥2

platelet count usually decreases substantially during the second and third trimesters. Therefore, at present, low-risk pregnant patients with ET or PV might be managed the same way as their nonpregnant counterparts. In high-risk disease, α-IFN is the drug of choice in women of childbearing age wishing to be pregnant, because of the theoretical risk of teratogenicity associated with the use of other cytoreductive agents.

Myelofibrosis

Both myeloablative and reduced intensity conditioning (RIC) transplant have been employed in patients with MF [27]. Regarding the former, a retrospective study of 66 patients revealed 5-year survival of 62% in patients younger than 45 years of age and 14% in those that were older, although other investigators have reported better survival figures in older patients [27]. In the most recent communication of RIC transplant in MF, 1-year mortality was 19%, and 32% of the patients experienced chronic graft versus host disease [27]. The 3-year overall survival, event-free survival, and relapse rate were 70%, 55%, and 29%, respectively. Taken together, it is reasonable to consider ASCT in high-risk MF: full myeloablative conditioning in patients below 45 years of age and RIC in older patients (Table 14.4).

Drugs for PMF-associated anemia include androgens, prednisone, erythropoiesis stimulating agents, and danazol [28]. Also, low-dose thalidomide in combination with prednisone has recently been identified as an effective approach for MF-associated anemia, thrombocytopenia, and splenomegaly, with approximately a 50% overall response rate [28]. Lenalidomide, a thalidomide analog, has also been evaluated in MF, and a 20–30% response rate in both anemia and splenomegaly was documented [28]. Lenalidomide response rates were higher and quality of responses most impressive in MF patients with the del(5q) abnormality.

Hydroxyurea is the current drug of choice for controlling splenomegaly, leukocytosis, or thrombocytosis in PMF [28]. Other drugs that have been used in a similar setting include busulfan, melphalan, and 2-chlorodeoxyadenosine. In contrast, α-IFN has limited therapeutic value in MF. Drug-refractory symptomatic splenomegaly may necessitate splenectomy that often alleviates mechanical symptoms and may also benefit approximately 25% of patients with transfusion-dependent anemia [28]. However, the procedure might be associated with 9% mortality and 25% morbidity, in the form of accelerated hepatomegaly and extreme thrombocytosis. Radiation therapy is most useful in the treatment of non-hepatosplenic extramedullary hematopoiesis. Finally, in less than 3 years from the first description of *JAK2*V617F, and in accordance with the CML-imatinib paradigm, small molecule JAK2 inhibitor drugs have been developed and are already undergoing clinical trials [28].

Management of thrombosis and bleeding in MPN

Recommendations for the acute and chronic management of thrombosis and bleeding in MPN are usually based on personal experience and not on hard evidence. I manage venous thrombotic complications in the usual manner with standard dose and schedule of systemic anticoagulant therapy. However, systemic anticoagulation alone is not sufficient, and myelosuppressive therapy should be added as soon as possible. I recommend lifelong therapy with warfarin in most cases of venous thrombosis in PV or ET, in the absence of overt contraindications. I also recommend the use

of aspirin in combination with systemic anticoagulation, again in the absence of conditions that preclude its use. I usually do not use systemic anticoagulation in most cases of arterial thrombosis and instead rely on aspirin and cytoreductive drug therapy. However, one must be careful in using aspirin in patients with extreme thrombocytosis (platelet count $>1000 \times 10^9$/L). In such instances, one must rule out the possibility of clinically relevant AVWS (e.g. ristocetin activity of $<30\%$) prior to instituting treatment with aspirin.

Finally, platelet count reduction to below 1000×10^9/L is the most effective means of controlling symptomatic, MPN-associated AVWS. Although definitive therapy in such instances requires cytoreductive drugs, urgent management might involve platelet pheresis. Because the beneficial effect of platelet pheresis is generally brief, it is recommended that cytoreductive therapy be initiated as soon as possible, to provide long-term control of the platelet count.

References

1 Tefferi A, Vardiman JW. Classification and diagnosis of myeloproliferative neoplasms: the 2008 World Health Organization criteria and point-of-care diagnostic algorithms. *Leukemia* 2008;22:14–22.

2 Levine RL, Pardanani A, Tefferi A, Gilliland DG. Role of JAK2 in the pathogenesis and therapy of myeloproliferative disorders. *Nat Rev Cancer* 2007;7: 673–83.

3 Fenaux P, Simon M, Caulier MT, Lai JL, Goudemand J, Bauters F. Clinical course of essential thrombocythemia in 147 cases. *Cancer* 1990;66:549–56.

4 Cortelazzo S, Viero P, Finazzi G, D'Emilio A, Rodeghiero F, Barbui T. Incidence and risk factors for thrombotic complications in a historical cohort of 100 patients with essential thrombocythemia. *J Clin Oncol* 1990;8:556–62.

5 Colombi M, Radaelli F, Zocchi L, Maiolo AT. Thrombotic and hemorrhagic complications in essential thrombocythemia. A retrospective study of 103 patients. *Cancer* 1991;67:2926–30.

6 Besses C, Cervantes F, Pereira A, et al. Major vascular complications in essential thrombocythemia: a study of the predictive factors in a series of 148 patients. *Leukemia* 1999;13:150–4.

7 Jensen MK, de Nully Brown P, Nielsen OJ, Hasselbalch HC. Incidence, clinical features and outcome of

essential thrombocythaemia in a well defined geographical area. *Eur J Haematol* 2000;65:132–9.

8 Chim CS, Kwong YL, Lie AK, et al. Long-term outcome of 231 patients with essential thrombocythemia: prognostic factors for thrombosis, bleeding, myelofibrosis, and leukemia. *Arch Intern Med* 2005;165:2651–8.

9 Wolanskyj AP, Schwager SM, McClure RF, Larson DR, Tefferi A. Essential thrombocythemia beyond the first decade: life expectancy, long-term complication rates, and prognostic factors. *Mayo Clin Proc* 2006;81:159–66.

10 Campbell PJ, Scott LM, Buck G, et al. Definition of subtypes of essential thrombocythaemia and relation to polycythaemia vera based on JAK2 V617F mutation status: a prospective study. *Lancet* 2005;366: 1945–53.

11 Polycythemia vera: the natural history of 1213 patients followed for 20 years. Gruppo Italiano Studio Policitemia. *Ann Intern Med* 1995;123:656–64.

12 Passamonti F, Brusamolino E, Lazzarino M, et al. Efficacy of pipobroman in the treatment of polycythemia vera: long-term results in 163 patients. *Haematologica* 2000;85:1011–8.

13 Marchioli R, Finazzi G, Landolfi R, et al. Vascular and neoplastic risk in a large cohort of patients with polycythemia vera. *J Clin Oncol* 2005;23:2224–32.

14 Carobbio A, Finazzi G, Guerini V, et al. Leukocytosis is a risk factor for thrombosis in essential thrombocythemia: interaction with treatment, standard risk factors and Jak2 mutation status. *Blood* 2007;109:2310–3.

15 Passamonti F, Rumi E, Pungolino E, et al. Life expectancy and prognostic factors for survival in patients with polycythemia vera and essential thrombocythemia. *Am J Med* 2004;117:755–61.

16 De Stefano V, Za T, Rossi E, et al. Recurrent thrombosis in patients with polycythemia vera or essential thrombocythemia: efficacy of treatment in preventing rethrombosis in different clinical settings. *Blood* 2006;108:Abstract #119.

17 Gangat N, Wolanskyj AP, Tefferi A. Abdominal vein thrombosis in essential thrombocythemia: prevalence, clinical correlates, and prognostic implications. *Eur J Haematol* 2006;77:327–33.

18 Kiladjian JJ, Cervantes F, Leebeek FW, et al. The impact of JAK2 and MPL mutations on diagnosis and prognosis of splanchnic vein thrombosis: a report on 241 cases. *Blood* 2008;111:4922–9.

19 Pardanani A, Lasho TL, Hussein K, et al. JAK2V617F mutation screening as part of the hypercoagulable work-up in the absence of splanchnic venous thrombosis or overt myeloproliferative neoplasm: assessment of value in a series of 664 consecutive patients. *Mayo Clin Proc* 2008;83:457–9.

20 Tefferi A, Elliott M. Thrombosis in myeloproliferative disorders: prevalence, prognostic factors, and the role of leukocytes and JAK2V617F. *Semin Thromb Hemost* 2007;33:313–20.

21 Fabris F, Casonato A, Grazia del Ben M, De Marco L, Girolami A. Abnormalities of von Willebrand factor in myeloproliferative disease: a relationship with bleeding diathesis. *Br J Haematol* 1986;63:75–83.

22 Landolfi R, Marchioli R, Kutti J, et al. Efficacy and safety of low-dose aspirin in polycythemia vera. *N Engl J Med* 2004;350:114–24.

23 Cortelazzo S, Finazzi G, Ruggeri M, et al. Hydroxyurea for patients with essential thrombocythemia and a high risk of thrombosis. *N Engl J Med* 1995;332:1132–6.

24 Tefferi A, Gangat N, Wolanskyj AP. Management of extreme thrombocytosis in otherwise low-risk essential thrombocythemia; does number matter? *Blood* 2006;108:2493–4.

25 Harrison CN, Campbell PJ, Buck G, et al. Hydroxyurea compared with anagrelide in high-risk essential thrombocythemia. *N Engl J Med* 2005;353:33–45.

26 Passamonti F, Randi ML, Rumi E, et al. Increased risk of pregnancy complications in patients with essential thrombocythemia carrying the JAK2 (617V>F) mutation. *Blood* 2007;110:485–9.

27 Kroger N, Mesa RA. Choosing between stem cell therapy and drugs in myelofibrosis. *Leukemia* 2008;22:474–86.

28 Tefferi A. Essential thrombocythemia, polycythemia vera, and myelofibrosis: current management and the prospect of targeted therapy. *Am J Hematol* 2008;83:491–7.

15 Arterial thrombosis

Gordon D.O. Lowe and R. Campbell Tait

Introduction

Arterial thrombosis is a common cause of hospital admission, death, and disability in developed countries (and increasingly in developing nations because of global epidemics of smoking, obesity, and diabetes). It usually follows spontaneous rupture of an atherosclerotic plaque, and may:

- be clinically silent;
- contribute to atherosclerotic progression resulting in coronary stenosis and stable angina, or lower limb artery stenosis and claudication;
- be present as acute ischemia in the heart (acute coronary syndromes: unstable angina, myocardial infarction), brain (transient cerebral ischemic attack or stroke), or limb (acute limb ischemia).

There is now good evidence that patients with acute ischemic syndromes have lower morbidity and mortality if they are promptly diagnosed, admitted as soon as possible to specialist acute units (coronary care, acute stroke, or peripheral vascular), undergo risk stratification, and receive appropriate treatment. This includes antithrombotic drugs (e.g. aspirin, heparin) and consideration of thrombolysis, thrombectomy, angioplasty, or vascular reconstruction in the acute phase and early, multidisciplinary rehabilitation.

Traditional risk factors (Table 15.1) remain the most important markers for arterial disease and together account for up to 90% of population attributable risk [1–3]. In patients with nonvalvular atrial fibrillation, the risk of stroke can be estimated by a variety of scoring systems, of which the CHADS$_2$ index [4], developed from an amalgamation of the Atrial Fibrillation Investigators and Stroke Prevention in Atrial Fibrillation schemes, is the most widely used and validated (Table 15.2).

Primary and secondary prevention of arterial thrombosis is everybody's business. All health care professionals, including hematologists, should take the opportunity to encourage their patients to adjust their lifestyles (when appropriate) and to consider pharmacologic prevention in all high-risk patients and in all with clinical evidence of arterial disease (Table 15.3).

Hematologists are commonly asked to develop or revise local hospital or area guidelines for investigations in thrombosis and antithrombotic therapies and their monitoring. In addition, they are often referred patients with arterial thrombosis that is premature, recurrent, or which occurs at multiple or unusual sites. Such referrals have increased in recent years, probably because general practitioners and physicians expect that (as with venous thromboembolism) hematologists may define underlying thrombophilias that may require specific management. This review therefore focuses on appropriate hematological investigation of patients with arterial thrombosis and appropriate antithrombotic therapy in various patient groups.

Evidence in this field is changing rapidly; hence, hematologists should keep up-to-date with systematic reviews and evidence-based national guidelines, such as those produced by the British Society for Haematology/British Committee for Standards in Haematology (http://www.bcshguidelines.com), the Scottish Intercollegiate Guidelines Network (SIGN; http://www.sign.ac.uk), and the National Institute for Health and Clinical Excellence (NICE).

Table 15.1 Traditional risk factors for cardiovascular disease [3].

Risk factor	Adjusted odds ratio	95% CI
Dyslipidemia	3.25	2.81–3.76
Current smoker	2.87	2.58–3.19
Diabetes	2.37	2.07–2.71
Hypertension	1.91	1.74–2.10
Abdominal obesity	1.62	1.45–1.80
Psychosocial factors	2.67	2.21–3.22
Daily fruit and vegetables	0.70	0.62–0.79
Regular exercise	0.86	0.76–0.97
Alcohol intake	0.91	0.82–1.02

Table 15.2 $CHADS_2$ risk stratification index for patients with nonvalvular atrial fibrillation [4].

$CHADS_2$ Score*	No. of patients (% of cohort)	Adjusted stroke rate per 100 patient years[†]	95% CI
6	5 (0.3)	18.2	10.5–27.4
5	65 (3.8)	12.5	8.2–17.5
4	220 (12.7)	8.5	6.3–11.1
3	337 (19.4)	5.9	4.6–7.3
2	523 (30.2)	4.0	3.1–5.1
1	463 (26.7)	2.8	2.0–3.8
0	120 (6.9)	1.9	1.2–3.0

*Two points are assigned for the history of prior cerebral ischemia and one point for the presence of each of the other risk factors: history of hypertension, diabetes mellitus, age ≥75 years, recent (<6 months) congestive heart failure.
[†] Adjusted stroke rates based on no antithrombotic therapy.

Routine laboratory investigations

Table 15.4 outlines routine and specialist investigations that are applicable to patients with arterial thrombosis or ischemia. These include:
• full blood count as a screen for anemia, polycythemia, hyperleukocytic leukemias, and thrombocytosis [5];
• erythrocyte sedimentation rate (ESR) or plasma viscosity as a screen for hyperviscosity syndromes and connective tissue disorders and/or vasculitis (e.g.

Table 15.3 Summary of lifestyle advice and pharmacologic prevention of cardiovascular disease.

Lifestyle advice
(primary and secondary prevention)
Stop or reduce smoking (cigarette, cigar, or pipe)
Take regular exercise (e.g. walk 30 minutes most days per week)
Lose weight if overweight (BMI >25 kg/m^2) or obese (BMI >30 kg/m^2)
Diet: reduce salt and saturated fat; increase fruit, vegetables, and fish
Moderate alcohol consumption (<16 units/week for women, <24 units/week men); avoid binge drinking

Pharmacologic
(primary prevention in high-risk patients: annual risk of CHD or stroke ≥2%; and secondary prevention in all patients with clinical cardiovascular disease)
Blood pressure reduction (if not achieved by lifestyle advice) to a target of 140/85 mm Hg
Beta-blocker following acute myocardial infarction (unless contraindicated)
ACE inhibitor following acute myocardial infarction if LV dysfunction
Cholesterol reduction (usually with a statin at dose of proven efficacy in cardiovascular reduction)
Aspirin (75 mg/day, loading dose 300 mg in acute coronary syndromes or acute ischemic stroke; 300 mg/day following coronary artery bypass grafting)

or

Clopidogrel (75 mg/day) in secondary prevention if aspirin contraindicated or not tolerated

or

Dipyridamole slow-release (200 mg b.d.) in patients with ischemic stroke or TIA, in addition to aspirin
Aspirin 75 mg/day and clopidogrel 75 mg/day for at least 3 months in acute coronary syndromes or following percutaneous coronary angioplasty ± stenting
Consider oral anticoagulation (usually with warfarin, target INR 2.0–3.0) in patients with atrial fibrillation with previous history of ischemic stroke or other thromboembolic event; or at high risk of thromboembolism ($CHADS_2$ score ≥ 2). Aspirin (75 mg/day) in other patients with atrial fibrillation, or if balance of benefit over risk of warfarin is uncertain, or if warfarin contraindicated or in patients who elect not to take warfarin

Abbreviations: ACE, angiotensin-converting enzyme; BMI, body mass index; CHD, coronary heart disease; INR, international normalized ratio; LV, left ventricle; TIA, transient ischemic attack.

Table 15.4 Summary of laboratory tests in persons with arterial thromboembolism.

Routine
Full blood count
    anemia (promotes ischemia)
    polycythemia
    hyperleukocytic leukemias
    thrombocytosis
ESR/plasma viscosity
    hyperviscosity syndromes
    vasculitis/connective tissue disorders
Cholesterol
    total cholesterol or LDL:HDL ratio predicts arterial disease

Specialized
Homocysteine
    if arterial thrombosis at age <30 years
Sickle cell screening
    in persons at ethnic risk
Lupus anticoagulant and anticardiolipin antibodies
    if arterial events at age under 50 years, without prominent
        clinical risk factors
Congenital thrombophilias
    utility unproven
Coagulation factors
    utility unproven
Fibrin D-dimer
    utility unproven
Fibrinolytic factors
    utility unproven
Platelet function studies
    utility unproven (e.g. aspirin resistance)

Abbreviations: ESR, erythrocyte sedimentation rate; HDL, high-density lipoprotein; LDL, low-density lipoprotein.

temporal arteritis, systemic lupus erythematosus, or polyarteritis nodosa). Hyperviscosity syndromes may be a medical emergency, requiring urgent plasma exchange, plasmapheresis, or cytapheresis; vasculitis may require urgent steroid or cytotoxic therapy and biopsy [5].

Acute elevations in white cell count and platelet counts, ESR or plasma viscosity, and other acute phase reactants, such as C-reactive protein and fibrinogen, are common in acute ischemic syndromes; but persistent elevations (e.g. more than 1 month) that are unexplained by complications, such as infections, limb necrosis, or venous thromboembolism, should raise the suspicion of underlying connective tissue disorder or malignancy.

Routine biochemical investigations should include:
• a lipid profile, specifically low-density lipoprotein and high-density lipoprotein cholesterol;
• glucose, or another measure of insulin resistance; and
• a thyroid screen for evidence of underlying thyrotoxicosis in patients with atrial fibrillation.

Careful control of diabetes and reduction of cholesterol have proven value in reduction of both primary and secondary vascular disease in affected individuals.

Specialized investigations

These should be reserved for patients in whom clinical assessment suggests a reasonable expectation of finding a "thrombophilia" that may alter clinical management. Over-investigation will result in identification of "abnormalities" that are irrelevant to clinical management and a source of confusion and anxiety to patients, family members, carers, and health care professionals [6]. Table 15.4 summarizes indications for particular tests in adults.

Thrombosis in childhood (apart from that associated with central venous catheters) is uncommon and requires specialist assessment by a pediatric hematologist.

Homocysteine measurement
This is indicated in all patients with premature (e.g. age under 30 years) arterial thrombosis, to exclude homocysteinuria. Such patients may be managed by regional specialists in metabolic medicine.

In recent years, epidemiologic studies have associated high-normal plasma homocysteine levels (and the common underlying MTHFR mutation, suggesting causality) with increased risk of arterial thrombosis (coronary, cerebral, and lower limb) as well as venous thrombosis [6–10]. Although vitamin supplementation (vitamin B_{12}, folate, vitamin B_6) reduces plasma homocysteine levels, to date randomized trials of secondary prevention (after ischemic events) have been negative for all vascular outcomes [6,10]. Further trials of vitamin supplementation are in progress.

Meanwhile, the use of screening for hyperhomocysteinemia in secondary prevention of arterial thrombosis in patients aged over 30 years is unproven. If high homocysteine levels are found, folate supplementation is reasonable because it is cheap and nontoxic (provided vitamin B_{12} levels are normal). It may be that folate supplementation of cereals (as practiced in the USA) or the folate component of a "polypill" (folic acid, antihypertensives, a statin, and possibly aspirin) [11] may be the most clinically effective and cost-effective strategy to reduce cardiovascular risk if homocysteine is shown to have a causal role in arterial (or venous) thrombosis.

Sickle cell screening

This may be appropriate in persons at ethnic risk, although in practice, a diagnosis of sickle cell disease (SCD) will usually have been made long before adulthood. Large- and small-vessel arterial thromboses are responsible for the protean manifestations of SCD. Sickle erythrocytes appear to induce a hypercoagulable state through a variety of mechanisms as assessed by increased platelet activation, increased thrombin generation, and decreased levels of anticoagulant proteins. However, measurement of such parameters has no proven use in the management of SCD, and clinical studies of long-term antiplatelet agents and anticoagulants have yet to show any beneficial effect on the incidence of vaso-occlusive events. Furthermore, it seems likely that the hypercoagulability is a secondary phenomenon to the sickling process, because treatment with hydroxyurea (which increases HbF levels and reduces sickling) is associated with a reduction in measures of hypercoagulability [12].

Screening for lupus anticoagulant and anticardiolipin antibodies

This is appropriate in all patients with premature (e.g. age under 50 years) cerebral or limb thrombosis or ischemia, and in other indications [13]. Management of the antiphospholipid syndrome is considered in Chapter 17.

Screening for congenital thrombophilias

The factor V Leiden and prothrombin G20210A mutations show modest but statistically significant associations with coronary heart disease (CHD), stroke, and peripheral arterial events, especially in younger persons (age under 55 years) and in women [9,14]. These findings may be relevant to the increases in risk of coronary and stroke events during pregnancy or with use of combined oral contraceptives or oral hormone replacement therapy (each of which increases resistance to activated protein C).

There is little evidence that other congenital thrombophilias are associated with increased risk of arterial disease, and the clinical use of screening for such abnormalities in patients with arterial thrombosis is at present unproven [15]. Furthermore, there is no evidence that secondary prevention with oral anticoagulants in such patients is more effective than routine antithrombotic prevention with aspirin (Table 15.3).

Ischemic stroke is often associated with a right-to-left cardiac shunt (e.g. patent foramen ovale, atrial septal defect) in younger patients, suggesting the possibility of "paradoxical" cerebral arterial embolism from venous thrombosis. Whether such an event is associated with thrombophilias is unknown, as are the relative benefits and risks of prophylaxis with aspirin, oral anticoagulants, or shunt closure [16].

Coagulation factors

Plasma fibrinogen is associated with CHD, stroke, and peripheral arterial events; the risks increase by 30–40% per 1-g/L increase [17]. Although there are several plausible biologic mechanisms through which increased circulating fibrinogen levels might promote such risk (atherogenic, thrombogenic, and rheological through increased plasma and blood viscosity), the lack of association of functional genetic polymorphisms with risk of CHD argues against causality. The association of fibrinogen with arterial risk may therefore be coincidental (because of mutual associations with multiple risk factors) or consequential (reverse causality, resulting from effects of atherosclerosis on plasma fibrinogen). The clinical use of plasma fibrinogen assessment in management of arterial thrombosis is unproven [6].

Von Willebrand factor (VWF) is weakly associated with risk of CHD [18]; there are few reported studies of functional polymorphisms.

Carriers of hemophilia A (or B) who have plasma levels of factor VIII or factor IX, which on average are 50% lower than female noncarriers, have an approximately 35% lower risk of CHD. Together with the 80% lower risk of CHD in male hemophiliacs compared with male non-hemophiliacs, these findings suggest that increasing levels of factor VIII (or factor

IX) increase the risks of arterial thrombosis, as well as of venous thrombosis [19].

The clinical use of assessment of plasma levels of VWF, factor VIII, or factor IX (or other clotting factors) in management of arterial thrombosis is unproven.

Coagulation activation markers

Plasma fibrin D-dimer levels are associated with increased risks of incident CHD and stroke, including studies of patients with atrial fibrillation [20–22]. Although D-dimer levels might therefore be useful in prediction of stroke in atrial fibrillation, and hence in stratifying choice of antithrombotic therapies, further management studies are required.

Fibrinolytic tests

Circulating levels of tissue plasminogen activator antigen, but not of plasminogen activator inhibitor type 1, are associated with increased risk of CHD in population studies. This association is markedly reduced after adjustment for associated CHD risk factors (obesity and other markers of insulin resistance) [23]. The clinical use of plasma components of the fibrinolytic system in management of arterial thrombosis is unproven.

Platelet function tests

Platelet aggregation studies and measures of platelet activation are not useful in prediction of arterial thrombosis. Although there is increasing evidence that aspirin resistance (defined as a laboratory measure of the failure of aspirin to inhibit platelet synthesis of thromboxane A_2, platelet aggregation, or the skin bleeding time) is associated with increased risk of recurrent cardiovascular events, further work is required to define the place of such laboratory measures in clinical practice [24].

Treatment

Primary and secondary prevention therapies for all patients with cardiovascular disease primarily involve antiplatelet agents and are summarised in Table 15.3. There have been recent advances in acute management of myocardial infarction and other acute coronary syndromes using aditional anticoagulant (low-molecular-weight heparins or fondaparinux) or antiplatelet (specific platelet glycoprotein IIb/IIIa

inhibitors) agents [25]; this is discussed in more detail in Chapter 18. In patients with recurrent events despite aspirin, possible empirical approaches are to add a second antiplatelet agent, to increase the dose of aspirin, or to change to oral anticoagulant therapy (after considering the increased bleeding risk and the logistical problems of long-term anticoagulant monitoring).

Combination therapy with vitamin K antagonists and antiplatelet agents

An increasingly problematic issue in clinical practice has been determining the risk:benefit ratios for combination treatment, either in patients already receiving a vitamin K antagonist (VKA) who develop an indication for aspirin (e.g. a patient being treated for recent DVT who then suffers an acute coronary syndrome), or a patient on aspirin who develops an indication for a VKA (e.g. a patient with previous myocardiol infarction developing atrial fibrillation). Management of such patients has to be individualized, considering the patient's thrombotic and bleeding risks. However, there is evidence in the literature that can inform decisions:

• In patients with atrial fibrillation, the combination of aspirin + clopidogrel is inferior to VKA (INR 2-3) in terms of stroke prevention, and is associated with similar bleeding rates [26].

• In patients with atrial fibrillation, the addition of aspirin (to VKA) is associated with a higher risk of major bleeding [27].

• In patients with peripheral arterial disease treated with aspirin, the addition of VKA does not reduce the cardiovascular event rate, but does increase the rate of life-threatening bleeding [28].

• In patients with stable coronary artery disease, a VKA is as effective as aspirin at reducing the risk of further ischemic events, albeit with an increased risk of major bleeding. Aspirin plus VKA is not significantly better than VKA alone [29].

• In high thrombotic risk patients with prosthetic heart valves (e.g. metal prosthetic valves, tissue prosthesis plus atrial fibrillation, or previous stroke), the benefit of adding aspirin to VKA, in terms of greater reduction in cardiovascular thrombotic events, outweighs the increased risk of major bleeding [30].

Therefore it would seem reasonable to treat with VKA alone in stable coronary artery disease patients who have an indication for VKA (e.g. atrial fibrillation

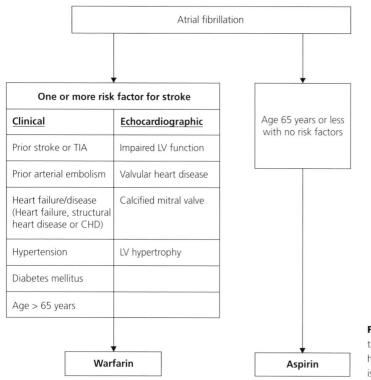

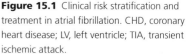

Figure 15.1 Clinical risk stratification and treatment in atrial fibrillation. CHD, coronary heart disease; LV, left ventricle; TIA, transient ischemic attack.

or venous thrombosis). The problem arises in acute coronary syndromes and the use of coronary artery stents where there is insufficient evidence comparing the relative efficacies and safeties of aspirin plus clopidogrel against VKA alone. A pragmatic approach is required: using bare metal stents where possible (requiring shorter exposure to combination antiplatelet therapy); using VKA plus single-agent antiplatelet therapy in lower thrombotic risk patients; and short-term triple therapy with VKA + aspirin + clopidogrel in patients at highest thrombotic risk [31].

Conclusions

At present, risk stratification for arterial disease continues to rely on assessment of traditional clinical (age, sex, smoking, blood pressure, obesity) and routine laboratory (cholesterol) risk factors.

The role of thrombophilia screening in patients with arterial disease is unproven, although selective testing for homocysteinuria and antiphospholipid syndrome is indicated in patients with premature arterial thrombosis, especially in the absence of traditional risk factors.

The mainstay of treatment is control, or eradication, of risk factors, coupled with antithrombotic therapy: primarily antiplatelet agents or anticoagulation for patients with atrial fibrillation and additional risk factors (Fig. 15.1).

References

1 Lowe GDO, Danesh J, eds. Classical and emerging risk factors for cardiovascular disease. *Semin Vasc Med* 2002;2:229–445.

2 Emberson J, Whincup P, Morris R, Walker M, Lowe G, Rumley A. Extent of regression dilution for established and novel coronary risk factors: results from the British Regional Heart Study. *Eur J Cardiovasc Prev Rehab* 2004;11:125–34.

3 Yusuf S, Hawken S, Ounpuu S, et al. Effect of potentially modifiable risk factors associated with myocardial infarction in 52 countries (the INTERHEART study): case-control study. *Lancet* 2004;364:937–52.

4 Gage BF, Waterman AD, Shannon W, Boechler M, Rich MW, Radford MJ. Validation of clinical classification schemes for predicting stroke: results from the national registry of atrial fibrillation. *JAMA* 2001;285: 2864–70.

5 Lowe GDO, ed. Blood rheology and hyperviscosity syndromes. *Baillieres Clin Haematol* 1987;3:597–867.

6 Lowe GDO. Can haematological tests predict cardiovascular risk? The 2005 Kettle Lecture. *Br J Haematol* 2006;133:232–50.

7 Homocysteine Studies Collaboration. Homocysteine and risk of ischemic heart disease and stroke: a meta-analysis. *JAMA* 2002;288:2015–22.

8 Klerk M, Verhoef P, Clarke R, et al. MTHFR 677C-T polymorphism and risk of coronary heart disease: a meta-analysis. *JAMA* 2002;288:2023–31.

9 Kim RJ, Becker RC. Association between factor V Leiden, prothrombin mutation G20120A, and MTHFR C677T mutations and events of the arterial circulatory system: a meta-analysis of published studies. *Am Heart J* 2003;146:948–57.

10 Toole JF, Malinow MR, Chambless LE, et al. Lowering homocysteine in patients with ischemic stroke to prevent recurrent stroke, myocardial infarction, and death. *JAMA* 2004;291:565–75.

11 Wald NJ, Law MR. A strategy to reduce cardiovascular disease by more than 80%. *Br Med J* 2003;326:1419.

12 Ataga KI, Orringer EP. Hypercoagulability in sickle cell disease: a curious paradox. *Am J Med* 2003;115: 721–8.

13 Greaves M, Cohen H, Machin SJ, Mackie I, on behalf of the British Committee for Standards in Haematology. Guidelines on the investigation and management of the antiphospholipid syndrome. *Br J Haematol* 2000;109:704–15.

14 Ye Z, Liu EHC, Higgins JPT, et al. Seven haemostatic gene polymorphisms in coronary disease: meta-analysis of 66 155 cases and 91 307 controls. *Lancet* 2006;367:651–8.

15 Walker ID, Greaves M, Preston FE, on behalf of the Haemostasis and Thrombosis Task Force, British Committee for Standards in Haematology. Guideline: Investigation and management of heritable thrombophilia. *Br J Haematol* 2001;114:512–28.

16 Wu LA, We LA, Lidar DA, et al. Patent foramen ovale in cryptogenic stroke: current understanding and management options. *Arch Intern Med* 2004;164:950–6.

17 Danesh J, Lewington S, Thompson SG, Lowe GDO, Collins R (writing committee). Fibrinogen Studies Collaboration. Plasma fibrinogen level and the risk of major cardiovascular diseases and non-vascular mortality: an individual participant meta-analysis. *JAMA* 2005;294:1799–1809.

18 Danesh J, Wheeler JG, Hirshfield GM, et al. C-reactive protein and other circulating markers of inflammation in the prediction of coronary heart disease. *N Engl J Med* 2004;350:1387–97.

19 Sramek A, Kriek M, Rosendaal FR. Decreased mortality of ischaemic heart disease among carriers of haemophlia. *Lancet* 2003;362:351–4.

20 Danesh J, Whincup P, Walker M, et al. Fibrin D-dimer and coronary heart disease: prospective study and meta-analysis. *Circulation* 2001;103:2323–7.

21 Vene N, Mavri A, Kosmelj K, Stegnar M. High D-dimer levels predict cardiovascular events in patients with chronic atrial fibrillation during oral anticoagulant therapy. *Thromb Haemost* 2003;90:1163–72.

22 Lowe GDO. Fibrin D-dimer and risk of cardiovascular events? *Semin Vasc Med* 2005;5:387–398.

23 Lowe GDO, Danesh J, Lewington S, et al. Tissue plasminogen activator antigen and coronary heart disease: prospective study and meta-analysis. *Eur Heart J* 2004;25:252–9.

24 Hankey GJ, Eikelboom JW. Aspirin resistance. *Br Med J* 2004;328:477–9.

25 Scottish Intercollegiate Guidelines Network (SIGN). Acute Coronary Syndromes. A national clinical guideline (SIGN93). Edinburgh: SIGN2007. Available from: http://www.sign.ac.uk.

26 Connolly S, Yusuf S, Camm J, et al. Clopidogrel plus aspirin versus oral anticoagulation for atrial fibrillation in the Atrial fibrillation Clopidogrel Trial with Irbesartan for prevention of Vascular Events (ACTIVE W): a randomised controlled trial. *Lancet* 2006;367:1903–12.

27 Douketis JD, Arneklev K, Goldhaber SZ, Spandorfer J, Halperin F, Horrow J. Comparison of bleeding in patients with nonvalvular atrial fibrillation treated with ximelagatran or warfarin. *Arch Intern Med* 2006;166:853–9.

28 The Warfarin Antiplatelet Vascular Evaluation Trial Investigators. Oral anticoagulant and antiplatelet therapy and peripheral arterial disease. *N Engl J Med* 2007;357:217–27.

29 Hurlen M, Abdelnoor MPH, Smith P, Erikssen J, Arnesen H. Warfarin, aspirin, or both after myocardial infarction. *N Engl J Med* 2002;347:969–74.

30 Little SH, Massel DR. Antiplatelet and anticoagulation for patients with prosthetic heart valves. *Cochrane Database Syst Rev* 2003;4:CD003464.

31 Eikelboom JW, Hirsh J. Combined antiplatelet and anticoagulant therapy: clinical benefits and risks. *J Thromb Haemost* 2007;5(Suppl 1):255–63.

Gualtiero Palareti and Benilde Cosmi

Introduction

Administration of coumarin drugs, also called vitamin K antagonists (VKAs), has been the mainstay of anticoagulation for more than 50 years. A great and increasing number of subjects receive this treatment all over the world because it has been shown to be effective on the basis of randomized clinical trials in many clinical conditions.

New anticoagulant drugs, based on a completely different mecchanism of action, are being introduced. Candidate for prolonged treatment, some of them are, at the moment, in advanced phases of clinical experimentation and are expected to be available for current clinical use in the near future.

Indications for anticoagulant treatment

A number of clinical trials provided evidence that anticoagulation with VKAs is indicated in several conditions as a formidable tool for primary or secondary prevention of thrombotic complications [1]. Although properly designed clinical trials are still lacking, anticoagulation with VKAs is widely accepted in several other conditions (see Table 16.1).

For the majority of indications, a moderate anticoagulant effect [international normalized ratio (INR) 2.0–3.0] is effective [2]. No adequate studies have been conducted on the efficacy of oral anticoagulants (OACs) for the secondary prevention in ischemic cerebrovascular disease, in retinal vein thrombosis, or in peripheral arterial disease. In the latter condition, VKAs are indicated in patients with venous infrainguinal bypasses at high risk of occlusion.

Contraindications for treatment

A reliable laboratory, an expert clinician, and a compliant patient are three essential components for appropriate therapy with VKAs. Before starting oral anticoagulation, patients should be carefully evaluated for compliance, absolute contraindications, and conditions with a higher risk of complications (see Table 16.1).

VKAs cross the placental barrier and can produce both bleeding and a teratogenic effect in the fetus (embryopathy with nasal hypoplasia and stippled epiphyses in the first trimester and central nervous system abnormalities at any time during pregnancy). They could be considered relatively safe after the first trimester up to 36 weeks of gestation. In the last 6 weeks, exposure to VKAs could increase the risk of bleeding at the time of delivery [3]. Nursing mothers can be treated with VKAs, as warfarin does not induce an anticoagulant effect in the breastfed infant.

Major bleeding is an absolute contraindication to VKAs for at least 1 month after the event.

Relative medical contraindications to VKAs are severe hepatic or renal insufficiency (which increase the risk of bleeding), severe hypertension, severe heart failure, esophageal varices, bleeding diathesis, recent central nervous system (CNS) surgery or trauma, recent hepatic or renal biopsy, active peptic ulcer, bacterial endocarditis, pericarditis, recent CNS hemorrhage, chronic bowel inflammatory disease, menorrhagia, thyrotoxicosis, and cerebral aneurysms.

Conditions of noncompliance of the patient, such as psychiatric disorders, dementia, and chronic alcoholism, can also be considered relative contraindications for VKAs.

Table 16.1 Indications and contraindications (absolute or relative) for anticoagulant treatment with VKAs.

Proven indications	- Primary and secondary prevention of venous thromboembolism - Prevention of systemic embolism in atrial fibrillation or in patients with tissue or mechanical heart valves - Prevention of stroke or death in patients with acute myocardial infarction - Prevention of acute myocardial re-infarction in men at high risk
Other accepted indications	Prevention of thrombotic complications in high-risk patients with: - prosthetic heart valves - mitral stenosis - systemic embolism of unknown etiology - intraventricular thrombosis - dilated cardiomyopathy
Absolute contraindications	- Pregnancy between the 6th and 12th week - Major bleeding (within 30 days)
Relative contraindications	All the conditions that increase the risk of bleeding or of insufficient quality of treatment - severe hepatic or renal insufficiency - severe uncontrolled hypertension - severe heart failure - bleeding diathesis - recent central venous system surgery or trauma - active peptic ulcer or bowel inflammatory disease - bacterial endocarditis or pericarditis - tendency to fall - chronic alcoholism - poor compliance - psychiatric disorders or dementia (if not supported by family or social services)

Oral anticoagulant drugs: clinical pharmacology and genetic control

VKAs are 4-hydroxycoumarin compounds, which were developed in the 1940s–1950s and introduced in the treatment of thrombotic disorders in the 1950s. Warfarin, acenocoumarol, and phenprocoumon are the compounds currently in clinical use. Warfarin is the most prescribed anticoagulant worldwide.

Warfarin is administered as a racemic compound containing equal amounts of the R and S enantiomers. The S enantiomer is three to five times as potent as the R enantiomer and accounts for about 60–70% of the anticoagulation effect of the racemic compound. The metabolism of (S)-warfarin is almost exclusively mediated by the activity of the enzyme CYP2C9, which accounts for ~85% of its catabolism. Several genetic polymorphisms of CYP2C9 have been identi-

fied, and two of them—CYP2C9*2 and CYP2C9*3—relatively frequent among Caucasians, are clinically relevant because subjects carrier of these variants are expected to metabolize (S)-warfarin in a lower rate than carriers of the wild-type allele (CYP2C9*1) and require lower warfarin doses [4].

In 2004, the gene encoding for vitamin K epoxide reductase subunit 1 (VKORC1) was identified [5]. Subsequently, numerous polymorphisms were found to induce a different sensitivity, highly increased or reduced, of the enzyme to action of VKAs [6].

VKAs exert their effect by interfering with the vitamin K-dependent hepatic synthesis of coagulation factors II, VII, IX, and X as well as the coagulation inhibitors proteins C and S. Vitamin K-dependent posttranslational carboxylation is critical for coagulation factors to acquire the calcium-mediated ability to bind to negatively charged phospholipid surfaces [7].

Carboxylation of vitamin K-dependent coagulation factors depends on a carboxylase that requires a reduced form of vitamin K (vitamin KH2), oxygen, and carbon dioxide. During this reaction, vitamin KH2 is oxidized to vitamin K epoxide, which is reduced to vitamin K by epoxide reductase and then to vitamin KH2 by vitamin K reductase. VKAs inhibit vitamin K epoxide reductase and possibly vitamin K reductase. As a result, intracellular depletion of vitamin KH2 takes place, and only partially carboxylated and decarboxylated proteins are secreted. The antagonizing effect on vitamin K with the resulting production of biologically inactive coagulation factors is the basis for the therapeutic use of VKAs.

The effect of VKAs is delayed because time is required for the normal coagulation factors to be cleared from plasma and replaced by partially carboxylated or decarboxylated factors. This delay in the onset of VKAs effect varies according to the coagulation factor's half-life, which is only 6–7 hours for factor VII or 60–72 hours for prothrombin.

Animal studies have shown that the reduction of prothrombin and possibly of factor X is more important than the reduction of factor VII and IX for the in vivo antithrombotic effect of VKAs. As a result, the initial effect of VKAs as measured by the prolongation of the prothrombin time:

- Reflects the reduction of factor VII.
- The antithrombotic effect is only observed after the reduction of prothrombin, which requires 60–72 hours.
- In addition, in the first days of treatment with VKAs, a reduction of the levels of protein C and protein S is also observed as the synthesis of these natural anticoagulants is also vitamin K-dependent. Protein C half-life is similar to that of factor VII; as a result, in the initial phase of treatment with VKAs, the levels of protein C can be reduced significantly before the achievement of an efficient antithrombotic effect of treatment. This can result in warfarin-induced skin necrosis (Fig. 16.1).
- The delayed onset of the antithrombotic effect of VKAs and the potentially prothrombotic effect in the first 24–48 hours provide the rationale for overlapping heparin with VKAs for 4–5 days until their full antithrombotic effect is obtained.

OACs can be safely started on the first instead of the fifth day of heparin treatment of deep vein thrombo-

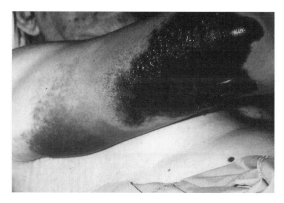

Figure 16.1 Skin necrosis of the elbow in a patient who just started warfarin.

sis (DVT). Although in the past, unfractionated heparin was the agent primarily used during the overlap, low-molecular-weight heparin is now the drug of choice (discussed in Chapter 13). Heparin can be safely stopped after a stable therapeutic INR range is reached (i.e. after 2 consecutive days of INR above 2.0).

Initiation and dosing of warfarin anticoagulation

Before starting warfarin anticoagulation, it is recommended that the following are performed:

- a baseline INR;
- a full blood and platelet count; and
- assessment of renal function.

Historically, large-loading warfarin doses were used at the start of anticoagulation. More recently, this practice has been abandoned as a result of the demonstration that initiating warfarin at a dosage close to that likely required for maintenance therapy not only produces therapeutic anticoagulation in most patients but is also less risky for complications [7].

The use of nomograms

There is clear evidence that use of nomograms to guide warfarin initiation is of great help in rapidly and safely achieving therapeutic anticoagulation levels in comparison with a physician-guided warfarin initiation, also resulting in shorter hospital stays for some patients. The use of nomograms may also reduce the need for anticoagulant monitoring in the first days of treatment.

A variety of nomograms for the initial days of warfarin therapy have been devised. Nomogram use requires that baseline INR is normal or near normal (not more than 1.4). A nomogram to start warfarin anticoagulation in children with thrombosis has also been proposed, with an initial dosage of 0.2 mg/kg. One of the first and most widely adopted nomograms to be used for adult patients was that proposed by Fennerty and colleagues, using 10-mg loading doses [8]. More recently, nomograms suggesting that warfarin be initiated with a 5-mg dose were proposed, with subsequent doses determined by the INR response, which can be checked on the third or fourth day [9].

Advantages of the 5-mg dose

It has been shown that the rate of lowering of prothrombin levels was similar when warfarin was started with either a 5- or 10-mg loading dose. However, the larger loading dose produced a more rapid reduction in protein C levels and a higher frequency in overanticoagulation (INR >3.0). A smaller loading dose of warfarin might therefore be less likely to produce a potentially prothrombotic effect in the first 24–48 hours of treatment.

Advantages of the 10-mg dose

In contrast to the data suggesting that a low initial warfarin dose is effective and safe, some authors have reported that higher initial doses are better [10]. Patients who receive a 10-mg initial dose of warfarin achieve a therapeutic INR earlier than patients initially treated with 5 mg, and more patients (83%) in the 10-mg group achieve a therapeutic INR by day 5, compared with the 5-mg group (46%). Also, fewer INR assessments are performed in the 10-mg group. There were no significant differences between the two groups in recurrent events or major bleeding. The authors concluded that 10-mg warfarin initiation nomogram is superior to the 5-mg nomogram because it allows more rapid achievement of a therapeutic INR.

Disadvantages of the 5-mg dose

It has recently been shown that starting anticoagulation with 5 mg warfarin in patients with DVT, entirely treated out of hospital, caused a prolongation of low-molecular-weight heparin treatment likely caused by a reduced number of INR determinations in outpatients. It has been suggested that either more frequent INR determination should be performed or higher initial dose of warfarin should be adopted in patients younger than 60 years.

Varying dose because of age or diagnosis

Some authors have demonstrated that the initial doses of warfarin should be different according to the age of patients because a reduced dose is required in the elderly.

Patients starting oral anticoagulation after heart valve replacement are more sensitive to warfarin than nonsurgical patients, and initial warfarin doses lower than 5 mg are indicated in some.

Guidance during anticoagulation

The effects of VKAs are highly variable both within and between individuals. Even though the average daily dose of warfarin is approximately 5 mg, individual patients may require much larger or smaller doses (the daily dose may range between 0.5 and 60 mg). Furthermore, OACs have a narrow therapeutic window, and over- or underdosage can result in overanticoagulation, with increased risk of hemorrhage, or under-anticoagulation, with increased risk of thrombosis, respectively.

The quality of monitoring anticoagulated patients is certainly an important factor influencing the risk of bleeding or thrombotic complications. Guiding VKA therapy requires some skill and practice [7]. Techniques to reduce the risk of inappropriate warfarin regimens include:

• warfarin regimen nomograms;
• computer-generated warfarin regimens; and
• dedicated anticoagulation clinics.

Several nomograms have been proposed to help warfarin regimens either during the induction phase or during the stabilized phase of anticoagulation. Some nomograms were specifically designed to guide warfarin treatment in some particular types of patients, such as in post-orthopedic surgery patients or in post-partum women.

Computer-guided dosing

Evidence is now available that computer-guided dosing is effective in helping doctors to prescribe therapeutic regimens, both during long-term maintenance and in the early, highly unstable phase of treatment. The use of computer-guided dosing increases the amount of time spent in the therapeutic range, compared with exclusive management by doctors. The safety and effectiveness of the computer-assisted dosage versus manual dosage on bleeding and thrombotic events was assessed in a randomized study conducted at 32 European centers with established interest in oral anticoagulation in 13 European countries (European Action on Anticoagulation) [11]. So far, this is the largest trial performed on oral anticoagulation, in which 6503 patients were randomized to medical staff and 6716 to computer-assisted dosage. Clinical events with computer dosage were lower (5.5% vs. 6% in the manual dosage arm), although the difference did not reach statistical significance. "Time in target INR range" was significantly improved by computer assistance compared with medical staff dosage at the majority of centers. This is the first study showing an advantage of computer dosage on clinical events, and it also provides an update and accurate description of event rate in centers dedicated to anticoagulation in Europe.

Dedicated anticoagulation clinics

It is a general experience, confirmed by some studies, that the quality of anticoagulation control is higher and the rate of bleeding lower when patients are monitored by dedicated anticoagulation clinics [12]. In the dedicated clinic, the specialized training and experience of medical and paramedical staff, proper patient education, and the use of computer programs help to ensure optimization of anticoagulant therapy.

Patients with highly unstable response to VKAs

Some patients may have a highly unstable response to VKAs, although universally accepted criteria for instability of response to VKAs are lacking. Some criteria have been proposed [13]: (1) less than 50% of INR results within the intended therapeutic range, with the other INR results both above or below the range, and/or (2) weekly dose changes (at least 15% of the previously prescribed coumarin weekly dose) in at least 40% of visits during the previous 4 months.

There are data indicating that instability is more frequently associated with working status (people who work vs. pensioners), use of acenocoumarol, and distribution of CYP2C9. Instability is more frequent in patients with insufficient score at Abbreviated Men-

tal Test administered to assess the degree of attention, and with lack of awareness of reasons for VKAs and of the mechanisms and possible side effects of VKAs [14].

Patient education and knowledge of VKAs and its management is a primary determinant of the quality of anticoagulation control, and appropriate education and information of patients is one of the most important tasks of anticoagulation clinics [15,16]. The distribution of patient education brochures at the beginning of anticoagulant treatment, often written in terms that are beyond the comprehension of many patients, may not be sufficient, and further education by personal interview should be considered for unstable patients [17].

Fluctuations in dietary vitamin K intake are also known to lead to changes in the INR. Additionally, patients with fluctuating INRs have a lower oral vitamin K intake than patients with stable INRs. Some patients on OACs have fluctuating INRs that cannot be explained by changes in concomitant medications, intercurrent illnesses, or obvious dietary changes. Supplementation with oral vitamin K in such patients is sometimes used in clinical practice, and some studies have shown that vitamin K supplementation (500 μg) daily decreases INR variability. INR decreased 2–7 days after vitamin K was initiated, and it took 2–35 days for INRs to return to the therapeutic range [18].

Complications of anticoagulation with VKAs: Bleeding

Bleeding is the most important complication and is a major concern for both physicians and patients, limiting the more widespread use of oral anticoagulation.

The risk of bleeding on VKAs in prospective studies has been reported to be:

• 0.1–1.0% patient-years of treatment for fatal episodes;

• 0.5–6.5% for major episodes; and

• 6.2–21.8% for minor bleeding.

Differences in the adopted classification of bleeding events (see Table 16.2) and in the composition of the cohorts studied may explain the wide range of bleeding rates reported in clinical studies. Although the criteria for major bleeding were different in

Table 16.2 Classification of bleeding complications.

Major bleeding (according to the Control of Anticoagulation Subcommittee of the ISTH [29])	- Fatal bleeding - Symptomatic bleeding in a critical area or organ, such as intracranial, intraspinal, intraocular, retroperitoneal, intra-articular or pericardial, or intramuscular with compartment syndrome - Bleeding causing a fall in hemoglobin level of 20 g/L or more, or leading to transfusion of two or more units of whole blood or red cells
Minor bleeding	Any overt hemorrhage not included among the major bleeds

Note: Bruising, small ecchymoses, nosebleed (not requiring tamponade), occasional hemorrhoidal bleeding, and microscopic hematuria should not be considered as clinically relevant bleeds.

different studies, in all studies, the most consistent risk factors for major bleeding were:
• intensity of anticoagulation;
• age; and
• the first 90 days of treatment.

An INR >4.5 increases the risk of hemorrhage six-fold, and the risk of major hemorrhage increases by 42% for each one point increase in INR. The intended intensity, and especially the actually achieved intensity, of anticoagulation is the major determinant of anticoagulation-induced bleeding. In prospective observational studies, such as the Italian ISCOAT study [19], the following have been shown:
• The lowest rate of bleeding is associated with INR results in the 2.0–2.9 INR range.
• Many bleeding events occur at a very low anticoagulation intensity (<2.0 INR).
• The increase in bleeding incidence becomes exponential for INR values >4.5.

The risk of bleeding for INR values >7.0 is 40 times greater than that associated with an INR of 2.0–2.9 and 20 times greater than that when the INR is 3.0–4.4. The risk of death in subjects on oral anticoagulation is strongly related to the INR level, with a minimum risk at 2.2 INR. High INR values are associated with an excess mortality: for one unit INR increase above 2.5, there is a two-fold risk increase [20].

Intracranial hemorrhage

Intracranial hemorrhage (Fig. 16.2) has a high mortality and morbidity [21]. The rate of intracranial hemorrhage in randomized trials of atrial fibrillation and postmyocardial infarction was 0.3%, whereas it was 0.5–0.6% in observational studies of patients on VKAs for arterial and venous thromboembolic indications.

The rate of intracranial bleeding was 1.15 per 100 patient-years in a meta-analysis evaluating studies in patients taking oral anticoagulant therapy for venous thromboembolism [22].

Risk factors for intracranial bleeding are:
• Older age;
• Intensity of anticoagulation: the risk increases four-fold for each unit increase in the prothrombin time ratio, and is particularly high for INR >4.0;
• Ischemic cerebrovascular disease; and
• Hypertension.

Various neurologic pathologies, such as arterial vasculopathies, predispose to intracerebral bleeding.

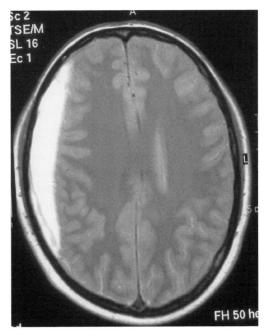

Figure 16.2 Subdural hematoma in a patient on warfarin.

Leukoaraiosis defines a diffuse white matter abnormality seen on computed tomography or magnetic resonance, and a dose–response relationship between such abnormality and intracranial hemorrhage has been demonstrated. Amyloid angiopathy increases with age and is associated with asymptomatic microhemorrhages and with spontaneous lobar intracerebral hemorrhage in the elderly [23]. This vasculopathy is a contributing factor to intracranial hemorrhage related to oral anticoagulation.

Extracranial hemorrhage

The rate of major extracranial hemorrhage in randomized trials of patients with atrial fibrillation and post-myocardial infarction was between 0.4% and 1.4% per year. It was 0.9–2.0% per year in observational studies of patients on VKAs for arterial and venous thromboembolic indications.

Management of over-anticoagulation and bleeding

Reversal of anticoagulation

Temporary withdrawal of coumarin drug administration

The coumarin drugs have very different half-lives: acenocoumarol has the shortest, phenprocoumon the longest, and warfarin is in between. Discontinuing coumarin drug intake will result in a slow reversal of anticoagulation, proportional to their half-lives. The majority of over-anticoagulated patients (INR >4.5) will take 3 days to return to the therapeutic range. For subjects already within the therapeutic range, it will take 3–5 days for the anticoagulation to be completely reversed. Temporary withdrawal of coumarin administration alone is useful in over-anticoagulated patients, especially if they are treated with acenocoumarol, are at low risk of bleeding, and in those anticoagulated patients who are due to undergo elective surgery. This option for treatment cannot be used alone in patients who are actively bleeding because of the long period necessary for the anticoagulation to be reversed.

Vitamin K administration

Administration of vitamin K (phytonadione) is the recommended mode of reversing the effects of coumarin drugs. However, a patient's response to vitamin K varies, depending on the pretreatment INR value, the route of administration, and the dose used. Vitamin K can be administered intravenously, orally, or subcutaneously. The intramuscular route is not recommended because of irregular, unpredictable absorption and the risk of intramuscular hematoma. It has been shown that higher doses and longer reversion times are needed with subcutaneous administration when compared with intravenous and oral administration. Vitamin K can be administered intravenously as a slow injection or infused in 5% glucose solution. Intravenous administration can cause anaphylaxis; however, this risk is much lower with the new vitamin K preparation, which is stabilized with a mixed micelle vehicle (Konakion® MM) instead of castor oil (Konakion®).

Vitamin K administration in anticoagulated patients is indicated in:
• cases of excessive over-anticoagulation, as recommended by the Eighth Consensus Conference of the American College of Chest Physicians [7], especially in patients at higher bleeding risk;
• patients who need to undergo invasive procedures that require an INR value >1.5; and
• cases with active major bleeding.

The oral route

In over-anticoagulated patients, oral vitamin K was demonstrated to be much more effective than placebo in correcting excessive INRs. Small amounts of vitamin K given orally can produce a major correction in the INR at 24 hours, but the correction is insufficient at 4 hours or for cases of major bleeding. In patients on acenocoumarol, administration of low-dose oral vitamin K offers no advantage to simple omission of a single dose of the drug and may result in an excessive risk of under-anticoagulation.

The intravenous route

Intravenous vitamin K administration leads to an effective reversal of anticoagulation within 6–8 hours and is therefore the treatment of choice in life-threatening bleeding. Intravenous vitamin K doses ranging between 0.1 and 3 mg have been shown to effectively reduce very high INR values in the absence of life-threatening bleeding. Higher doses may frequently result in subtherapeutic INR.

Fresh frozen plasma

Administration of fresh frozen plasma (FFP) is intended to correct the deficiency of factors II, VII, IX, and X resulting from the effect of coumarin drugs. The recommended FFP dose for warfarin reversal is 15 mL/kg body weight. However, several factors should be considered that limit the value of FFP as the best replacement treatment in this indication [24]:

• Large FFP volumes (e.g. approximately 1000 mL for an adult weighing 70 kg) are needed to be given rapidly to replace vitamin K-dependent factors, and this may be harmful, especially in patients with compromised cardiovascular conditions.

• FFP may not be virally inactivated and therefore a potential risk of viral infection cannot be excluded.

• The time needed to prepare the plasma, which is stored frozen at −20°C, is usually a cause of delay before transfusion.

• It has been shown that administration of the recommended dose of FFP fails to significantly correct the coumarin-induced coagulopathy, especially for persistently low factor IX levels.

Prothrombin complex concentrates

Concentrates of factors II, VII, IX, and X, called prothrombin complex concentrates (PCCs), are available and are highly effective in replacing clotting factors that are deficient in anticoagulated patients [25]. A dose of 30 U/kg is usually effective. The precise optimal dose of PCC remains to be defined, but the following have been suggested:

• 25 U/kg for patients with an INR of 2.0–3.9; and
• 35 U/kg for an INR of >4.0.

Potential adverse effects of PCC administration are viral infection and thrombogenicity. Despite all the precautions taken (selection of donors as well as specific viral inactivation procedures), an extremely small risk of viral infection can still persist. Thrombotic events have been reported after PCC transfusion in anticoagulated patients; however, this risk is also small, especially in preparations with added antithrombin and heparin. The potential risks of PCC indicate that their use should be reserved for patients with major bleeding, especially to those with intracranial hemorrhage in whom an immediate correction of the coagulopathy is highly recommended.

Clinical management of over-anticoagulation and bleeding

An unexpected condition of over-anticoagulation is not a rare finding during treatment with VKAs. The incidence rate of an INR >6.0 was found to be as high as 7.8 in 10,000 treatment days in prevalent users and 22.5 in 10,000 treatment days in incident users. Because it is known that the risk of bleeding increases sharply in association with very high INR values, it is desirable for a patient to spend as little time as possible in a condition of over-anticoagulation. In these cases, the clinical management should be as follows:

• Patients with very high INR values (>7.0), or with more moderately high INR values but at high risk of bleeding, should receive 1–2 mg vitamin K orally; the INR should be measured the following day and oral vitamin K given again if necessary.

• In patients with an INR of 4.5–6.9, and in those treated with acenocoumarol whatever the INR, withholding the coumarin drug for 1–2 days followed by a reduction of the weekly dose is usually sufficient.

• All patients with minor bleeding and an INR over the therapeutic range should receive intravenous vitamin K, which will reduce the high INR values within 6–8 hours.

• In cases with major, although not life-threatening, bleeding, a complete reversal of anticoagulation with intravenous vitamin K is advisable.

• A complete and rapid reversal of anticoagulation is recommended in patients with life-threatening bleeding. PCC infusion will completely correct the coagulopathy within 5–10 minutes. A dose of 5–10 mg vitamin K should also be administered intravenously.

• Please note the lack of recommendation to use FFP.

Management of patients treated with VKAs who require surgery or invasive procedures

There are no universally accepted guidelines for the management of anticoagulated patients requiring surgery or invasive procedures. Clear indications are lacking because of different patients, procedures, anticoagulant regimens, event definition and duration of follow-up, as well as the absence of randomized clinical trials in this setting. However, the increasing

Table 16.3 Strategies to manage patients treated with VKAs who require surgery or invasive procedures.

Continuation of VKA treatment	*In conditions at low risk of bleeding complications:* Punctures and catheterization of veins and arteries (e.g. femoral artery and Seldinger catheter) Sternal punctures and bone marrow aspirates Skin biopsies, minor dermatologic surgery, biopsy of mucosa that is easily accessible and explorable (oral cavity, vagina), minor eye surgery Endoscopic examinations without surgery Simple tooth extraction
Temporary discontinuation of VKA treatment	*In patients with low risk of thrombotic complications in conditions at risk of bleeding:* Major elective surgery, general or specialist Explorative cavity punctures (thoracocentesis, paracentesis) Biopsies of deep tissues (liver, kidney, bone) or mucosa (gastroenteric, respiratory, genital) not accessible Epidural anesthesia
Perioperative anticoagulant bridging therapy	*In patients with high risk of thrombotic complications:* Prosthetic heart valves Atrial fibrillation with high/moderate $CHADS_2$ score (especially if with previous systemic embolism) Recent (within 30 days) or at high risk of recurrence venous thromboembolism Multiple risk factors

number of patients undergoing oral anticoagulation demands practical recommendations in spite of the lack of evidence on the efficacy and safety of the recommended procedures.

The general strategy for the management of VKA treatment in patients undergoing invasive procedures requires the careful evaluation of three elements [26]:
• the thromboembolic risk of the individual patient in case of interruption of OAC, in relation to its indications and to the risk of postoperative thromboembolic complications;
• the bleeding risk of the procedure per se and in case anticoagulation is continued; and
• the necessity of alternative anticoagulant drugs (bridging therapy) and their relative efficacy and safety.

The substantial difference between the consequences of major bleeding events and thromboembolic complications should also be taken into account. Permanent disability and death are common after arterial thromboembolism, especially in cases of cerebrovascular events (70–75%), whereas they are less frequent in cases of venous thromboembolic complications (4–10%) or major postoperative hemorrhage (1–6%). It is also crucial to consider the attitude of the specialist who performs the procedure, who is gen-

erally more concerned about any bleeding resulting from the procedure if oral anticoagulation is continued rather than the risk of thromboembolism if oral anticoagulation is stopped. In the absence of certain indications, a careful evaluation by several specialists is warranted (hematologist, internist, cardiologist, surgeon, and anesthesiologist). There are three possible choices (see Table 16.3) [27].

Continuation of VKA treatment

In procedures associated with a low risk of bleeding, such as traumas of superficial tissues where local hemostatic measures (e.g. pressure, antifibrinolytics, fibrin glue) can be applied, VKAs can be continued:
• punctures and catheterization of superficial veins and arteries (e.g. femoral artery and Seldinger catheter);
• Sternal punctures and bone marrow aspirates;
• skin biopsies, minor dermatologic surgery, biopsy of mucosa that is easily accessible and explorable (oral cavity, vagina), minor eye surgery;
• endoscopic examinations without surgery; and
• simple tooth extraction in the absence of infection or surgical incisions. In the latter cases, it is recommended to use local hemostatic agents, suturing of alveolar edges, and mouth rinses with a 5%

tranexamic acid solution, 4–5 minutes every 6 hours for 5–6 days, combined with antibiotic therapy.

In these cases, it is it is advisable to lower the INR to approximately 2.0 to decrease the hemorrhagic risk without an increase in the thromboembolic risk. If the expected risk of bleeding is higher (e.g. multiple teeth extractions in the presence of infection, closed biopsy, endo-ocular surgery, or cataract with retrobulbar anesthetic) and the risk of thromboembolism is not high (in most cases, excluding patients with prosthetic heart valves or cardiac endocavitary thrombosis), VKAs can be temporarily reduced, aiming at INR values between 1.5 and 2.

Patients being treated with VKAs should be told to avoid, whenever possible, intramuscular injections so to avoid the risk of hematomas (especially if the patient needs many injections).

Temporary discontinuation of VKA treatment

This is recommended in conditions associated with a significant risk of bleeding (such as cases of trauma to deep tissues not easily accessible to local hemostatic measures; see Table 16.3) in patients with non-high risk of thrombotic complications.

Perioperative bridging therapy

This strategy is indicated in patients who are at high risk of thrombotic complications (see Table 16.3). In these patients, the goal is to minimize risk by reducing the duration of the bridging therapy to the minimum and by administering bridging therapy for the duration of subtherapeutic INR. If the procedure is elective, no immediate reversal of VKAs is required and VKAs can be discontinued 3–4 days before the procedure (in case of therapeutic INR), as the INR is expected to fall to subtherapeutic values in 3–4 days. The bridging therapy can be commenced 60 hours after the last warfarin dose (third morning after last evening dose). The INR should be measured the day before surgery to determine whether it is below 1.5–1.7. If not, 1 mg vitamin K can be given orally and the INR repeated on the day of surgery.

The bridging therapy can be conducted with unfractionated heparin (subcutaneous or intravenous) when the INR falls below 2.0. Bridging therapy can be started with prophylactic unfractionated heparin (5000 U every 8–12 hours subcutaneously). Those at very high

risk of thromboembolic complications (previous systemic embolism in atrial fibrillation, prosthetic heart valves, multiple risk factors) can also be given bridging therapy by administering adjusted dose heparin (subcutaneous in outpatients or by continuous intravenous infusion in case of hospital admission) to maintain an APTT value equal to 1.5–2 times the normal value of control.

Bridging therapy can also be administered with low-molecular-weight heparin subcutaneously as out- or inpatient for 2–3 days preoperatively, using doses recommended for prophylaxis or, in patients at very high risk of thrombosis, therapeutic doses once (150–200 U/kg) or twice (100 U/kg) daily.

Drug administration immediately prior to surgery must be avoided in these cases:
- Subcutaneous unfractionated heparin should be discontinued 12 hours before surgery.
- Intravenous heparin should be discontinued 6 hours before surgery.
- Low-molecular-weight heparin should be discontinued no less than 8–10 hours at prophylaxis dose or 18 hours preoperatively with treatment doses, with an additional 6-hour interval in case of planned neuroaxial anesthesia.

In venous thromboembolism, the risk of recurrence is the highest in the first month after the acute event (40%). As a result, invasive procedures should be deferred, if possible, for at least 1 month and preferably 3 months after the acute event. If surgery is necessary within 2 weeks from an acute event, patients should have an inferior vena cava filter inserted preoperatively or intraoperatively.

Postoperative management of anticoagulation

VKAs may be resumed only after evaluating each case very carefully as a function of the time needed for tissues to heal and in the absence of bleeding complications. Intravenous heparin should be resumed after 12 hours postoperatively at a rate of no more than 18 U/kg, and it has the advantage of rapid elimination if discontinued and of neutralization with protamine. If subcutaneous low-molecular-weight heparin is preferred, twice daily doses are recommended, started 24 hours postoperatively and only after hemostasis has been achieved. In patients with a very high bleeding risk (e.g. after neurosurgery or prostatectomy), heparin is resumed only after clinical evaluation and in general after at least 48–72 hours. VKAs can be resumed postoperatively as soon as the patients can take solid foods, overlapping with heparin until an INR >2 is obtained for two consecutive days. In case of emergency surgery, oral anticoagulation must be reversed as soon as possible.

Spinal or epidural anesthesia

Regional anesthesia in association with perioperative prophylaxis or heparin therapy is safe and efficacious with an adequate selection of patient and anesthesiologic technique. There are no controlled studies evaluating the risk of spinal hematoma in the course of therapy or with heparin prophylaxis.

The following can be suggested with intravenous (IV) or subcutaneous (SC) unfractionated heparin:
• Perform the spinal puncture or the positioning of the catheter at least 1 hour before starting heparin IV, or more than 4 hours after the suspension of the heparin IV and after the administration of the heparin SC.
• Maintain APTT value not more than 1.5 times the control value.
• Remove the catheter only after normalization of the APTT.

The following are suggestions for the use of prophylactic dose low-molecular-weight heparins:
• Perform spinal puncture or positioning of the catheter 10–12 hours after the last dose;
• Remove the catheter at least 10–12 hours after the last dose, and administer the successive dose at least 2 hours after removal.

In any case it must be remembered:
• Do not administer drugs that interfere with the hemostasis.
• Defer the operation in the presence of a bloodstained spinal tap.
• Constant patient surveillance is essential for the onset of signs or symptoms of medullary compression (sphincteric alterations, progression of paresthesia, and limb weakness).
• In the case of spinal hematoma, emergency decompressive laminectomy is mandatory (<6 hours from the onset of the symptoms).

Cataract surgery

With modern techniques, which rely on limited incision of the cornea (nonvascularized tissue), the risk of bleeding from surgery itself is practically null. Possible bleeding complications are linked to the type of anesthesia. Cases have been reported of retro- and peribulbar hematomas in patients on VKAs following retro- and peribulbar anesthesia. Despite the lack of exact data on the incidence of these complications, it should be borne in mind that retro- and peribulbar anesthesia requires normal blood hemostasis and hence discontinuation of VKAs, so it should be contraindicated in patients on VKAs in whom the thrombotic risk following a suspension of treatment is high. In contrast, cataract surgery can be performed without anticoagulant suspension in all those subjects in whom a topical or general anesthesia can be used. Evaluating the risk–benefit and cost–benefit ratios of the different options (e.g. surgery without VKAs suspension vs. surgery with retrobulbar anesthesia and VKAs suspension) should be carried out in each patient on the basis of a general consideration of the risk factors (thrombotic and hemorrhagic).

New anticoagulants

The complexities of oral anticoagulation treatment have prompted the search for improved anticoagulants [28]. The ideal anticoagulant should be effective, with minimal complications/side effects and convenient administration (i.e. oral for outpatients), with rapid absorption and fast on- and offset action, predictable pharmacokinetics, no interactions with food or drugs, no need of coagulation monitoring, and availability of an antidote.

New anticoagulants have been developed that target a single coagulation factor and have predictable dose–response relationships. These include direct thrombin inhibitors and factor Xa inhibitors. Two parenteral direct thrombin inhibitors, lepirudin and argatroban, have FDA approval for the management of heparin-induced thrombocytopenia (HIT). Bivalirudin is a parenteral direct thrombin inhibitor that is licensed for patients undergoing percutaneous coronary interventions and for those with HIT who require percutaneous coronary interventions. Ximelagatran, an oral prodrug of the direct thrombin inhibitor melagatran, showed efficacy in the prevention and treatment of venous thromboembolism as well as stroke prevention in patients with atrial fibrillation. However, due to nonhematologic safety concerns, it did not receive FDA approval in the US. Fondaparinux is a synthetic pentasaccharide, which is highly selective for antithrombin with exclusive anti-Xa activity, with a predictable dose response due to the absence of aspecific binding to plasma proteins, and with virtually absent risk of HIT. The effectiveness of fondaparinux has been shown in phase III studies in the prophylaxis and treatment of venous thromboembolism, and it is now available for clinical use in Europe. Idraparinux is a modified pentasaccaride with a long half-life, which can be administered by injection once weekly. In Phase III studies, idraparinux has been shown to be as effective as warfarin in the treatment of venous thromboembolism, albeit with a higher risk of bleeding.

An oral direct thrombin inhibitor, dabigatran etexilate, has been recently approved for clinical use in Europe for the prophylaxis of venous thromboembolism in major orthopedic surgery. Dabigatran etexilate has a molecular weight of 628 Da, with a half-life of 14–17 hours and time to peak level of 2 hours, with prevalent renal excretion. Dabigatran etexilate can be administered orally without laboratory monitoring at a dose of 110 mg at 1–4 hours after surgery and then at full dose of 220 mg once daily for 10 days after knee prosthesis and 28–35 days after hip surgery; the dose should be reduced at 150 mg once daily in case of age greater than 75 years and in case of chronic renal failure. Phase III studies are ongoing in the treatment of venous thromboembolism with the aim of replacing warfarin. Two oral direct factor Xa inhibitors, rivaroxaban and apixaban, are undergoing evaluation in phase III studies in the prevention and treatment of venous thromboembolism. In spite of the potential advantages of the newer oral anticoagulant drugs, their main limitation is the lack of an antidote.

References

1 Baglin TP, Keeling DM, Watson HG. Guidelines on oral anticoagulation (Warfarin): third edition – 2005 update. *Br J Haematol* 2006;132:277–85.

2 Hirsh J, Dalen JE, Anderson DR, et al. Oral anticoagulants: Mechanism of action, clinical effectiveness, and optimal therapeutic range. *Chest* 2001;119:8S–21S.

3 Chan WS, Anand S, Ginsberg JS. Anticoagulation of pregnant women with mechanical heart valves: a systematic review of the literature. *Arch Intern Med* 2000;160:191–6.

4 Margaglione M, Colaizzo D, D'Andrea G, et al. Genetic modulation of oral anticoagulation with warfarin. *Thromb Haemost* 2000;84:775–8.

5 Rost S, Fregin A, Ivaskevicius V, et al. Mutations in VKORC1 cause warfarin resistance and multiple coagulation factor deficiency type 2. *Nature* 2004;427:537–41.

6 Rieder MJ, Reiner AP, Gage BF, et al. Effect of VKORC1 haplotypes on transcriptional regulation and warfarin dose. *N Engl J Med* 2005;352:2285–93.

7 Ansell J, Hirsh J, Hylek E, et al. Pharmacology and management of the vitamin K antagonists. *Chest* 2008;133:160S–198S.

8 Fennerty A, Dolben J, Thomas P, et al. Flexible induction dose regimen for warfarin and prediction of maintenance dose. *Br Med J* 1984;288:1268–70.

9 Crowther MA, Ginsberg JB, Kearon C, et al. A randomized trial comparing 5-mg and 10-mg warfarin loading doses. *Arch Intern Med* 1999;159:46–8.

10 Kovacs MJ, Rodger M, Anderson DR, et al. Comparison of 10-mg and 5-mg warfarin initiation nomograms together with low-molecular-weight heparin for outpatient treatment of acute venous thromboembolism. A randomized, double-blind, controlled trial. *Ann Intern Med* 2003;138:714–9.

11 Poller L, Keown M, Ibrahim S, et al. An international multicenter randomized study of computer-assisted oral anticoagulant dosage vs. medical staff dosage. *J Thromb Haemost* 2008;6:935–43.

12 Chiquette E, Amato MG, Bussey HI. Comparison of an anticoagulation clinic with usual medical care: anticoagulation control, patient outcomes, and health care costs. *Arch Intern Med* 1998;158:1641–7.

13 Vandermeer FJM, Briet E, Vandenbroucke JP, et al. The role of compliance as a cause of instability in oral anticoagulant therapy. *Br J Haematol* 1997;98:893–900.

14 Palareti G, Legnani C, Guazzaloca G, et al. Risks factors for highly unstable response to oral anticoagulation: a case-control study. *Br J Haematol* 2005;129:72–8.

15 Barcellona D, Contu P, Marongiu F. Patient education and oral anticoagulant therapy. *Haematologica* 2002;87:1081–6.

16 Tang EO, Lai CS, Lee KK, et al. Relationship between patients' warfarin knowledge and anticoagulation control. *Ann Pharmacother* 2003;37:34–9.

17 Estrada CA, Hryniewicz MM, Higgs VB, et al. Anticoagulant patient information material is written at high readability levels. *Stroke* 2000;31:2966–70.

18 Ford SK, Misita CP, Shilliday BB, et al. Prospective study of supplemental vitamin K therapy in patients on oral anticoagulants with unstable international normalized ratios. *J Thromb Thrombolysis* 2007;24:23–7.

19 Palareti G, Leali N, Coccheri S, et al. Bleeding complications of oral anticoagulant treatment: an inception- cohort, prospective collaborative study (ISCOAT). Italian Study on Complications of Oral Anticoagulant Therapy. *Lancet* 1996;348:423–8.

20 Oden A, Fahlen M. Oral anticoagulation and risk of death: a medical record linkage study. *Br Med J* 2002;325:1073–5.

21 Fang MC, Go AS, Chang YC, et al. Death and disability from warfarin-associated intracranial and extracranial hemorrhages. *Am J Med* 2007;120:700–5.

22 Linkins LA, Choi PT, Douketis JD. Clinical impact of bleeding in patients taking oral anticoagulant therapy for venous thromboembolism: a meta-analysis. *Ann Intern Med* 2003;139:893–900.

23 Rosand J, Hylek EM, Odonnell HC, et al. Warfarin-associated hemorrhage and cerebral amyloid angiopathy: a genetic and pathologic study. *Neurology* 2000;55:947–51.

24 Makris M, Watson HG. The management of coumarin-induced over-anticoagulation. *Br J Haematol* 2001;114:271–80.

25 Hellstern P, Halbmayer WM, Kohler M, et al. Prothrombin complex concentrates: Indications, contraindications, and risks: a task force summary. *Thromb Res* 1999;95:S3–S6.

26 Kearon C, Hirsh J. Current concepts: management of anticoagulation before and after elective surgery. *N Engl J Med* 1997;336:1506–11.

27 Kearon C. Management of anticoagulation in patients requiring invasive procedures. *Semin Vasc Med* 2003;3:285–93.

28 Bates SM, Weitz JI. The status of new anticoagulants. *Br J Haematol* 2006;134:3–19.

29 Schulman S, Kearon C. Definition of major bleeding in clinical investigations of antihemostatic medicinal products in non-surgical patients. *J Thromb Haemost* 2005;3:692–4.

17 Antiphospholipid syndrome

Henry G. Watson and Beverley J. Robertson

Introduction

The antiphospholipid syndrome (APS) is an acquired prothrombotic or thrombophilic state that is also associated with adverse outcome of pregnancy. An association of antiphospholipid antibodies with a variety of disorders has been made since the first report in patients with systemic lupus erythematosus (SLE), and the clinicopathological criteria for the diagnosis of APS have been agreed internationally [1]. In spite of this, our understanding of the pathogenesis of the condition is limited, particularly with respect to the complications of pregnancy for which there is no compelling evidence of an ischemic pathogenesis. Because the manifestations of the APS are common in the population, differentiation between those individuals with and without the syndrome is heavily dependent on laboratory assays to detect persistent antiphospholipid antibodies. The laboratory-based diagnosis, however, is a subject of serious concern with disappointing quality assurance data for all tests. This is very important because the diagnosis of APS changes clinical management significantly in those affected. For example, anticoagulation following a first episode of venous thromboembolism should probably be prolonged in those with APS, whereas it is appropriate in other groups of patients to consider periods of 3–6 months only. However, whereas there are good data to inform on the management of venous thromboembolism, the same is not true for arterial thrombosis. Finally, there are conflicting views on the treatment of women with adverse pregnancy outcome attributable to APS.

Definition of APS

The APS describes a clinicopathologic entity. APS is an acquired prothrombotic state that probably has an immune-mediated pathogenesis, and its diagnosis requires the coexistence of clinical manifestations (thrombosis or adverse pregnancy outcome) with laboratory evidence of antiphospholipid antibodies.

The Sapporo diagnostic criteria for APS were revised in 2005 by an International Consensus Panel (Table 17.1) [2]. A variety of other clinical abnormalities, which are frequently observed in association with antiphospholipid antibodies, are not included in the internationally agreed definition of APS. The most common of these are thrombocytopenia and livedo reticularis, which are frequently found in patients who do not otherwise fulfil the criteria for APS (Table 17.2). Identification of these other associated conditions should lead to consideration of a diagnosis of APS. It is not clear whether thrombosis is implicated in the pathogenesis of these conditions, and the role of antithrombotic medicines is even less clear.

Clinical features of APS

The main clinical presentation of APS is either with thrombosis or pregnancy failure. However, the condition is heterogeneous (as are the implicated antibodies), and most individuals do not suffer from all the clinical features of the syndrome. Interestingly, although a combination of venous and arterial thrombotic events may predate the development of a

Table 17.1 Diagnostic criteria for APS.

Clinical criteria

Thrombosis
Venous, arterial, or small-vessel thrombosis involving any organ
or tissue

Pregnancy
Unexplained death of a morphologically normal fetus at or
after 10 weeks' gestation
Three or more consecutive unexplained abortions before 10
weeks' gestation
Severe pre-eclampsia or placental insufficiency before 34
weeks' gestation

Laboratory criteria
LA
IgG or IgM anticardiolipin antibodies at moderate or high titer
IgG or IgM anti-β_2–glycoprotein 1 antibodies in titer >99th
centile

Note: To fulfill the diagnosis of APS, there must be at least
one clinical and one laboratory criterion present. The detection
of antiphospholipid antibodies must have been performed on
two occasions at least 12 weeks apart.

history of pregnancy failure in some women, especially those with SLE, most women who present with
adverse pregnancy outcome tend to have this as a sole
manifestation.

Table 17.2 Some conditions associated with
antiphospholipid antibodies but not included in the definition
of APS.

Thrombocytopenia
Livedo reticularis
Allograft failure
Transverse myelopathy
Chorea
Multifocal central nervous system syndrome resembling multi-
ple sclerosis
Skin necrosis
Pulmonary hypertension
Sensorineural deafness
Cardiac valve disease (vegetations, valve thickening and dys-
function)
Nephropathy (small-vessel vasculopathy)

Thrombosis

Thrombosis may involve both the arterial and the venous systems. The most common presentation is with
lower limb deep vein thrombosis, sometimes with
clinically significant pulmonary embolus. Other sites
for venous thrombosis such as cerebral vein, axillary
and subclavian vein, and intra-abdominal veins, including the portal, hepatic, and mesenteric veins, are
less common but well recognized in APS. Patients
tend to be young individuals with unprovoked venous
thromboembolism, thrombosis at unusual sites, and
an absence of a family history of thrombophilia.

Stroke and transient cerebral ischemia are the most
common presentations of arterial thrombosis in APS.
Myocardial infarction appears rare, although the reason for this is not clear. Embolic thrombus from sterile
endocarditis and cardiac valve vegetations are also described.

Microvascular thrombosis is uncommon but is described in the extremely rare "catastrophic antiphospholipid syndrome" that presents with multiorgan failure and which usually progresses unabated in spite of
all forms of therapy (Plate 17.1).

Pregnancy failure

This is now the most common presentation that results
in a diagnosis of APS being made. This is in part because of the wish (and pressure) to investigate women
who are distressed by this presentation. Recurrent
early fetal loss is most commonly seen, although otherwise unexplained fetal death after the first trimester
and severe pre-eclampsia before 34 weeks are also recognized features.

The emotive nature of these cases may result in
the inappropriate investigation of women with only
one or two early miscarriages, which can result in a
chance finding of an innocent antiphospholipid antibody. Having detected antiphospholipid antibodies
in these women who do not fulfill the APS criteria
[3], clinicians find it difficult to withhold treatment,
resulting in some women spending the whole of subsequent pregnancies on aspirin and low-molecular-
weight heparin (LMWH), based on very little
evidence.

Most proponents of this approach argue that
waiting for a third early loss in these women is
inappropriate and add that the therapy has so few side

effects that this is not an issue. However, side effects, although few, are seen and the costs of clinic time and drugs are significant. This practice also converts normal women into patients for the duration of their pregnancy while skewing the perception of benefit for intervention.

Antiphospholipid antibodies

These are a heterogeneous group of antibodies, which are detected because of their capacity to react with phospholipid either in phospholipid-dependent coagulation assays in the case of a lupus anticoagulant (LA) or bound to enzyme-linked immunosorbent assay (ELISA) plates in the case of anticardiolipin and anti-β_2-glycoprotein 1 antibodies.

The earliest descriptions of antiphospholipid antibodies were in individuals with SLE who had false-positive tests for syphilis. Further investigation of these patients indicated that they had circulating antibodies that were capable of binding to the negatively charged phospholipid, cardiolipin. This gave rise to the nomenclature *anticardiolipin antibodies.*

About the same time, it was noted that some subjects with SLE had prolonged blood-clotting times in in vitro test systems but had no evidence of a bleeding diathesis. The prolonged clotting in phospholipid-dependent tests could not be reversed by addition of normal plasma, indicating the presence of an inhibitor, the so-called *lupus anticoagulant.*

Paradoxically, the presence of the LA was associated with an increased risk of thrombosis in patients with SLE, and when it became apparent that the presence of either of these antibodies was associated with an increased thrombosis risk, the concept of an acquired prothrombotic or thrombophilic state was proposed.

Antiphospholipid antibodies with features of APS may be found either in isolation as a *primary antiphospholipid syndrome* or in association with SLE and other autoimmune conditions, such as Sjögren syndrome as a *secondary antiphospholipid syndrome.*

Although they are called antiphospholipid antibodies, it is now clear that the antigenic targets for most of these antibodies are not phospholipid per se, but instead are proteins that bind to phospholipid (Table 17.3). The best known of these is β_2-glyco-

Table 17.3 Antigenic targets of antiphospholipid antibodies.

β_2-glycoprotein 1
Prothrombin
Protein C
Protein S
Annexin V
Factors XI and XII

protein 1, a circulating protein of unknown function which avidly binds negatively charged phospholipid. β_2-Glycoprotein 1 is considered the most important antigenic target for antiphospholipid antibodies. The molecule has five domains, and antibodies against domain 1 have been shown to be the pathogenic antibodies that cause the LA effect and associate most strongly with thrombosis. It has also been shown that the binding of β_2-glycoprotein 1 to phospholipid causes a conformational change in the molecule and the exposure of "cryptic epitopes." This may, in part, explain the formation of autoantibodies [4].

Other antigen targets for antiphospholipid antibodies include prothrombin, factor XI, proteins C and S, and annexin V, all proteins involved in hemostatic pathways that might be relevant in explaining the thrombotic complications associated with these antibodies. In response to these findings, ELISA assays that have β_2-glycoprotein 1 and prothrombin as antigen are now commercially available.

Despite this knowledge, the pathogenesis of thrombosis and pregnancy failure in APS remains unclear. Laboratory findings combined with the outcome of clinical studies indicate that the pathological manifestations of APS are caused by a prothrombotic state with little evidence that overt histological inflammation contributes significantly to the process. No single mechanism has been shown to underlie the prothrombotic tendency, and this is perhaps not surprising given the varied sites of thrombosis and the range of target antigens for antiphospholipid antibodies.

Whether antiphospholipid antibodies are indeed directly pathogenic is debated. IgG from serum of patients with APS has been shown to be pathogenic in animal models of thrombosis and pregnancy loss. Laboratory experiments have assessed the effects of antiphospholipid antibodies on many of the processes involved in hemostasis, thrombosis, inflammation, and fibrinolysis.

There are data to support that antiphospholipid antibodies may induce tissue factor expression by monocytes, inhibit the function of the natural anticoagulants activated protein C and protein S, induce endothelial cell apoptosis and activation, and induce platelet activation by binding via the Fc receptor. All, none, or, more likely, a combination of these mechanisms may contribute to the disease process [4]. Although the criteria for diagnosis of APS state that histological evidence of inflammation excludes the diagnosis, there is increasing experimental evidence that antiphospholipid antibodies may induce an inflammatory state. Up-regulation of adhesion molecules, such as VCAM-1 and E-selectin, and secretion of interleukin-6 has been observed in endotheial cells incubated with antiphospholipid antibodies. Increased leukocyte adhesion to endothelium with associated release of tissue factor could perceivably be involved in the pathogenesis of the condition.

The pathogenesis of pregnancy failure in APS is even more difficult to explain. Knowledge of the possible prothrombotic mechanisms has led to the inference that placental ischemia is the main mechanism resulting in pregnancy failure in APS (Plate 17.2). The evidence from clinical studies suggesting improved outcome in patients treated with antithrombotic medicines, such as heparin and aspirin, is felt by many to support this hypothesis. However, overt placental ischemia is rare, and the observation that the most common manifestation of APS in pregnancy is miscarriage before 10 weeks (i.e. prior to development of the placental circulation) suggests that other mechanisms must contribute. Complement activation by antiphospholipid antibodies has been linked to early pregnancy loss, and antiphospholipid antibodies have been shown to inhibit trophoblastic proliferation and spiral artery invasion in vitro. Interestingly, these effects may be inhibited by heparin, which suggests that at least part of any benefit for heparin may relate to an anti-complement effect and/or improved implantation.

Other work has suggested that antiphospholipid antibodies may act by displacing the natural anticoagulant annexin V from endothelial cell surfaces, resulting in a procoagulant state. However, as normal expression of annexin V has been demonstrated in affected pregnancies, the importance of these observations remains unclear.

Diagnosis of APS

APS is a clinicopathologic entity that depends on the identification of a clinical diagnosis combined with demonstration of appropriate antiphospholipid antibodies (Table 17.1). Although criteria for diagnosis have been internationally agreed, the diagnosis of APS is still complicated by two main problems:
• Many antiphospholipid antibodies are nonpathological and are not associated with APS.
• The standardization of assays for LA and immunologically detectable antiphospholipid antibodies, such as anticardiolipin antibodies and β_2-glycoprotein 1 antibodies, is unfortunately very poor.

Transient and nonpathological antiphospholipid antibodies

Both LAs and anticardiolipin antibodies, alone or together, are found in a significant number of normal subjects. Like the finding of a positive direct antiglobulin test in approximately 1 in 10,000 blood donors, the finding is of little consequence to the individual, but it does generate further investigation and anxiety in the patient if handled badly. One common source of this type of scenario is in the recruitment of healthy ward and laboratory personnel as normal controls. On some occasions, the antiphospholipid antibody is transient, but persistent high-titer anticardiolipin antibodies and strong positive LAs are not uncommon. Some series report the finding of antiphospholipid antibodies, most often anticardiolipin, in up to 5% of normal subjects.

Perhaps the most common cause of transient antiphospholipid antibodies is infection (Table 17.4). This is mostly seen following viral infection but may complicate bacterial and parasitic infections also. Although these antibodies are not typically associated with significant disease, purpura fulminans resulting from acquired protein S deficiency due to antiphospholipid antibodies, is a well-documented complication of varicella infection in children. Some infections, such as HIV, hepatitis C, leprosy, syphilis, leptospirosis, leishmaniasis, and malaria, are associated with

Table 17.4 Infections associated with antiphospholipid antibodies.

Viral
HIV
Hepatitis C
Varicella

Bacterial
Helicobacter pylori
Syphilis
Leprosy
Leptospirosis

Parasitic
Malaria
Leishmaniasis

persistent antiphospholipid antibodies. These are rarely linked with the development of clinical features of APS (Table 17.1).

The use of certain common drugs is also associated with the development of antiphospholipid antibodies. The association with chlorpromazine is the best documented, and although these antibodies are not typically said to be associated with the development of thrombosis, it may be that this underlies the recent reported association of psychoactive drugs with an increased risk of venous thromboembolism.

Laboratory assays

Correct diagnosis of APS is ultimately dependent on the availability of accurate diagnostic assays. A vast amount of work has been carried out to try to standardize assays for anticardiolipin and LA. Although internationally agreed guidelines have been drawn up to address this, the intricacies of the assays and the plethora of nonstandardized reagents available make this a difficult area. Summarized below are the key features that require attention in detecting antiphospholipid antibodies.

Lupus anticoagulants

The Scientific and Standardization Committee of the International Society of Thrombosis and Hemostasis

recommends that the laboratory diagnosis of LAs should be carried out on double-centrifuged plasma following a four-step procedure adhering to these principles [5]:

1 Prolongation of a phospholipid-dependent coagulation test.
2 Evidence of inhibitory activity on mixing tests.
3 Evidence of phospholipid dependence.
4 Lack of specificity for any one coagulation factor.

This process allows the detection of inhibitory activity in the plasma and then facilitates differentiation of LA from specific inhibitors of coagulation, which are more rare. As the management of patients with antiphospholipid antibodies often involves antithrombotic medication, while patients with acquired inhibitors of coagulation harbor an often life-threatening bleeding diathesis, differentiation is of paramount importance.

Some laboratories perform LA screening tests, such as a dilute prothrombin time and activated partial thromboplastin time (APTT) tests, using reagents with a high sensitivity to LA. Others screen requests for clinical detail and perform fewer, more specific tests, such as dilute Russell viper venom time or kaolin clotting time, to investigate suspected cases.

It is widely agreed that the use of more than one coagulation based test is essential to detect LA. Mixing studies are performed to demonstrate inhibitor activity in test plasma. Errors arising in the mixing procedure relate to the quality of the normal plasma, particularly its platelet content, and to the level of dilution employed. Platelet contamination, even to levels as low as 1000/μL, can result in quenching of the inhibitory effect and therefore to a false-negative result.

Confirmation of the phospholipid dependence of the inhibitor is assessed by adding excess phospholipid to the test system. The rationale for this is that the excess phospholipid neutralizes or bypasses the LA effect. Platelet membrane particles or purer forms of phospholipid may be used for this purpose.

Platelet membrane preparations suffer from significant batch-to-batch variability that does not lend itself to standardization.

Specific coagulation factor assays may help to confirm the nature of an inhibitor. They are probably indicated when there is concern about a bleeding diathesis or when there is discordance in the earlier stages of detecting a LA. Simultaneous reduction of more than one coagulation factor may indicate the presence of a LA.

When using this method to detect a LA, factor assays should be performed at numerous plasma dilutions. Unlike the situation where a specific coagulation factor inhibitor is present, the apparent coagulation factor activity rises with greater dilution in the presence of a LA; that is, the assay curves are non-parallel. The results from these assays may vary with different reagents.

Anticardiolipin assays

A great deal of effort has gone toward producing new, more specific assays to measure anti-β_2- glycoprotein 1 and anti-prothrombin activity in the hope that this would improve diagnostic accuracy. A direct anti-β_2-glycoprotein 1 antibody ELISA should theoretically be more specific than traditional standard assays, which use cardiolipin-coated plates with β_2-glycoprotein 1 as a cofactor for antibody binding. In addition, an international standard for units to measure anticardiolipin antibodies and terminology for the reporting of results has been developed. However, in spite of this, problems in measuring and interpreting anticardiolipin and anti-β_2-glycoprotein 1 assays persist.

Significant numbers of patients have low-titer anticardiolipin antibodies, and in an attempt to address this and to try to more clearly delineate pathological antibodies, the diagnostic criteria state that, to fulfil a diagnosis of APS, patients must have moderate or high titers of antibody (>40 GPL or MPL). However, this does not resolve all clinical scenarios. Furthermore, although assay performance has been improved by these changes, interassay comparability is still poor, and it appears that the new specific assays may be no more sensitive for the diagnosis of APS than standard anticardiolipin and LA tests.

Quality assurance

Quality assurance is a major issue for laboratories attempting to identify and quantify antiphospholipid antibodies. Although national and international standards and guidelines have been prepared (and are adhered to), recent quality assurance exercises still indicate that there are major problems.

A European Concerted Action on Thrombophilia survey indicated that plasma containing a 10 Bethesda unit inhibitor of factor VIII was wrongly identified as a LA in approximately 20% of 128 participating laboratories.

Likewise, a quality assurance exercise report on detection of anticardiolipin antibodies indicated an interlaboratory coefficient of variation of more than 50% in 74% of tests performed, leaving the authors to conclude that, in the majority of cases, the laboratories could not decide whether a sample was positive or negative.

Practical approach to diagnosis

A physician must be aware of these limitations when making a diagnosis of APS. From published literature, it has been shown that some antiphospholipid antibodies correlate better with thrombotic risk than others. LAs are stronger risk factors for thrombosis than anticardiolipin antibodies, and IgG anticardiolipin antibodies are more significant than IgM. The correlation between anti-β_2-glycoprotein 1 antibodies and thrombosis and pregnancy morbidity is still debated, and their clinical value in this context has not been clearly established. As a rule, high-titer antibodies have shown a better correlation with thrombosis than low titer, and positivity for more than one antibody adds to the significance.

Finally, testing for APS should be considered only when there is a reasonable clinical suspicion of the diagnosis and when the results will impact on management, for example, in a young patient with no risk factors for stroke or in unprovoked venous thromboembolism. Unselected screening for antiphospholipid antibodies in all patients with thrombotic events is inappropriate and will result in false-positive tests and misdiagnosis. Interpretation of results should always be individualized.

Management of APS

Thrombosis

The initial management of venous or arterial thrombosis in a patient with APS is, on the whole, no different to the management applied to similar cases without APS. Instead of discussing these in detail, it is more relevant to discuss issues that are specific to management of patients with APS. These relate to:

- choice of antithrombotic medication;
- intensity and duration of anticoagulation; and
- monitoring of anticoagulants.

Patients presenting with a first episode of unprovoked deep vein thrombosis or pulmonary embolus have a risk of thrombosis recurrence after discontinuation of anticoagulation of approximately 10% per annum, which seems to plateau after 3 years. Based on these data and on considering the risks of life-threatening or fatal hemorrhage associated with warfarin at 1% and 0.25–0.5%, respectively, most physicians treat these cases with warfarin for 6 months at an international normalized ratio (INR) target of 2.5. In contrast, the reported rates of recurrence of thrombosis in patients with APS is as high as 30–50% per annum, and as a result, many physicians offer long-term anticoagulation after a first unprovoked event in these cases. This change in management has major ramifications for the patient, and this emphasises the implications of making a diagnosis of APS in this clincal scenario.

Previous retrospective data suggested that an INR target of 3.5 provided better thromboprophylaxis than a target of 2.5, but recent prospective data from Crowther and colleagues [6] indicate that, certainly for prevention of recurrence of venous thromboembolism, an INR target of 2.5 is optimal.

In all of these cases, the likely benefit and risk to the patient has to be considered, and additional risk factors for bleeding on anticoagulants, such as increasing age, anemia, previous stroke, and history of gastrointestinal bleeding diabetes mellitus, and renal impairment have to be considered.

For patients who present with arterial thrombosis as a manifestation of APS, there are differences in approach to management. In the UK, in patients in whom there is no source of cardioembolic stroke, such as valvular heart disease or atrial fibrillation, it is usual to offer antiplatelet therapy with aspirin or dipyridamole to patients with ischemic stroke or transient cerebral ischemia. The Antiphospholipid Antibodies and Stroke Study found no benefit of warfarin over aspirin in prevention of recurrent stroke in patients positive for antiphospholipid antibodies at the time of stroke [7]. However, this study did not test for persistence of antibody and found a higher than expected incidence of antibodies in the elderly control cohort, suggesting a high detection rate of transient or clinically insignificant antibodies. Antiplatelet therapy alone seems to be effective for patients with low-titer or transient antiphospholipid antibodies, but is probably *not appropriate* for patients with clearly defined APS (i.e. persistently posisitive LA or high-titer anticardiolipin antibodies). These patients should be considered for warfarin and, in the absence of good data to indicate a benefit for more intense anticoagulation, should maintain an INR target of 2.5 [6].

The final issue for consideration is of the effect of LAs on monitoring of anticoagulation. Although the use of unfractionated heparin has been largely superseded by LMWHs, where the former is still used, there may be problems monitoring the APTT. Solutions to this are to use an APTT reagent that is not sensitive to LA (e.g. Actin FS) or to use a thrombin time or anti-Xa assay for heparin monitoring. Few LAs produce significant prolongation of the prothrombin time. If this does occur, using a low ISI thromboplastin, which has been locally calibrated prior to use, can usually circumvent it. The recent trend toward the use of point-of-care devices for the GP-based or home-based management of patients with antiphospholipid antibodies has highlighted issues of significant discrepancy between laboratory-based and point-of-care assays. In such cases, where point-of-care testing is desirable, appropriate collaboration with a local laboratory is required to ensure that safe monitoring can be performed.

Pregnancy failure

Pregnancy failure is often the only manifestation of disease in patients with primary APS, and although the evidence for a prothrombotic state is still not overwhelming, the main focus of therapy over the past 10 years has been to assess the effects of antithrombotic medication. Studies of immunosuppression using prednisolone have shown deleterious effects on pregnancy outcome for both mother and child. Intravenous immunoglobulin has been shown to have no benefit over aspirin and LMWH in a randomized trial. As such, the mainstay of therapy for those women who fulfill the criteria for APS consists of intensive antenatal care combined with aspirin with or without low-dose heparin.

Since 1997, when Rai and colleagues published a significant study of intervention in APS, there has been a trend toward the combined use of low-dose aspirin and heparin in pregnant women with APS [8]. However, two further studies at least challenge the validity of these conclusions:

• In a randomized study of 98 subjects, the outcomes for aspirin alone were the same as for aspirin and heparin in combination (pregnancy failure rates 28% vs. 22%) [9].

• A second study reported similar outcomes for patients randomized to supportive care only or to aspirin and supportive care (pregnancy failure rates 15% vs. 20%) [10].

In comparison with these data, the earlier studies, which purported to demonstrate a benefit for combined heparin and aspirin, reported pregnancy failure rates for the aspirin only groups of approximately 60%.

In clinical practice, it may be difficult to convince women with a history of pregnancy loss of the validity of treating only those who fulfil the diagnostic criteria, and for those who present with an Internet search in hand, discouraging heparin may be difficult.

References

1 Wilson WA, Gharavi AE, Koike T, et al. International consensus statement on preliminary classification criteria for definite antiphospholipid syndrome: report of an international workshop. *Arthritis Rheum* 1999;42: 1309–11.

2 Miyakis S, Lockshin AD, Atsumi T, et al. International consensus statement on an update of the classification criteria for definite antiphospholipid syndrome (APS). *J Thromb Haemost* 2006;4:295–306.

3 Creagh MD, Malia RG, Cooper SM, et al. Screening for lupus anticoagulant and anticardiolipin antibodies in women with fetal loss. *J Clin Pathol* 1991;44:45–7.

4 Urbanus RT, Derksen RHMW, de Groot PG. Current insight into the diagnosis and pathophysiology of the antiphospholipid syndrome. *Blood Rev* 2008;22: 93–105.

5 Brandt JT, Triplett DA, Alving B, et al. Criteria for the diagnosis of lupus anticoagulants: an update. On behalf of the Subcommittee on lupus anticoagulant/antiphospholipid antibody of the scientific and standardization committee of the ISTH. *Thromb Haemost* 1995;74:1185–90.

6 Crowther MA, Ginsberg JS, Julian J, et al. A comparison of two intensities of warfarin for the prevention of recurrent thrombosis in patients with the antiphospholipid antibody syndrome. *N Engl J Med* 2003;349: 1133–8.

7 Levine SR, Brey RL, Tilley BC, et al. Antiphospholipid antibodies and subsequent thrombo-occlusive events in patients with ischemic stroke. *JAMA* 2004;291: 576–84.

8 Rai R, Cohen H, Dave M, Regan L. Randomized controlled trial of aspirin and aspirin plus heparin in pregnant women with recurrent miscarriage associated with phospholipid antibodies (or antiphospholipid antibodies). *Br Med J* 1997;314:253–7.

9 Farquharson RG, Quenby S, Greaves M. Antiphospholipid syndrome in pregnancy a randomized controlled trial of treatment. *Obstet Gynecol* 2002;100: 408–13.

10 Pattison NS, Chamley LW, Birdsall M, et al. Does aspirin have a role in improving pregnancy outcome for women with the antiphospholipid syndrome? A randomized controlled trial. *Am J Obstet Gynecol* 2000;183:1008–12.

18 Cardiology

Jeffrey S. Berger and Richard C. Becker

Introduction

A balance between thrombosis, as the determining substrate for clinical phenotypes in coronary atherothrombosis, and excess bleeding (a well-known adverse effect from antithrombotic therapy) is a fundamental paradigm for practicing clinicians.

This chapter summarizes the pathobiological mechanisms of coronary atherothrombosis, including, as a platform for understanding pharmacotherapies and evidence-based treatment strategies, its development, natural history, and the clinical expression of disease. The classic model establishes platelets, and their complex interactions with inflammatory cells, activated endothelial cells, smooth muscle cells, apoptotic cells, oxidized low-density lipoprotein (LDL) cholesterol, and coagulation proteins, at the epicenter of initiating events.

Over time, atherosclerotic plaques may either progress to the point of coronary luminal narrowing or lose intrinsic architectural stability, predisposing them to rupture. Rupture of a vulnerable plaque is a potentially catastrophic event that serves as a sudden stimulus for blood flow and myocardial tissue perfusion-limiting thrombosis.

Pharmacotherapies directed against platelets and one or more coagulation proteins have advanced the care of patients with and those at risk for coronary atherothrombosis, owing to their well-documented ability to prevent clinical events, including myocardial infarction, reinfarction, and, in some instances, cardiovascular death. The development of direct, selective, and targeted therapies in conjunction with a better understanding of their inherent pharmacokinetic and pharmacodynamic properties will foster safe and effective treatments.

Pathophysiology of thrombosis

Progressive atherosclerosis is the primary mediator for development of thrombotic complications, such as acute coronary syndromes.

Atherogenesis begins in early childhood with the development of fatty streaks involving endothelial cells, vascular smooth muscle cells, and inflammatory cells and platelets [1].

Inflammatory mediators promote endothelial dysfunction and damage, stimulating accumulation and oxidation of LDL cholesterol within the artery wall [2].

Increased expression of cellular adhesion molecules leads to monocyte and platelet recruitment and subsequent migration of monocytes into the arterial wall, where they differentiate into macrophages.

The proinflammatory state stimulates migration and proliferation of smooth muscle cells and the accumulation of intracellular lipid deposits and/or extracellular lipids by macrophages, and thereby the transition to lipid-laden foam cells during fatty streak formation [3].

As these lesions expand, more smooth muscle cells migrate into the arterial wall; and deposition of extracellular matrix macromolecules, such as collagen and elastin, accompanies cellular accumulation and proliferation, leading to atherosclerotic plaque formation [4].

A mature plaque contains a core of lipid droplets, foam cells, and smooth muscle cells within a collagen-rich matrix.

In the setting of ongoing inflammation, there is a shift toward apoptosis and matrix degradation, leading to accumulation of necrotic material within the atheroma. Both inflammation and accelerated degradation of the matrix promote thinning of the protective fibrous cap surrounding the atherosclerotic plaque, thereby increasing the likelihood of plaque rupture [4], exposing the thrombogenic core to the circulating blood pool, stimulating platelet activation, and thrombus formation.

The most drastic complication occurs when plaque rupture causes arterial occlusion, leading to myocardial infarction in the heart, ischemic stroke in the brain, or critical ischemia in peripheral tissues.

In cases where plaque rupture and thrombosis do not lead to arterial occlusion, the thrombotic response plays an important role in the progression of atherosclerosis. Repetitive nonocclusive plaque rupture, thrombosis, and fibrotic healing accelerate progressive luminal narrowing and increase smooth muscle proliferation within the atheroma. The healing process after plaque rupture and thrombosis restores the integrity of the injured intima, re-endothelialization, and thus an increase in lesion size [2].

Acute coronary syndromes

The term acute coronary syndrome (ACS) has evolved as a useful description of the spectrum of patients presenting with angina pectoris caused by myocardial infarction or unstable angina. The underlying pathological mechanism for the development of ACS is a vulnerable atherosclerotic plaque with either plaque rupture or plaque ulceration leading to thrombosis. Rupture or ulceration of the atherosclerotic plaque exposes the subendothelial matrix to formed elements of circulating blood, leading to activation of platelets, thrombin generation, and ultimately thrombus generation.

Completely occlusive

The dynamic process of plaque rupture may evolve to a completely occlusive thrombus with ST elevation on the electrocardiogram, known as an ST elevation myocardial infarction (STEMI), or new left bundle branch block (LBBB). If left untreated, such occlusive thrombi lead to a large zone of necrosis involving the full or nearly full thickness of the ventricular wall.

Less obstructive thrombi

These typically produce ST segment depression or T wave changes on the electrocardiogram. If prolonged, this may result in the release of cardiac enzymes and may be diagnosed as non-ST elevation myocardial infarction (NSTEMI).

Unstable angina

Less prolonged and/or less flow-limiting thrombi may not cause release of cardiac enzymes and is therefore called unstable angina.

Therapies for ACS

The ACS spectrum follows a common pathophysiological substrate and is useful for developing therapeutic strategies.

Fibrinolytic therapy
The goal of fibrinolytic therapy is rapid restoration of flow in an occluded vessel achieved by accelerating fibrinolysis of a coronary arterial thrombus. Mechanistically, fibrinolytic drugs accelerate the conversion of plasminogen to plasmin, a serine protease that degrades the insoluble fibrin clot matrix.

Large, placebo-controlled clinical trials have consistently demonstrated improved ventricular function, decreased infarct size, and reduced mortality in patients receiving fibrinolytic therapy *within 6 and potentially upto 12 hours of the onset of STEMI*. Several agents are available and approved for use in STEMI [5].

Complications of fibrinolytic therapy
The most serious is intracerebral hemorrhage, which occurs in between 0.5% and 1.0% of patients. Major risk factors for intracranial hemorrhage include:
- age greater than 75,
- hypertension,
- low body weight,
- female gender, and
- coagulopathy.

Table 18.1 Fibrinolytic therapy recommendations.

- In patients who present with STEMI ≤6–12 hours, and when primary PCI is not readily available, fibrinolytic therapy is recommended.
- In patients who are candidates for fibrinolytic therapy, administration as soon as possible (ideally within 30 minutes) is recommended.
- If possible, prehospital administration of fibrinolytic therapy is recommended.
- Fibrinolytic therapy is not recommended in patients with a history of intracranial hemorrhage, or with a history of head trauma, or with ischemic stroke within the past 6 months.

Because of this significant increased risk, primary percutaneous coronary intervention is preferred when performed in a timely fashion. Nevertheless, the relative advantages and limitations of each therapy should be considered for each individual patient.

In comparison, fibrinolytic therapy has not been effective in patients with NSTEMI or unstable angina (Table 18.1).

Anticoagulation

Anticoagulants are used widely by cardiologists. Anticoagulation therapies interfere with the clotting cascade and therefore reduce the risk of atherothrombosis.

In the setting of ACS, patients are treated with an anticoagulant to suppress the risk of recurrent cardiovascular events and systemic thromboembolism. The heparins (unfractionated heparin, low-molecular-weight heparin, and fondiparinux), direct thrombin inhibitors (bivalirudin), and vitamin K antagonists (warfarin) are the most commonly used agents (Table 18.2); however, newer agents are being developed and studied in clinical trials [6].

Following ACS, long-term therapy with anticoagulation must be balanced by the excess bleeding risk.

Unfractionated heparin (UFH)

Compared with aspirin alone, UFH (plus aspirin) reduces non-fatal cardiovascular events in the setting of ACS. Major limitations specific to UFH include the

need for frequent monitoring, and a narrow therapeutic window. Other limitations of UFH include heparin-induced thrombocytopenia (HIT) and a reduced ability to inactivate thrombin bound to fibrin.

Low-molecular-weight heparins (LMWHs)

LMWHs have pharmacological and biological advantages over heparin that render them more convenient to administer and less likely to cause HIT [7]. They lack the nonspecific binding affinities of UFH and, as a result, have more predictable pharmacokinetic and pharmacodynamic properties. Typically, LMWHs are given in weight-adjusted doses without monitoring. However, monitoring may be warranted in obese patients, in those with renal insufficiency, and when therapeutic doses of LMWHs are required during pregnancy.

The most frequently studied LMWH in ACS is enoxaparin. Compared with UFH, enoxaparin provides clinical benefit. In a meta-analysis of 12 randomized trials in the setting of ACS [8], enoxaparin versus UFH was associated with a significant 16% reduction in the rate of death or myocardial infarction with a small but significant increase in the risk of major bleeding.

Fondaparinux

This synthetic pentasaccharide selectively inhibits factor Xa. Fondaparinux shares all the pharmacological and biological advantages of LMWHs over UFH. Two large trials have addressed the role of fondaparinux in ACS: OASIS (Organization to Assess Strategies for Ischemic Syndromes)-5 in non-ST elevation ACS and OASIS-6 in STEMI [9,10]. OASIS-5 successfully demonstrated noninferiority for fondaparinux, compared with enoxaparin with respect to efficacy, and a lower rate of major bleeding.

Among STEMI patients, compared with "usual care," fondaparinux was effective in reducing death and reinfarction. The downside of fondaparinux is the small but heightened risk of catheter thrombosis, which makes it an unattractive anticoagulant option during percutaneous coronary intervention.

Thrombin inhibitors

As the name implies, direct thrombin inhibitors bind to thrombin and block its interaction with substrates.

Table 18.2 Antithrombotic drugs used in cardiovascular disease.

Agent	Route of administration	Plasma half-life	Clearance	Indications
Anticoagulants				
UFH	Intravenous or subcutaneous	30–60 minutes	Reticuloendothelial system*	Venous thromboembolism; ACS
LMWH	Intravenous or subcutaneous	3–6 hours	Renal	Venous thromboembolism; ACS
Fondaparinux	Subcutaneous	17–21 hours	Renal	Venous thromboembolism; ACS (not in patients undergoing PCI)
Bivalirudin	Intravenous	25 minutes	20% renal	PCI; HIT
Warfarin	Oral	36–42 hours	Liver	Venous thromboembolism; atrial fibrillation; mechanical prosthetic heart valve; long-term anticoagulation
Antiplatelets				
Aspirin	Oral and intravenous	15–20 minutes	Reticuloendothelial system	ACS, stroke, PCI, peripheral artery disease, primary prevention, secondary prevention
Ticlopidine	Oral	24–96 hours	Liver	ACS, stroke, PCI
Clopidogrel	Oral	8 hours	Liver	ACS, stroke, PCI, peripheral artery disease, secondary prevention
Abciximab	Intravenous	30 minutes	Reticuloendothelial system	ACS, PCI
Eptifibatide	Intravenous	2 hours	Renal/hepatic	ACS, PCI
Tirofiban	Intravenous	1.6 hours	Renal	ACS, PCI

*A slower, nonsaturable mechanism of clearance is renal.

The most commonly used agent in this class, bivalirudin, has recently been tested in several studies [11].

The overall conclusion from the bivalirudin studies is that it is an effective anticoagulant in patients, with ACS undergoing percutaneous coronary intervention [12]. Compared with other anticoagulants, its major benefit is its reduction in major bleeding.

Vitamin K antagonists (VKAs)

The coumarins (such as warfarin) are competitive inhibitors of vitamin K. They exert their anticoagulant effect by interfering with the γ-carboxylation reactions required for synthesis of the vitamin K-dependent coagulation factors II, VII, IX, and X. Importantly, VKAs also inhibit the vitamin K-dependent γ-carboxylation of proteins C and S. Environmental factors, such as drugs and diet, can importantly alter the pharmacokinetics and pharmacodynamics of VKAs. The prothrombin time assay is sensitive to the inhibition of factors II, VII, IX, and X, the carboxylation of which is inhibited by VKAs, and has been used for decades to monitor the intensity of oral anticoagulant therapy.

Complications of VKAs

Bleeding is the most serious and common complication of oral anticoagulation. The risk is related primarily to:
- patient characteristics (e.g. older),
- the intensity of the anticoagulation (measured by INR), and
- length of therapy (short or long term).
- concomitant antithrombotic drugs

Risk factors for bleeding include older age, recent surgery or trauma, previous gastrointestinal bleeding, renal disease, hypertension, cerebrovascular disease, and use of drugs with potentiating activity. The intensity of anticoagulation as reflected by the INR is the most important predictor of bleeding risk which dramatically increases once the INR supersedes the therapeutic range. Despite an increased absolute risk early after treatment initiation, the cumulative risk of bleeding increases with duration of therapy.

Initiating warfarin therapy following STEMI can reduce reinfarction and cerebrovascular accidents and may reduce mortality [13]. Following STEMI, warfarin is considered in patients:

• at high risk for embolization, including left ventricular thrombus or aneurysm;
• with left ventricular ejection fraction below 30%; and
• with a history of thromboembolism and atrial fibrillation.

In comparison, data concerning the possible role of oral anticoagulation therapy with warfarin in NSTEMI or unstable angina are limited and of uncertain applicability to current practice. Because of the increased risk of bleeding, the relative advantages and risks of this therapy need to be considered (Table 18.3).

Anti-platelet therapies

Therapies aimed at disrupting platelet activity (Fig. 18.1) are successful in decreasing cardiovascular morbidity and mortality. In the largest investigation to date, the Antiplatelet Trialists' Collaboration (ATC), a systematic overview of trials of antiplatelet therapy, demonstrated a reduction in myocardial infarction, stroke, and death with antiplatelet therapies among a wide range of patients at risk of occlusive vascular events [14].

Aspirin

Aspirin is one of the most widely used cardioprotective drugs. Although its use has been available for centuries, only during the latter part of the 20th century was it recognized for its cardiovascular protection. Since then, there have been numerous studies demonstrating its benefit in the prevention and treatment of cardiovascular disease.

Mechanistically, aspirin irreversibly inhibits platelet cyclooxygenase (COX)-1, thereby impairing prostaglandin metabolism and thromboxane (TX) A_2 synthesis (Fig. 18.2). As a result, aspirin irreversibly blocks platelet function. Because platelets cannot generate new COX, the effects of aspirin last for the duration of the life of the platelet ($\approx$7–10 days).

Table 18.3 Anticoagulation therapy recommendations (based on the 2008 ACCP).

ST elevation ACS [5]
Antithrombin therapy is recommended for those patients receiving thrombolysis, primary PCI, or patients receiving no reperfusion therapy.
For patients undergoing primary PCI, UFH is recommended (versus no UFH therapy).
For patients receiving fibrinolytic therapy with preserved renal function, enoxaparin (versus UFH) is recommended for up to 8 days.
For patients receiving fibrinolytic therapy, fondaparinux is recommended (versus no therapy).
For patients not receiving reperfusion therapy, fondaparinux is recommended (versus no therapy).

Non-ST elevation ACS [12]
For all patients, anticoagulation with UFH or LMWH or bivalirudin or fondaparinux is recommended (versus no anticoagulation).
For patients undergoing early invasive strategy, we recommend:

1. UFH versus either LMWH or fondaparinux.
2. Bivalirudin versus UFH in patients with moderate–high risk features and scheduled for very early (<6 hours) coronary angiography.

For patients undergoing a conservative or delayed invasive strategy, we recommend:

1. Fondaparinux versus enoxaparin (if the patient undergoes PCI, UFH should be added at the time of the procedure).
2. LMWH versus UFH.

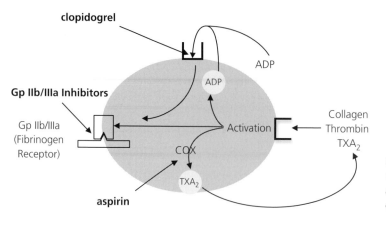

Figure 18.1 An overview of the mechanism of benefit for various antiplatelet agents. ADP, adenosine diphosphate; COX, cyclooxygenase; TXA_2, thromboxane A_2.

The benefits of aspirin [15]

In the acute setting of STEMI, aspirin (162.5 mg/day) reduced 5-week mortality by 23%. In addition, aspirin significantly reduced nonfatal reinfarction and nonfatal stroke [16].

In patients presumed to have an ischemic stroke, aspirin therapy reduced the risk of early recurrent ischemic stroke and improved long-term outcomes.

Among patients with stable vascular disease, low-dose aspirin was found to significantly reduce the risk of cardiovascular events, as well as each individual endpoint of myocardial infarction, stroke, and death [17].

When comparing the effect of aspirin to other cardioprotective drugs, such as statins and ACE-inhibitors, aspirin is comparable in its protective effect.

In patients without established vascular disease, based on a meta-analysis of 6 trials (including more than 90,000 men and women), low-dose aspirin was found to significantly reduce a composite of myocardial infarction, stroke, or cardiovascular death in women and men [18]. Interestingly, women were noted to have their greatest benefit via a reduction in the risk of stroke, whereas men tended to have their greatest benefit in the reduction in the risk of myocardial infarction.

Adverse events of aspirin

Despite aspirin's demonstrated effectiveness in reducing fatal and nonfatal vascular disease, adverse effects need to be mentioned [15]. Aspirin is responsible for minor and major gastrointestinal bleeding. Although rare, several studies have suggested that aspirin increases the risk of hemorrhagic stroke. Other side effects are gastric ulcers, renal insufficiency, and allergic reactions.

Although the benefits of prolonged aspirin use are well known, the optimal dose of aspirin is somewhat controversial [19]. There is evidence to support dosages that range from 81 to 325 mg (75 to 300 mg in UK). Nevertheless, because of the increased risk with an increased dose, most situations require use of 75–81 mg/day. Exceptions include the acute setting of a myocardial infarction or stroke, where 162–325 mg is the preferred dose.

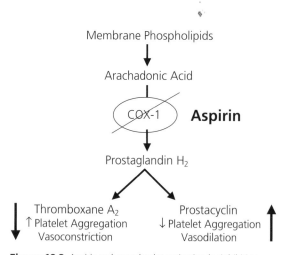

Figure 18.2 Aspirin reduces platelet activation by inhibiting COX-1, limiting the synthesis of thromboxane A_2, a potent platelet agonist.

Table 18.4 Antiplatelet therapy recommendations (based on the 2008 ACCP).

ST elevation ACS

For all patients, we recommend aspirin (162–325 mg) versus no aspirin at initial evaluation, and this should be followed indefinitely (75–162 mg/day).

For all patients, we recommend clopidogrel in addition to aspirin.

In patients undergoing primary PCI, an initial loading dose of at least 300 mg should be used.

In patients receiving fibrinolytic agents or conservative therapy, 300 mg should be used in patients <75 years (75 mg should be used in patients >75):

GPIIb/IIIa inhibitors should not be used with fibrinolytic therapy,

For patients undergoing primary PCI, we recommend the use of abciximab.

Non-ST elevation ACS

For all patients without a clear allergy to aspirin, we recommend aspirin (162–325 mg) at initial evaluation, and this should be followed indefinitely (75–162 mg/day).

For all patients with an aspirin allergy, we recommend immediate treatment with clopidogrel (300 mg load) followed by 75 mg daily.

For patients at moderate or greater risk and who will undergo an early invasive strategy, we recommend:

1. Early treatment with clopidogrel or a small-molecule IV GPIIb/IIIa inhibitor,
2. Both early clopidogrel or a small-molecule IV GPIIb/IIIa inhibitor.

For patients at moderate or greater risk and who will undergo a conservative or a delayed invasive strategy, we recommend:

1. Early treatment with clopidogrel,
2. Both early clopidogrel or a small-molecule IV GPIIb/IIIa inhibitor.

For patients who undergo PCI, we recommend both clopidogrel and an IV GPIIb/IIIa inhibitor

Thienopyridines

The thienopyridines ticlopidine and clopidogrel inhibit adenosine diphosphate (ADP) receptor-mediated platelet activation; they are more potent platelet inhibitors than aspirin. Because ticlopidine has been associated with thrombocytopenic purpura and neutropenia, clopidogrel has emerged as the drug of choice [20].

In randomized trials, clopidogrel has been shown to reduce cardiovascular events in the treatment of cardiovascular conditions [15]. This includes the use of clopidogrel as:

• adjunct therapy in the acute management of STEMI,
• the invasive and conservative management of ACS without ST-segment elevation,
• as adjunct therapy following percutaneous coronary intervention (PCI), and
• as lone therapy in the secondary prevention of atherosclerotic heart disease [15].

Recent data suggest that clopidogrel, in addition to aspirin for primary prevention, is of no additional benefit and only increases the risk of bleeding.

Glycoprotein IIb/IIIa inhibitors

Activation of the platelet-surface glycoprotein (GP) IIb/IIIa receptor is the final common pathway in the process leading to platelet aggregation and, eventually, thrombus formation. The intravenous GPIIb/IIIa receptor inhibitors have been established as effective therapy for the reduction of ischemic events when used in both the management of ACS and as adjunctive therapy during PCI [21,22]. Because of its increased potency as an antiplatelet agent, bleeding is a major side effect that needs to be considered with its use.

Novel antiplatelet therapies

Important limitations, including response variability, irreversible inhibitory effects, and length of time required for maximal platelet inhibition, exist among the current antiplatelet agents, and therefore, a pressing need for the development of improved antiplatelet agents exists. Three ADP receptor antagonists currently under investigation (prasugrel, AZD6140, and cangrelor) in clinical trials for the treatment of ACS appear promising [23]. Prasugrel is a new thienopyridine compound with a much faster onset of action than clopidogrel. In the recently reported TRITON trial [24], prasugrel therapy was associated with significantly reduced rates of ischemic events, but with an increased risk of major bleeding, including fatal bleeding. This study validated the hypothesis that greater degrees of adenosine diphosphate-mediated platelet inhibition are associated with a greater suppression of clinical ischemic events. Two direct and reversible P2Y antagonists [15], cangrelor, which can only be given intravenously, and AZD6140, which can be given orally, have rapid onset and reversal of platelet inhibition, which make them attractive alternatives to thienopyridines, especially when rapid inhibition of platelet aggregation or its quick reversal is required (Table 18.4).

Combination therapy of VKA and antiplatelet therapy

Although mechanistically sound, the combination of VKAs and antiplatelet therapy has not been convincingly shown to have a favorable benefit/risk profile for the long-term management of coronary heart disease patients. Aspirin increases the risk of warfarin-associated bleeding. The size of this increased risk depends on the intensity of anticoagulation as well as on the daily dose of aspirin.

A number of trials have evaluated the efficacy of warfarin plus aspirin versus aspirin alone following ACS [25]. A large meta-analysis that evaluated 14 trials involving over 25,000 patients found no significant difference in the overall risk of myocardial infarction, stroke, or all-cause mortality, but increased the risk of major bleeding. However, a combined strategy of aspirin plus warfarin at INR values of 2–3 was superior to aspirin alone in preventing major adverse events. Importantly, the applicability of these results is not known in patients treated with aspirin plus clopidogrel, the currently recommended regimen in most patients following ACS.

References

1 Fuster V, Stein B, Ambrose JA, Badimon L, Badimon JJ, Chesebro JH. Atherosclerotic plaque rupture and thrombosis. Evolving concepts. *Circulation* 1990;82:II47–59.

2 Croce K, Libby P. Intertwining of thrombosis and inflammation in atherosclerosis. *Curr Opin Hematol* 2007;14:55–61.

3 Libby P. Multiple mechanisms of thrombosis complicating atherosclerotic plaques. *Clin Cardiol* 2000;23(Suppl 6):VI-3–7.

4 Virmani R, Burke AP, Farb A, Kolodgie FD. Pathology of the vulnerable plaque. *J Am Coll Cardiol* 2006;47:C13–18.

5 Goodman SG, Menon V, Cannon C, Steg G, Ohman EM, Harrington RA. Aute ST-Segment Elevation Myocardial Infarction: American College of Chest Physicians evience-based clinical practice guidelines (8th edition). *Chest* 2008;133:708S–75S.

6 Hirsh J, Bauer K, Donati M, Gould M, Samama M, Weitz J. Parenteral anticoagulants: American College of Chest Physicians evience-based clinical practice guidelines (8th edition). *Chest* 2008;133:141S–59S.

7 Weitz JI. Low-molecular-weight heparins. *N Engl J Med* 1997;337:688–98.

8 Petersen JL, Mahaffey KW, Hasselblad V, et al. Efficacy and bleeding complications among patients randomized to enoxaparin or unfractionated heparin for antithrombin therapy in non-ST-Segment elevation acute coronary syndromes: a systematic overview. *JAMA* 2004;292:89–96.

9 Fifth Organization to Assess Strategies in Acute Ischemic Syndromes I, Yusuf S, Mehta SR, et al. Comparison of fondaparinux and enoxaparin in acute coronary syndromes. *N Engl J Med* 2006;354:1464–76.

10 Yusuf S, Mehta SR, Chrolavicius S, et al. Effects of fondaparinux on mortality and reinfarction in patients with acute ST-segment elevation myocardial infarction: the OASIS-6 randomized trial. *JAMA* 2006;295:1519–30.

11 Direct Thrombin Inhibitor Trialists' Collaborative G. Direct thrombin inhibitors in acute coronary syndromes: principal results of a meta-analysis based on individual patients' data. *Lancet* 2002;359:294–302.

12 Harrington RA, Becker RC, Cannon C, et al. Antithrombotic therapy for non-ST-segment elevation acute coronary syndromes: American College of Chest Physicians evience-based clinical practice guidelines (8th edition). *Chest* 2008;133:670S–707S.

13 Smith P, Arnesen H, Holme I. The effect of warfarin on mortality and reinfarction after myocardial infarction. *N Engl J Med* 1990;323:147–52.

14 Antithrombotic Trialists C. Collaborative meta-analysis of randomised trials of antiplatelet therapy for prevention of death, myocardial infarction, and stroke in high risk patients. *Br Med J* 2002;324:71–86.

15 Patrono C, Baigent C, Hirsh J, Roth G. Antiplatelet drugs: American College of Chest Physicians evience-based clinical practice guidelines (8th edition). *Chest* 2008;133:199S–233S.

16 Anonymous. Randomised trial of intravenous streptokinase, oral aspirin, both, or neither among 17,187 cases of suspected acute myocardial infarction: ISIS-2. ISIS-2 (Second International Study of Infarct Survival) Collaborative Group. *Lancet* 1988;2:349–60.

17 Berger JS, Brown DL, Becker RC. Low-dose aspirin in patients with stable cardiovascular disease: a meta-analysis. *Am J Med* 2008;121:43–9.

18 Berger JS, Roncaglioni MC, Avanzini F, Pangrazzi I, Tognoni G, Brown DL. Aspirin for the primary prevention of cardiovascular events in women and men: a sex-specific meta-analysis of randomized controlled trials. *JAMA* 2006;295:306–13.

19 Campbell CL, Smyth S, Montalescot G, Steinhubl SR. Aspirin dose for the prevention of cardiovascular disease: a systematic review. *JAMA* 2007;297:2018–24.

20 Quinn MJ, Fitzgerald DJ. Ticlopidine and clopidogrel. *Circulation* 1999;100:1667–72.

21 Anderson JL, Adams CD, Antman EM, et al. ACC/AHA 2007 guidelines for the management of patients with unstable angina/non ST-elevation myocardial infarction: a report of the American College of Cardiology/American Heart Association Task Force on Practice Guidelines (Writing Committee to Revise the 2002 Guidelines for the Management of Patients With Unstable Angina/Non ST-Elevation Myocardial Infarction): developed in collaboration with the American College of Emergency Physicians, the Society for Cardiovascular Angiography and Interventions, and the Society of Thoracic Surgeons: endorsed by the American Association of Cardiovascular and Pulmonary Rehabilitation and the Society for Academic Emergency Medicine. *Circulation* 2007;116:e148–304.

22 King SB 3rd, Smith SC Jr, Hirshfeld JW Jr, et al. 2007 focused update of the ACC/AHA/SCAI 2005 guideline update for percutaneous coronary intervention: a report of the American College of Cardiology/American Heart Association Task Force on Practice guidelines. *J Am Coll Cardiol* 2008;51:172–209.

23 Weitz JI, Hirsh J, Samama M. New antithrombotic drugs: American College of Chest Physicians evience-based clinical practice guidelines (8th edition). *Chest* 2008;133:234S–56S.

24 Wiviott SD, Braunwald E, McCabe CH, et al. Prasugrel versus clopidogrel in patients with acute coronary syndromes. *N Engl J Med* 2007;357:2001–15.

25 Andreotti F, Testa L, Biondi-Zoccai GG, Crea F. Aspirin plus warfarin compared to aspirin alone after acute coronary syndromes: an updated and comprehensive meta-analysis of 25,307 patients. *Eur Heart J* 2006;27:519–26.

Cardiothoracic surgery

Denise O'Shaughnessy and Ravi Gill

The importance for surgeons to understand the normal hemostatic mechanisms cannot be overemphasized. Hemostasis is a balance protecting the integrity of the vascular system after tissue injury and maintaining the fluidity of blood. Excessive bleeding can be due to surgical causes, a derangement of hemostasis, or, more often, a combination of both, of which cardiothoracic surgery is a prime example [1].

As the incidence of heart disease continues to rise, the consequent demand for coronary artery bypass surgery also increases: with 400,000 in USA, over 100,000 in Europe, and 30,000 in UK per annum. Most of these procedures, together with major heart surgery on congenital defects and valvular heart disease, are performed on beating hearts supported by cardiopulmonary bypass (CPB).

During surgery on the heart, it is common to stop the heart to make it easier to suture the bypass grafts onto the coronary arteries, which are only 1.5 mm in diameter. During this time, the function of the heart and lungs is taken over by a heart–lung or CPB machine.

The heart can be stopped using several different methods. In general, a mixture of potassium and magnesium with some other chemicals is infused into the coronary arteries. This mixture can be carried in either blood (preferred) or a clear saline-like solution. These solutions are called cardioplegia and are referred to as either blood or crystalloid cardioplegia, respectively. The heart can also be stopped electrically, and this is referred to as cardiac arrest with ventricular fibrillation.

In conventional coronary artery bypass grafting (CABG), operations are performed after cardioplegic arrest. The pericardium is usually opened longitudinally to allow unrestricted access to underlying heart and proximal great vessels. The pericardium is usu-

ally left open. A second incision in the posterior pericardium allows drainage through chest tube.

Cardiac surgery without CPB

CABG can now be performed with or without CPB. These minimally invasive procedures restore healthy blood flow to the heart without having to stop the beating heart [2].

It was thought that off-pump coronary artery bypass (OPCAB) would have a lower risk of complications, such as stroke, acute lung injury, renal dysfunction, neurocognitive outcome, and tranfusion rates. Although observational data have supported this, randomized clinical trials have proved disappointing.

Performing surgery on a beating heart is technically more difficult than working on a heart that has been stopped with the help of the heart–lung machine. In addition, the stress on the heart during the procedure may lead to more heart muscle damage, lower blood pressure, irregular heartbeat, and potentially, brain injury if blood flow to the brain is reduced for too long during surgery. In some cases (usually <10%), it is necessary to convert to conventional CABG methods on an emergency basis.

Currently there are three methods used:

Minimally invasive direct coronary artery bypass (MIDCAB)

This procedure is for patients with blockage(s) in the arteries on the front of the heart [the left anterior descending (LAD) artery and its branches]. A small incision is made on the patient's left chest to expose the heart. After muscles in the area are pushed apart and a small part of the front of the rib (costal cartilage) is removed, the surgeon temporarily closes off the artery that lies underneath and frees its lower end. An opening is made in the pericardium, and a device is attached to the heart to reduce its movement. Finally, the surgeon connects the artery below the blockage to the LAD artery or one of its branches. The procure takes 2–3 hours.

Unfortunately, due to the limited size of the incision, the procedure is limited to only a few patients who have a blockage in one or two coronary arteries located on the front side of the heart, whether healthy or considered too high-risk for conventional bypass surgery or balloon angioplasty. However, for younger patients, for those who have small coronary arteries and need several bypasses, or for those whose heart will not tolerate being manipulated during the procedure, it may be preferable to use the traditional CABG technique.

Off-pump coronary artery bypass (OPCAB)

During this procedure, the chest is opened and grafts harvested conventionally. Like the MIDCAB procedure, a device is used to restrict movement of parts of the heart so that the surgeon can operate on it while it is still beating. The surgeon can repair four to five vessels on the beating heart during the same procedure. This procedure also takes 3–4 hours.

OPCAB has grown significantly because of its advantages over other procedures, such as fewer blood transfusions, possible decreased risk of stroke, shorter stay in the hospital, and return to normal activities more rapidly. OPCAB is suitable for patients with poor heart function (very low ejection fraction), severe lung disease (chronic obstructive pulmonary disease, COPD, and emphysema), and acute or chronic kidney disease. It is also suitable for those at high risk for stroke or for those who have a calcified aorta.

Robot-assisted coronary artery bypass (RACAB)

RACAB is the latest advance in heart surgery. Surgeons use a robot to perform the bypass. The breastbone does not need to be split open at all. Surgeons do not have direct contact with the patient, performing the operation while watching a videoscreen. As the technology becomes more advanced, the surgeon may perform coronary bypass from a distant site (i.e. from another room or another geographical location).

Trainee beating heart surgeon

Until a surgeon has performed up to 50 OPCAB procedures, he/she is advised to avoid: cardiomegaly, small or diffusely diseased vessels, hemodynamically unstable patients, critical left main disease, recent myocardial infarction, or severe left ventricular dysfunction [left ventricular ejection fraction (LVEF) <35%].

Expert beating heart surgeon

With experience, OPCAB can be performed safely in the vast majority of cases (>90%). However, it is not advisable to perform OPCAB if multiple unfavorable characteristics are present (e.g. cardiomegaly in a patient with LVEF 25% and small targets).

Anticoagulation used

The heparin dose (1–1.5 mg/kg) is one-third of the standard dose for CPB. The target activated clotting time (ACT) is >300 seconds. The ACT should be checked every 30 minutes with heparin supplemented as needed. Heparin reversal is not mandatory; some centers administer one-half the calculated protamine dose.

Cardiac surgery without CPB versus cardiac surgery with CPB

In a series of 17,401 isolated CABGs performed in Dallas, Texas, 7283 (41.9%) were OPCABs and 10,118 (58.1%) were conventional coronary artery bypass with CPB [3]. Factors determining selection of patients for OPCAB included female gender, pre-existing renal failure, and reoperations. Operative mortality was 2.8%.

Published data from the UK cardiac database in the financial years 2002–2003 ($n = 56,065$) demonstrated that <20% of CABG were performed off-pump, most being performed at 5 leading hospitals: St Marys, London (40%), Harefield Hospital, Sutton and Bristol Royal Infirmary (38%), Manchester, and Liverpool (30%).

Cardiopulmonary bypass

In 2002, 80% of all CABG surgery was performed on CPB; the figure now, in 2008, is still over 70%.

During CPB, blood is drained from the right atrium and returned to the aorta, creating a bloodless field for the cardiothoracic surgeon. This is achieved by administrating high doses of heparin to anticoagulate patients (monitored using the ACT or anti-Xa levels), and residual heparin is reversed by protamine at the end of surgery.

The process of CPB:

- activates fibrinolysis,
- disturbs platelet function,
- often reduces the platelet count, and
- reduces the concentration of clotting factors.

Reduction in volume of the CPB circuit and improvements in operative techniques, together with cell salvage and the use of antifibrinolytic drugs, have reduced the need for transfusion. Recent "near patient" coagulation testing devices have enabled much of this progress and include the Haemoscope Thrombelastograph® (TEG®).

Bleeding is usually manifest postoperatively, after protamine reversal of heparin, and shed into the mediastinal and pleural drains. There are two main causes of peri-operative bleeding:

- Surgical, due to failure to secure hemostasis at the operative site.
- Nonsurgical, due to failure of hemostatic pathways, and principally due to:

1 The procedure itself, in this case CPB (the circuit and its effect on hemostasis);

2 Incomplete reversal of heparin by protamine;

3 Antiplatelet drugs (Aspirin, Clopidrogel, IIb/IIIa inhibitors);

4 A pre-existing bleeding disorder (e.g. hemophilia, von Willebrand disease); or

5 Oral anticoagulation that has not been reversed completely.

Critical rates of blood loss are 500 mL in the first hour, 800 mL at 2 hours, 900 mL at 3 hours, 1000 mL at 4 hours, and 1200 mL by 5 hours.

The CPB circuit

Bigelow showed in dogs that circulatory arrest (CA) was possible, allowing simple operations without circulatory support, but only for 15 minutes. Originally invented by Gibbon in the 1930s, the pump oxygenator only worked successfully in the 1950s. Even then,

only one in four cases survived and 14–25 L of fresh blood prime was required. At the same time, Lillehei connected a patient to a volunteer donor (parent). He drained the blood from the superior vena cava (SVC) of the patient, and pumped this blood into the femoral vein of the donor. Blood was then returned from the femoral artery of the donor to the carotid artery of the patient. Forty-five patients (mostly children) had operations. The 63% survival, despite no reliable ventilators, blood gas or electrolyte analysis, pacemakers, or defibrillators, was remarkable. However, this was not a long-term solution.

The Gibbon Mayo pump in 1955 had bubble oxygenators, high-flow total cardiopulmonary support, but still required 10–14 U fresh blood prime. Adaptations over the next 60 years have reduced adult prime volumes to 1.5–2.5 L crystalloid and pediatric prime volumes to 400–1000 mL prime including some blood (depending on the size of the child), such that on bypass the hematocrit will not fall below 20%.

A representation of current CPB is shown in Fig. 19.1.

Hemostasis in CPB

Hemostasis is a dynamic and extremely complex process, involving many interactive factors. These include coagulation and fibrinolytic proteins, activators, inhibitors, and cellular elements (e.g. platelet cytoskeleton, cytoplasmic granules, and cell surfaces), as described in Chapter 1.

In order to measure any degree of hemostatic imbalance, we need to have the ability to measure the net product of the interactions, which is the three-dimensional clot matrix. Once the coagulation cascade is activated, thrombin is formed.

- Thrombin will cleave soluble fibrinogen into fibrin monomers, which polymerize to form protofibril strands and then undergo linear extension, branching, and lateral association, leading to the formation of a three-dimensional matrix of fibrin.

- This matrix is given rigidity by the anchoring platelet network, thus allowing resistance to shear. Platelet glycoprotein receptors (GPIIb/IIIa) bind the polymerized fibrin network to the actin cytoskeleton of the platelet. Actin is a muscle protein that has the ability to transmit contractility force, which is the major contributor to clot strength.

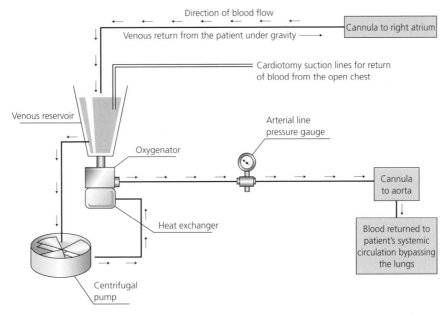

Figure 19.1 Cardiopulmonary bypass circuit.

It follows that, in order to adequately treat failures of the hemostatic system, we would need to evaluate and target this interaction of platelet and fibrin in order to assess the basic principles of functional hemostasis: activation, kinetics, contribution, and stability of clotting.

Conventional tests of coagulation

Until recently, hemostatic component therapies were guided by the results of conventional laboratory-based testing (see Chapter 2). These tests, which include the prothrombin time (PT), activated partial thromboplastin time (APTT), platelet count, and fibrinogen concentrations may be unrelated to both postoperative bleeding and the need for blood and component therapies after cardiac surgery.

Inappropriateness of component transfusion

The national blood service for England issues approximately 1.7 million units of blood per year (a 16% reduction in the past 4 years), of which 8% are still used in cardiac surgical units. There is a wide unexplained variation in the transfusion practice between different cardiac surgical units.

This was noticed first by Goodenough [4], who showed that approximately 50% of platelet and 30% of fresh frozen plasma transfusions, in a survey of patients undergoing routine heart surgery, did not conform to the American Association of Blood Banks published guidelines for transfusion practice.

Seven years later, Stover and colleagues [5] showed that little improvement had been made in relation to inappropriate ordering and administration of component products.

Finally, in a third study (unpublished at time of writing) conducted as a national benchmarking audit of blood and component use in primary myocardial revascularization in the UK (National Blood Service and Royal Brompton and Harefield NHS Trust), it was shown that a high degree of transfusion practice variability still existed, and it confirmed that the majority of platelet and fresh frozen plasma transfusions did not conform to national guidelines.

The need for near patient testing (NPT)

A number of possibilities exist to explain this poor compliance and wastage of resource. The most

Table 19.1 Blood components received by the patients.*

Blood component	LAG (*n* = 51)	POC (*n* = 51)	CD (*n* = 108)	*P* (χ^2) test
Red blood cells	35 (69)	34 (68)	92 (85)	0.01
Fresh frozen plasma	0	2 (4)	16 (15)	0.003
Platelets	1 (2)	2 (4)	14 (13)	0.02

*The table shows the number of patients (%) in each group that received transfusions.
Abbreviations: LAG, laboratory-guided algorithm; POC, point of care; CD, clinical discretion.

obvious to the clinician is the delay between receiving test results when the patient has already developed serious bleeding.

Avidan [6] published a comparison of 102 retrospective controls where decisions were made using clinical discretion, a laboratory-guided algorithm, and a group using point of care (see Table 19.1).

This demonstrated that using NPT or laboratory testing (in appropriate time frames) was better than no test at all. It would seem logical that, to improve performance and to reduce inappropriate exposure to component products, NPT is available, which is able to indicate an abnormal coagulation profile, when a patient is bleeding.

Early attempts at NPT

A number of suggestions and attempts have been made to develop point-of-care tests to fulfil these requirements. Early attempts at such devices included the use of machines to produce dedicated heparin/protamine response curves. Providing an individual solution for a specific patient was shown to be of benefit to reduce both bleeding and the requirement for red cells in patients undergoing heart surgery.

The potential failing in the concept of using a simple coagulation monitor as the only point-of-care test is shown in Fig. 19.2.

Standard laboratory tests (see Chapter 2)

PT and APTT

These tests use activators to initiate either intrinsic or extrinsic pathways of coagulation. The endpoint for these tests, whether performed in citrated plasma in the laboratory or whole blood in a point-of-care test, is the establishment of fibrin strands.

ACT

The ACT is a test in which whole blood is added to a tube containing an activator, such as kaolin, and is the test for measuring high doses of heparin (when on bypass). It cannot be used in cases of heparin resistance and is likely to be inaccurate if the patient has an inhibitor (e.g. lupus anticoagulant).

Anti-Xa

Heparin binds to and enhances the activity of antithrombin AT. Plasma containing heparin is incubated with AT and an excess of factor Xa. It is used primarily to monitor low-molecular-weight heparin (LMWH), which is not detectable by the APTT clotting test. It is a more accurate test for monitoring unfractionated heparin and is the test of choice if there is a lupus anticoagulant present or heparin resistance. There are NPT devices to measure anti-Xa available, but currently, these are used only in the US. When monitoring LMWH, testing should be performed 2–3 hours after the injection.

Prophylaxis LMWH	Therapy LMWH	CPB (large-dose UFH)
0.2–0.4 IU/mL	0.4–1.0 IU/mL	5–8 IU/mL

None of these standard laboratory tests attempt to go further in order to evaluate the kinetics, strength, or relative contribution (platelet to fibrin) of the clot and whether it remains stable over time.

Platelet count

Normal platelet numbers and function are required for normal hemostasis. A platelet count in patients undergoing surgery gives little information to the clinician.

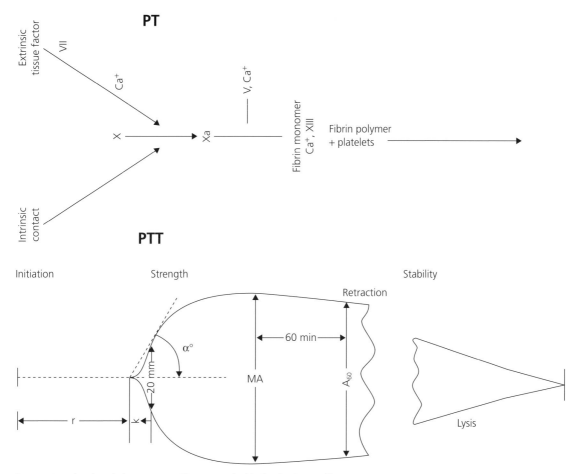

Figure 19.2 The thrombelastogram profile compared with the clotting profile.

A normal platelet count gives no indication as to the functional capacity of the platelet and therefore is of limited value within the decision-making process, especially as many patients who undergo CPB already present as, or become, thrombocytopenic.

Non-standard laboratory tests

Thrombelastography

The Haemoscope Thrombelastograph® Haemostasis System [7] uses its ability to measure the viscoelastic properties of blood to target hemostatic imbalance. It uses a simple premise: that the end result of the process of hemostasis is to create a single product (i.e. the clot) and that the physical properties of the clot (kinetics, strength, and stability) will determine whether the patient will have normal hemostasis, hemorrhage, or develop thrombosis.

The concept of coagulation analysis using the Haemoscope Thrombelastograph® was first described in Germany by Professor Hartert, in the 1940s. At this time, the device had two components: the mechanism for measuring clot formation and a mirror-galvanometer recording onto light-sensitive paper. The permanent record of activity was developed on this photographic paper and was available some hours, or days, later.

This somewhat slow, if highly innovative method, no longer takes this amount of time to produce data upon which the clinician can base treatment options. The new software, which can be networked, allows results to be seen anywhere in the hospital in real time and data which is useful to the clinician can be obtained within 10–15 minutes. A rigorous quality assurance program protects the validity of these results. However, despite these advancements, the principle of producing a trace that identifies a number of variables related to functional disturbances in the hemostatic system is still key to Thrombelastographic analysis.

Coagulation analysis: definitions of coagulation parameters using the Thrombelastograph

R = reaction time
• Time from sample placement into the cup until the tracing amplitude reaches 2 mm.
• This represents the rate of initial fibrin formation and is related functionally to plasma clotting factors and circulating inhibitor activity (i.e. PT and APTT).
• Prolongation of the R-value may be a result of coagulation factor deficiencies, anticoagulation (heparin), or severe hypofibrinogenemia.
• A reduced R-value may be present in hypercoagulability syndromes.

K = clot formation time
• Measured from R time to the point where the amplitude of the tracing reaches 20 mm.
• The coagulation time represents the time taken for a fixed degree of viscoelasticity to be achieved by the forming clot, as a result of fibrin build-up and cross-linking.
• It is affected by the activity of the clotting factors, fibrinogen, and platelets.

Alpha angle (α)
• This is a line tangent from the point at which clot formation begins to the peak of the curve. It denotes speed at which solid clot forms.
• Decreased values may occur with hypofibrinogenemia and thrombocytopenia affecting platelet function.

Maximum amplitude/G (MA/G)
• This is the greatest amplitude of the TEG® trace and is a reflection of the absolute strength of the clot. It is a direct function of the maximum dynamic properties of the interaction of fibrin and platelets via GP IIb/IIIa, and has been correlated to platelet aggregometry.
• Platelet abnormalities, whether qualitative or, if severe enough, quantitative, substantially disturb the maximum amplitude (MA). There is a significant, albeit complex, relationship between the MA of the TEG® trace and the platelet count. A significant relationship with the MA value and the aggregation responses to collagen and ADP has also been reported.

Clot lysis
• This can be expressed in a number of ways.
• Normal clot will retract with time, and thus, a certain amount of narrowing of the MA can be expected.
• The LY30 measures the amount of reduction in maximum amplitude at 30 minutes and may be predicted before this using the estimated percent lysis (EPL) parameter. These parameters represent lysis rather than retraction of the clot.
• Both measures reflect an abnormal decrease in amplitude as a function of time and reflect loss of clot integrity as a result of lysis.

A stylized thrombelastography trace is shown in Fig. 19.2 together with the standard clotting profile.

It is easy to recognise that thrombelastography can provide information on clot kinetics, strength, and stability, which are not available with conventional laboratory-based testing.

A unique attribute of thrombelastography is its ability to define previously unrecognized changes in certain clinical scenarios. It can be observed that the trace develops more vigorously and produces a more stable and strong clot in certain prothrombotic clinical conditions.

Hypercoaguability
Increased alpha angle and MA associated with a shorter R-value can be defined as hypercoagulability. This is an increasing focus of attention in many fields, largely due to the recognition of genetic determinants of increased likelihood of developing a thrombotic disease process, such as stroke, coronary artery, or deep vein thrombosis.

Development of inhibitor and activator reagents for the Haemoscope TEG® System

A now common development of thrombelastography is to use commercially available activator and inhibitor reagent technology to define specific parts of the coagulation system.

Kaolin

The effects of contact activation (equivalent to APTT) are assessed using kaolin.

Tissue factor

An equivalent to the PT is performed by the addition of tissue factor.

Heparinase

This enzyme is known to convert unfractionated heparin to a relatively inactive form. It therefore allows the use of thrombelastography to look at the underlying clotting in a patient who is fully heparinized, such as on CPB. It also reverses the effect of some LMWHs.

PlateletMapping® (ADP and arachidonic acid)

As more pharmacological interventions using platelet inhibitor agents are becoming evident, thrombelastography technology has addressed the issue by using reagent technology to assess the impact of such interventions. Two new assays have been developed using ADP and arachidonic acid agonists, generating modified MA values that measure the degree of inhibition caused by these antiplatelet agents (see "Extended Uses of TEG").

Functional Fibrinogen

This reagent contains a monoclonal antibody to the glycoprotein IIb/IIIa receptors on the platelet surface. When it is added to the system, it inhibits the platelet component (80%) of the clot strength shown in the MA, revealing the functional fibrinogen element of the clot (normally 20%). The results have been correlated to the laboratory gold standard Clauss method of fibrinogen determination and are generated automatically by the software.

RapidTEG™

This contains both tissue factor and kaolin to fully activate the sample and produces an ACT correlated result in seconds. It also allows for a quicker determination of the MA of a patient.

Thrombelastography-based transfusion algorithms

Some centers, such as Mount Sinai (New York), Southampton (UK), and Harefield Hospital (UK), have incorporated the TEG® system into their transfusion algorithms.

The Mount Sinai protocol

The measurements used were partly TEG-based (celite, with and without heparinase), in conjunction with platelet count and fibrinogen concentration from the laboratory [8].

• If the R-value in the non-heparinase sample was greater than twice that found in the heparinase sample, then the patient was given supplementary protamine.
• If the platelet count was <100,000 and the MA was <45 mm, then platelets were administered.
• Fresh frozen plasma (FFP) was given if the celite activated R-value, 10 minutes post protamine administration, was >20 mm.
• Low fibrinogen was treated with cryoprecipitate.
• Episilon aminocoproic acid (amicar) was given in the event of excess lysis.

Using this protocol, they showed significant reductions in the use of hemostatic products compared with their more conventional transfusion protocol.

The Harefield protocol

The concept of a TEG®-derived algorithm was taken a stage further, with measurements taken during the bypass phase in order to predict the need for component products [9]. A study was conducted in 60 patients who were considered to have a higher than average risk of bleeding and thus the need for hemostatic products, but were not given aprotinin or tranexemic acid. They were randomly allocated to have products ordered and administered based on either a TEG®-derived decision tree or the clinicians' discretion after the return of conventional laboratory-based testing results.

Results for the TEG® trace were available, on average, 70–90 minutes before conventional tests of coagulation, fibrinogen, and platelet count. This was considered significant in terms of logistical appropriateness. The TEG®-guided group also showed a 50% reduction in the number of patients given hemostatic products, with a reduction in the use of FFP from a total of 16 to 5 U in transfused patients. The use of platelet concentrates was reduced, with only one patient receiving a single platelet pool in the TEG®-guided group.

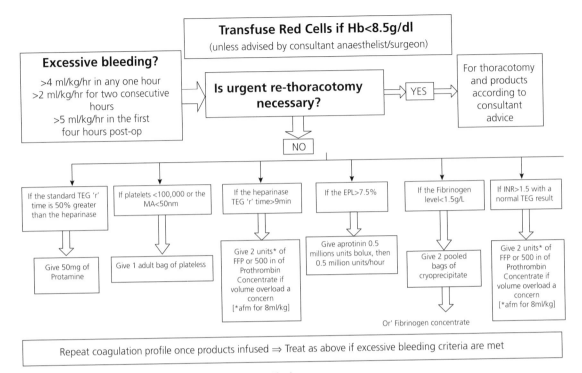

Figure 19.3 The Wessex Allogenic Blood Transfusion Protocol [10].

The Wessex protocol

This protocol was designed in Southampton (UK) with defined parameters to enable consistent use of blood and components, thus enabling trials comparing non-pharmacological and later different pharmacological agents. It incorporates both static test of coagulation (INR, APTR, platelet count, fibrinogen) and the dynamic results from a TEG (Fig. 19.3) [10].

Extended uses of TEG®

Previously, TEG has been performed on whole blood in many settings, but in particular cardiothoracic and liver surgery to distinguish between hemostatic and surgical causes of bleeding. Recent new reagents for the TEG system have allowed it to be used to assess platelet function ex vivo as part of the dynamic clot formation in response to certain agonists. Whereas standard kaolin-activated TEG assesses gross platelet function, the new reagents (PlateletMapping) assess specific pathways of activation [10].

Aspirin and clopidrogel

The antiplatelet agents exert their affect predominately by inhibiting arachadonic acid (AA) and ADP pathways, respectively, with aspirin inhibiting cyclooxygenase-mediated production of thromboxane A_2, and Clopidrogel selectively inhibiting ADP-induced platelet aggregation as well as inhibiting conformational change of platelet GPIIb/IIIa such that fibrinogen cannot bind.

It is well established that long-term use of aspirin in patients with vascular disease decreases morbidity and mortality from cardiovascular events by 25% and is a cornerstone of secondary prevention treatment in the setting of coronary artery disease. More recent studies demonstrate the efficacy of clopidrogel, particularly when given with aspirin.

Current guidelines recommend that aspirin and/or clopidrogel be stopped 5 days prior to surgery because of the excessive perioperative bleeding. However, there is marked individual variation in the degree of platelet inhibition [11].

Aspirin and clopidrogel resistance

Aspirin resistance is a well-recognized entity present in 20% of patients with stable coronary artery disease. Patients resistant to aspirin are at greater risk of cardiovascular and neurological events.

Clopidrogel resistance is reported to be 11%, although in one study of patients undergoing percutaneous coronary intervention, the incidence was recorded as 40%.

PlateletMapping®

NPT assessment of platelet function can help rationalize the management of patients who continue to take antiplatelet drugs up to the day of surgery as well as identify aspirin or clopidrogel resistance or noncompliance [12,13].

In standard kaolin-activated TEG, the MA is largely dependent on thrombin. Thrombin is a powerful activator and overwhelms the effect of the other less potent activators, such as AA and ADP. However, by taking blood into a heparin-containing tube, thrombin is inhibited. The subsequent addition of Activator F™ (reptilase and factor XIIIa) generates a fibrin network in which platelets can interact independent of thrombin. Without alternative sources of platelet activation, there is minimal activation, and therefore the response (MA) generated by the TEG is due to fibrin only.

However, other platelet activators like AA or ADP can be added and, in the absence of inhibition of their specific pathways of action (aspirin or clopidrogel), this increases the MA. Maximum platelet activation generates a curve similar to the kaolin-activated TEG in the presence of thrombin.

The effect of platelet medication can therefore be calculated by comparing:
• Maximum platelet activation MA (in presence of thrombin),
• Zero platelet activation (Activator F), and
• Residual activation due to AA or ADP stimulation (in presence of aspirin or clopidogrel)

The percentage inhibition is calculated automatically by the software (Fig. 19.4).

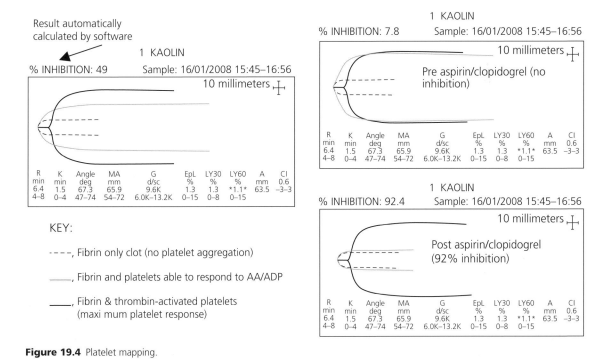

Figure 19.4 Platelet mapping.

Blood and hemostatic component management: future development

It is well recognized that postoperative bleeding and the subsequent need for reoperation to control bleeding is associated with an increase in morbidity and mortality following cardiac surgery. Replacement therapy using red cells and plasma-based hemostatic components may themselves be contributors to the morbidity and mortality.

Clinical indications to reduce exposure

The complex relationship between transfusion, mortality, and morbidity is ill defined. There is emerging evidence that blood transfusion is an independent risk factor for death after cardiac surgery. In addition, platelet transfusion is associated with an increased risk of organ dysfunction or death from uncertain causes. Immune modulation may play a role, because leukodepletion of blood may reduce mortality in the critically ill adult and neonate. Given the complexity of these issues, it would seem to be prudent to avoid transfusion unless necessary and to use simple, safe, available methods to reduce the chances of patients needing a transfusion during surgery.

Logistical indications to reduce exposure

The current donor pool is known to be decreasing at 6% per annum, and may well continue to decrease.

This trend is probably multifactorial; however, the ongoing public debate concerning variant Creutzfeldt-Jacob disease (vCJD) has to be considered a significant contributory element. Some estimates put the possible overall donor reduction at 50% due to the eventual inclusion of a screening test for vCJD. It remains to be seen whether this trend is capable of being reversed, even with the advent of increased public relations awareness and legislative measures introduced to lower the acceptable donor age limit. This must be viewed against a projected increase in demand for blood and hemostatic products of approximately 4.9% by 2008.

The true role for TEG® analysis is as a platform for an integrated approach to hemostasis management. Information is the key to this whole process, and any technology that fails to provide relevant information because of scientific or logistical failures only serves to further exacerbate an already complex clinical management task.

Methods to reduce blood loss

- Mechanical strategies [14],
- Pharmacological strategies,
- Preoperative methods, and
- Anesthetic methods.

Pharmacological methods

Pharmacotherapy is a component in minimizing blood loss and transfusion in cardiothoacic surgery. Nothing beats meticulous surgical technique, but some loss is inevitable. Both aprotinin and tranexamic acid are antifibrinolytic agents that have been used widely in this setting to reduce blood loss.

Aprotinin

This is a nonspecific serine protease inhibitor (inhibits plasmin at low dose, kallikrien at high dose, and inhibits activated protein C and thrombin); in addition to its antifibrinolytic properties, it may have effects on preventing platelet activation by blocking the thrombin activated protease-activated receptor 1 (PAR1) and appears to affect novel anti-inflammatory targets preventing transmigration of leukocytes.

Efficacy is dose-dependent over a wide range of surgery, and high-dose regime reduces blood requirements and perioperative bleeding by two-thirds; however, adverse events have been reported, and, as a result of the recent BART study, its routine use is now precluded.

Tranexamic acid

Tranexamic acid is a synthetically derived antifibrinolytic agent that has its effects by the prevention of the interaction between plasminogen with fibrin via interaction with lysine residues. It is has been shown to reduce blood loss and transfusion but not to the same extent as aprotinin. There is little evidence about the optimal or safe dose.

Studies comparing antifibrinolytic agents

Antifibrinolytic therapy has been extensively studied in cardiac surgical patients, with three major

Table 19.2 Results of study comparing blood-saving properties of antifibrinolytics.

Patients	Red blood cells	FFP	Platelets
Control	27	32	24
TEA	20	14	10
Aprotonin	8	4	3

Units	Red blood cells	FFP	Platelets
Control	101	80	38
TEA	60	32	16
Aprotonin	17	14	5

meta-analyses favoring their use in terms of reduction of exposure to allogenic blood and in reduction in postoperative blood loss. The Cochrane Collaboration identified seven studies that compared aprotinin with tranexamic acid. This showed a nonsignificant trend to benefit in the aprotinin group. Only one of these trials reported the use of cell salvage.

In Southampton, UK, 186 patients were randomized to one of 3 treatment groups in addition to ICS. The aprotonin treatment protocol was 2 million kallikrein inhibitor units (m kiu) at the start of surgery, 2 m kiu in the CPB prime, and 0.5 m kiu hourly; the TEA group received 5 g (Table 19.2) [10].

Adverse effects were no different between the groups, and the conclusion drawn was that the most effective intraoperative pharmacological regime to use with ICS was aprotinin. A simplified analysis of cost based on the prices of blood in the UK demonstrated that either of the antifibrinolytic drugs reduced the average cost per patient by approximately £150.

Recently, the Canadian trial "Blood Conservation Using Antifibrinolytics: A Randomized Trial in a Cardiac Surgery Population (BART)" suspended enrollment after more patients receiving aprotinin died within the first 30 days of the trial, as compared with patients taking the other antifibrinolytics, Epsilon-aminocaproic acid or Tranexamic acid [15]. This may be a particular problem of off-pump coronary surgery, but the jury is still out.

Recombinant factor VIIa

Factor VIIa (Novoseven) is approved for the treatment of hemophilia with inhibitors. In recent years, there has been increasing interest in using factor VIIa in major hemorrhage in nonhemophilia patients.

A total of 89% of patients with complex noncoronary surgery on CPB will have an allogeneic transfusion. FVIIa has been used on a named patient basis to terminate bleeding in patients with serious hemorrhage who already have had numerous units of blood and products [16].

Kartoutis designed the Toronto protocol for managing cardiac patients if there was over 2 L postoperative loss of blood or the patient received more than 4 U of red cells, had ongoing blood loss in theatre that precluded sternal closure, blood loss of >100 mL/mL/hour in ICU or blood loss refractory to conventional therapy [17].

Of 4630 patients who underwent CPB, 655 (14%) met the criteria, and within this group, 114 received at least one dose of FVIIa. The study cohort had a higher overall risk profile and more frequently underwent complex surgical procedures and longer bypass times. Those receiving ≤8 U of blood were classified as the early therapy group. The recorded adverse events were 24% in the untreated group, 30% in the early therapy, and 60% in the late therapy groups. However, there were many confounding effects, which, if taken into account, suggested that FVIIa may be associated with better outcomes if given early.

The conclusion was that definitive multicenter, randomized clinical trials are warranted. Similar audits have been published from Australia, Mount Sinai (New York), Illinois, and Chicago.

In the UK, Diprose and colleagues [18] describe a pilot study of 20 patients receiving complex surgery and highly likely to bleed excessively (Fig. 19.5). These were randomized to receive FVIIa or placebo after CPB and reversal of heparin. Only 2 of 10 patients in the FVIIa group were exposed to allogeneic transfusion compared with 8 in the placebo group ($P = 0.037$). In the FVIIa group, 13 U of blood or products were given compared with 103 U in the placebo group. Patients with coronary artery disease were excluded from the study. No adverse effects were found, but the cost of the drug would currently limit the use of FVIIa in this manner [18].

Prothrombin complex concentrates (PCCs)

Despotis [19] measured the relationship between hemostatic changes in platelets and clotting factors in

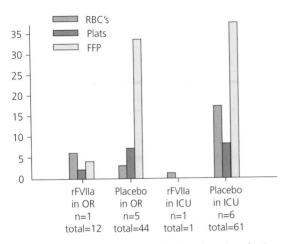

Figure 19.5 Type of product transfused. Total number of units transfused by group in the OR and ICU [18].

patients on CPB (Fig. 19.6). Non-bleeders had an average platelet count of over 100, and none of the vitamin K-dependent factors (II, VII, IX, and X) fell below 40%. Those with microvascular bleeding averaged 1 hour longer on CPB than those without microvascular bleeding, and their clotting factors were 10–30% lower.

The Wessex protocol therefore recommends measuring the INR as part of their protocol, advising the use of FFP or PCCs. PCCs are a low-volume concentration of factors II, VII, IX, and X, which is now recommended for the urgent reversal of oral anticoagulation (warfarin) and are increasingly being used

as a rapid low-volume replacement of FFP in cardiac surgery [20].

Preoperative assessment clinics

The prescribing clinician should anticipate and plan ahead for the situation that may necessitate transfusion and aim to reduce the chance that the patient will actually need to be given blood.

Assessment of patients specific to hemostasis should include:

1 *Diagnosis of any bleeding disorder*: Previously undiagnosed bleeding disorders are common and can lead to greater use of donor blood if not known about prior to surgery. Consider specific questions about bleeding history in standard presurgical assessment.

2 *Assessment of patient's current medication, its potential for increasing bleeding tendency and impact on recovery*: Commonly used drugs increase bleeding time (aspirin, NSAIDs, coumarins). Some of these drugs can be stopped prior to surgery; others may need to be continued, but the surgical team needs to be aware.

3 Identification of problems which may require specialist intervention (ITP, PTP).

4 Patient beliefs (e.g. Jehovah's Witnesses).

Diagnosis of a bleeding disorder

Although most hemostatic defects in hospitalized patients are acquired, underlying mild hereditary disorders may only manifest in the hospital setting, such as mild hemophilia A (deficient factor VIII),

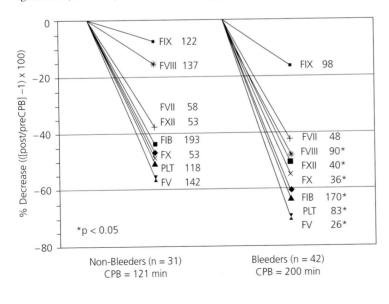

Figure 19.6 Reduction in coagulation proteins in CABG.

mild hemophilia B (deficient factor IX), and mild hemophilia C (deficient factor XI), all of which prolong the APTT. If patients are found to have hemophilia, it is essential that a hematologist advises on best treatment, which can vary from DDAVP preoperatively followed by an antifibrinolytic postoperatively to the giving of regular doses of a recombinant replacement factor that can be monitored with the TEG®. The latter may not be available in all hospitals out of hours without prior notice.

Assessment of current medication
Antiplatelet drugs
Clopidogrel causes platelet inhibition via a different mechanism to aspirin, and following coronary stenting, the two drugs are increasingly being prescribed together. There is growing evidence that the hemorrhagic risk is increased when the two drugs are taken concurrently. An increasing number of patients take antiplatelet agents. NSAIDs, dipyridamole, aspirin, and clopidogrel are all implicated in increased surgical blood loss. Ideally, these drugs should be stopped prior to surgery, to allow platelet function to return to normal.

The time required off the drug to ensure normal platelet function varies. NSAIDs provide reversible inhibition of cyclooxygenase, and their antiplatelet effects are half-life-dependent (usually hours). Aspirin and clopidogrel lead to irreversible inhibition of platelet aggregation for the lifespan of the platelet (~10 days). These drugs need to be stopped for 7 days to be confident of adequate platelet function. However, due consideration must be given to the risks associated with stopping these drugs in surgical patients.

Many patients are presenting for emergency coronary revascularization having had failed coronary stenting procedures. These patients have usually received aspirin and clopidogrel. Hemorrhage during the subsequent surgery may be a major problem. Use of the new TEG reagents is very useful here, as 15% of patients have normal platelet function despite therapy, and in others the degree of dysfunction is variable.

Clopidogrel is a pro-drug. The active metabolite circulates for approximately 18 hours after the last dose, and may permanently inhibit any platelets present during this time (whether endogenous or transfused). Surgery is best delayed for at least 24 hours after the last dose of clopidogrel.

Surgery in patients who have received clopidogrel in the last 7 days should, where possible, be postponed. If the surgery is a genuine emergency, platelets should be made available for transfusion, and consideration given to using aprotinin. Delaying for 24 hours after the last dose of clopidogrel will improve the response to platelet transfusion.

Warfarin
With a patient on oral anticoagulant therapy, it is sufficient to stop warfarin 3 days before surgery and restart the usual maintenance dose the evening of the surgery. If they have a mechanical heart valve or have had a venous thromboembolism in the past, this period should be covered by heparin. Having stopped warfarin, if the INR pre-op is over 2.5, small amounts of vitamin K (1–2 mg) may be given.

Anesthetic techniques to reduce blood loss
There are some basic things that the anesthetist and surgeon can do to reduce blood loss during surgery:
• Positioning of the anesthetized patient so as to minimize any venous congestion in the operating field.
• The use of local vasoconstrictors.
• The sequencing of a multistage procedure (e.g. a coronary artery bypass procedure where the saphenous vein is harvested by one member of the team as another is opening and preparing the chest. The vein harvester needs to close his operation site fully before ascending to assist with the chest).

There are also some specific procedures that may help in reducing blood loss, such as:
• preventing hypertension.
• minimizing the period of hypothermia, and
• controlled hypotension.

References

1 Bevan DH. A review of cardiac bypass haemostasis , putting blood through the mill. *Br J Haematol* 1999;104:208–19.
2 Van Dijk D, Nierich AP, Jansen EWL. Early outcome after off-pump vs on pump CABG, results from a randomised study. *Circulation* 2001;104:1761–6.
3 Mack MJ, Pfister A, Bachand D, et al. Comparison of coronary bypass surgery with and without cardiopulmonary bypass in patients with multivessel disease. *J Thorac Cardiovasc Surg* 2004;127:167–73.

4 Goodenough LT, Johnston MFM, Toy PTCY, and the Medicine Academic Award Group. The variability of transfusion practice in coronary artery bypass surgery. *JAMA* 1991;265:86–90.

5 Stover FP, Stegel IC, Parks R, et al. Variability in transfusion practice for coronary artery bypass surgery persists despite national consensus guidelines: a 24-institution study. *Anesthesiology* 1998;88(2):327–33.

6 Avidan MS, Alcock EL, Da Fonseca J, et al. Comparison of structured use of laboratory tests or near-patient assessment with clinical judgement in the management of bleeding after cardiac surgery. *Br J Anaesth* 2004;92(2):178–86.

7 Spiess BD. Thrombelastograph analysis and cardiopulmonary bypass. *Semin Thromb Hemost* 1995;21:S4.

8 Shore-Lesserson L, Manspeizer HE, Francis S, Deperio M. Intraoperative Thrombelastograph analysis (TEG r) reduces transfusion requirements. *Anesthesia Analg* 1998;86:S104.

9 Von Kier S, Royston D. Reduced hemostatic factor transfusion using heparinase-modified Thrombelastograph analysis (TEG) during cardioplumonary bypass. *Anesthesiology* 1998;89(3A):A911.

10 Diprose P, Herbertson MJ, O'Shaughnessy D, Deakin CD, Gill RS. A randomised double-blind placebo-controlled trial of antifibrinolytic therapies used in addition to intra-operative cell salvage. *Br J Anaesth* 2005;94(3):271–8.

11 Hobson AR, Agarwala RA, Swallow RA, Dawkins KD, Curzen NP. Thrombelastography: current clinical applications and its potential role in interventional cardiology. *Platelets* 2006;17(8):509–18.

12 Agarwal S, Coakely M, Reddy K, Riddell A, Mallett S. A comparison of the platelet function analyzer and modified TEG with light transmission platelet aggregometry. *Anaesthesiology* 2004;105(4):676–83.

13 Gwozdziewicz M, Nemec P, Zezula R, Novotny J. Platelet mapping in postoperative management of acute aortocoronary bypass thrombosis. *Kardiochirurgia I Torakochirurgia Polska* 2006;3(2):214–16.

14 McGill N, O'Shaughnessy D, Pickering R, Herbertson M, Gill R. Mechanical methods of reducing blood loss in cardiac surgery. A randomised controlled trial. *Br Med J* 2002;324:1299.

15 Fergusson MHA, Hébert PC, Mazer D, et al. A comparison of aprotinin and lysine analogues in high-Risk cardiac surgery: the BART Study. *N Engl J Med* 2008;358(22):2319–31.

16 Despotis G, Avidan M, Lublin DM. Off-label use of recombinant factor VIIa concentrates after cardiac surgery. *Ann Thorac Surg* 2005;80:3–5.

17 Kartoukis K, Yau TM, Riazi S, et al. Determinants of complications with recombinant factor VIIa for refractory blood loss in cardiac surgery. *Can J Anaesth* 2006;53(8):802–9.

18 Diprose P, Herbertson MJ, O'Shaughnessy D, Gill RS. Activated recombinant factor VII after CPB reduces allogeneic transfusion in complex non-coronary cardiac surgery: randomised double-blind placebo-controlled pilot study. *Br J Anaesth* 2005;95:596–602.

19 Despotis GJ, Joist JH, Goodenough LT. Monitoring of haemostasis in cardiac surgical patients: impact of point-of-care testing on blood loss and transfusion outcomes. *Clin Chem* 1997;43:1684–96.

20 Stuklis RG, O'Shaughnessy DF, Ohri SK. Novel approach to bleeding in patients undergoing cardiac surgery with liver dysfunction. *Eur J Cardiothorac Surg* 2001;19(2):219–20.

20 Neurology

Natalie Aucutt-Walter, Valerie Jewells, and David Y. Huang

Neurological complications of hematological disease can present in many ways. Examples include seizure triggered by cerebral ischemia or hemorrhage and headache in patients with sickle cell disease. The overwhelming majority of these neurologic complications are vascular in nature, owing to the fact that most hematological abnormalities lead to either thrombosis in the cerebral vasculature or brain hemorrhage. Associated cerebrovascular events include both ischemic and hemorrhagic strokes, as well as cerebral venous sinus thromboses.

Ischemic stroke

Ischemic stroke can be divided into two broad categories: embolic and lacunar. The characteristic clinical profile of acute embolic stroke is sudden onset of a maximal neurological deficit. Emboli often arise from the heart or from ulcerated carotid plaques. Atrial fibrillation, which predisposes patients to forming cardiac thrombi, is associated with a six-fold increased risk for stroke [1]. Cardiac emboli are highly correlated with large vessel ischemia. Warfarin is strongly recommended for stroke prevention in the presence of atrial fibrillation unless otherwise contraindicated. Thrombotic infarction, including lacunar infarction, is often preceded by transient ischemic attacks (TIAs) and may progress over hours or days in a stuttering fashion. TIAs correlate with carotid stenosis and often present with border zone or "watershed" ischemic injury distal to the area of critical stenosis. The prognosis of TIAs varies considerably. Up to 33% of patients who experience a TIA will develop a disabling stroke within 5 years. The incidence of stroke after TIA is 10–20% in the first 12 months and 5% each year thereafter [1]. Watershed territory infarcts may be seen with clinically significant drops in blood pressure. Lacunar infarcts are usually deep, small-vessel ischemic lesions <10 mm in diameter and account for between 10% and 25% of all ischemic strokes [1]. They are often found in patients with a long-standing history of hypertension, diabetes, hypercholesterolemia with atherosclerotic disease, and tobacco abuse. The pathophysiology is thought to be multifactorial and includes small-vessel lipohyalinosis and fibrinoid degeneration, decreased perfusion of the penetrating arteries, and atheromatous occlusion or embolism.

Acute management of suspected ischemic stroke involves rapid assessment of the patient's presenting symptoms by a neurovascular specialist or at the nearest emergency department. Patients who present <3 hours from symptom onset may be candidates for thrombolytic therapy with intravenous recombinant tissue plasminogen activator (IV-tPA). Prior to administering IV-tPA, the patient should have a noncontrast head CT to rule out intracerebral bleeding and laboratory tests, including coagulation studies, complete blood count (CBC), and serum glucose, must be checked. Contraindications and guidelines for IV-tPA administration are widely published and should be reviewed carefully prior to administering the drug [2]. Treatment is associated with a 6% risk of bleeding complications, including intracranial hemorrhage, and patients and/or their families should be counseled about the benefits and risks associated with thrombolytic therapy. Other acute treatments include intra-arterial thrombolytic therapy and mechanical endovascular clot retrieval using aspiration or evacuation devices, but such interventions are less well-studied and are limited to centers with experienced interventionalists.

Beyond the acute interventions, general management of ischemic stroke concentrates on rehabilitation and secondary prevention. All patients presenting with stroke or TIA symptoms should undergo a complete stroke evaluation to identify stroke ethnology and risk factors. Guidelines for the early management of patients with ischemic stroke were published by the American Stroke Association in 2003 [2].

Venous sinus thrombosis

Venous sinus thrombosis (VST) describes occlusion of one or more of the dural venous sinuses that drain the brain. In one series of 154 cases of VST, the transverse sinus was the most common site of thrombosis followed by the sagittal and sigmoid sinuses. Nearly half of the patients in this series had involvement of multiple sinuses [3]. VST may present as gradual onset of severe headache. Other presenting symptoms include seizure, somnolence, and cranial nerve palsies. Less frequently, VST may present with gradual neurological deficits when secondary venous infarcts or subarachnoid hemorrhage develop.

Magnetic resonance venography (MRV) is usually diagnostic for VST and readily reveals thrombosis in the major venous structures, including the superior (Fig. 20.1), transverse, and sigmoid sinuses as well as the veins of Labbe and Trolard. Thrombosis of the deep venous system (internal cerebral veins, straight sinus, and vein of Galen) can also be seen. Thrombosis of the deep venous structures typically results in thalamic infarcts. Head CT demonstrates up to 70% of lesions within 7 days, but MRV is more sensitive in the acute setting. Venous phase angiography is considered the gold standard for diagnosis and will show a contrast filling defect; however, this procedure is seldom performed with the greater availability of MRV. Etiologies associated with VST include:

- trauma,
- infection,
- pregnancy and post partum,
- oral contraceptives,
- volume depletion,
- dehydration,
- hyperosmolar states,
- hematologic disorders (myeloproliferative, sickle cell disease, DIC, hypercoagulable states),
- carcinoma,
- congestive heart disease,

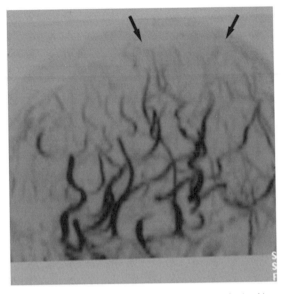

Figure 20.1 A sagittal 3D time-of-flight MRV was obtained in this patient presenting with headache and altered mental status. The superior sagittal sinus is absent due to thrombosis (arrows).

- chemotherapy,
- mastoiditis, and
- systemic lupus erythematosus (SLE).

Acute treatment is generally with intravenous heparin to an activated partial thromboplastin time of 60–80 seconds. This is followed by warfarin therapy for 3–6 months. Anticoagulation has been shown to be safe even in patients with secondary intracerebral hemorrhage. Good results from catheter-infused thrombolytic therapy at the site of thrombosis have been reported in many small series. However, thrombolysis is generally reserved for those patients who progress while on intravenous heparin, as the risk of hemorrhagic complications increases with intervention [4]. Patients who have seizures as a complication of VST should be treated with an anticonvulsant. However, prophylaxis with anticonvulsants in the absence of seizures is not a common practice.

Long-term prognosis of VST is good. In a prospective series of 624 patients followed for 16 months, approximately 10.5% were dead or severely disabled, but almost 80% had minor or no residual deficits. Multivariate predictors of death or dependence were:

- age >37 years,
- male sex,

- coma,
- mental status disorder,
- hemorrhage on admission CT scan,
- thrombosis of the deep cerebral venous system,
- central nervous system infection, and
- cancer [5].

Intracerebral hemorrhage

Intracerebral hemorrhage (ICH) is a bleed into brain parenchyma that accounts for 10% of all strokes and the majority of hemorrhagic strokes. ICH is typically of sudden onset with a smooth progression of symptoms. Unlike ischemic stroke, patients seldom awaken with symptoms. Nearly 40% of all cases are associated with severe headache, and 50% of patients have a change in mental status. Nausea and vomiting are common. The differential diagnosis for ICH includes:
- amyloid angiopathy (Fig. 20.2A, B),
- anticoagulation or bleeding diatheses,
- thrombolysis,
- sympathomimetic drugs,
- vascular malformations,
- brain tumor or metastasis,
- vasculitis, and
- venous thrombosis.

Hypertension is the predominant risk factor. Location of ICH in order of frequency is as follows:
- putaminal or basal ganglia (35–50%),
- subcortical white matter (30%),
- cerebellar (15%),
- thalamic (10–15%), and
- pontine (5–12%).

The duration of bleeding is usually minutes to hours, although hematoma expansion can continue for up to 24 hours. Clinical deterioration after 24 hours is usually due to secondary ischemia and hemorrhage-induced edema rather than recurrent bleeding. Mortality rates are as high as 30–40% in the first 30 days, with more than half of these deaths occurring within the first 48 hours. Independent predictors of poor prognosis include:
- low GCS (Glasgow Coma Scale),
- depressed level of consciousness,
- age >75,
- bleed volume >30 mL,
- intraventricular hemorrhage,

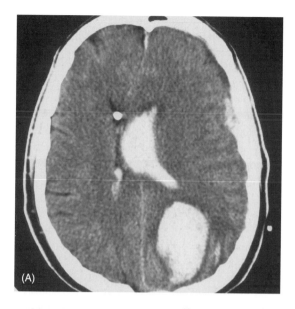

(A)

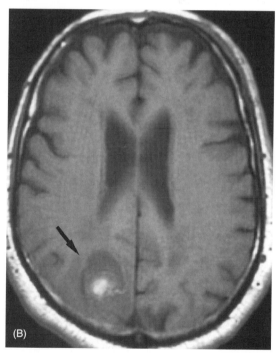

(B)

Figure 20.2 (A) This axial CT image demonstrates a large left parietal–occipital parenchymal hemorrhage in a patient with amyloid angiopathy, which extended into the left lateral ventricle and resulted in the patient's death. (B) An axial T1 noncontrasted image in another patient with amyloid angiopathy demonstrates a mirror image parenchymal hemorrhage with surrounding vasogenic edema (arrow).

- concurrent antiplatelet therapy,
- hyperglycemia, and
- infratentorial location.

Diagnosis is made by emergent head CT. Angiography may be necessary to evaluate for an underlying source of bleed, such as an arterial venous malformation, aneurysm, angioma, cavernoma (which is not seen with angiography, and is therefore called "cryptic"), or tumor. If initial angiography is unrevealing, it should be repeated in 3–4 months when the intraparenchymal blood has cleared.

Guidelines for the management of ICH were published in *Stroke* in 2007 [6]. ICH management includes control of blood pressure, seizure, infection, fever, glucose, and increased intracranial pressure (ICP). Aggressive blood pressure management remains controversial, and blood pressure guidelines vary. In general, patients are at increased risk for rebleeding and hematoma enlargement with systolic blood pressures >160 mm Hg [7]. However, blood pressure reduction should be balanced with the risk of concurrent ischemia, as blood pressures that are dramatically lower than the patient's baseline can lead to decreased cerebral perfusion pressure (CPP). This is of particular concern in patients with a large ICH, cerebral edema, or other factors that increase ICP [8]. When ICP is elevated (>20 mm Hg), blood pressure should be titrated to maintain a CPP of 60–80 mm Hg (CPP = mean arterial pressure – ICP). In the acute setting, pressures should be lowered with short-acting agents, such as intravenous labetalol, nitroprusside, or nicardipine, which allow for rapid titration.

When monitoring and treating cerebral edema and increased ICP, intraventricular pressure monitors should be placed in patients with a GCS <9 or with clinical deterioration in their neurological exam [8]. Approaches such as head-of-bed elevation and head positioning are simple and often effective for quickly lowering ICP. Other interventions should be limited to situations where herniation is of immediate concern. Patients with significant bleeding or intraventricular extension are at risk for obstructive hydrocephalus, and ventricular drain placement may be necessary. Hyperventilation to keep the PCO_2 between 28 and 30 torr is effective to reduce increased ICP, with peak effect within 30 minutes. However, the effect is transient and only lasts until the pH of cerebrospinal fluid equilibrates with systemic pH, usually within a few hours [6]. Osmotic agents such as mannitol and hypertonic saline may be used for short periods, but use for more than a few days can lead to rebound increases in ICP. Steroids should be avoided as they have not been shown to be effective.

There are few indications for surgical intervention in ICH. Indications for surgical intervention are generally limited to patients with:
- cerebellar hemorrhage >3 cm in size and brainstem compression,
- acute hydrocephalus, or
- neurological deterioration.

Patients with lobar clots within 1 cm of the cortex may also be considered for surgery based on a trend toward a positive effect of surgery over medical management for such patients in the International Surgical Trial for Intracerebral Hemorrhage (STICH) [9].

Hemostasis treatment using recombinant activated factor VII (rFVIIa) for ICH has been investigated in a phase 3 trial [10]. Compared with placebo, treatment with rFVIIa at 20 and 80 μg reduced hematoma growth but did not improve functional outcome. In addition, 80 μg of rFVIIa was associated with a nonsignificant but increased frequency of adverse arterial thromboembolic events compared with placebo. rFVIIa is not currently recommended for treatment of acute ICH.

Use of warfarin for anticoagulation to INR 2.5–4.5 increases the risk of ICH by up to 10-fold and doubles the mortality. Patients with ICH who are anticoagulated with warfarin should have their INR corrected as quickly as possible with prothrombin complex concentrate (PCC) or rFVIIa. Intravenous vitamin K should be administered without delay, because peak effect is dependent on protein synthesis, approximately 6–8 hours later. Although fresh frozen plasma (FFP) is commonly used, large volumes need to be given and only partial correction is observed.

Subarachnoid hemorrhage

Subarachnoid hemorrhage (SAH) is often the result of a ruptured saccular aneurysm but may also arise from head trauma, extension of ICH into the subarachnoid space, spinal arteriovenous malformation, or idiopathic causes. Aneurysmal ruptures account for 80% of all nontraumatic SAHs and are of greatest concern, given a high mortality rate of approximately 45%. Presenting symptoms include a sudden and severe "thunder clap" headache, with an acute change in mental status, in some cases leading to lethargy and coma. Sudden loss of consciousness occurs in up to 20% of patients. Meningeal signs, papilledema, and seizure are common at presentation. Increased size of the bleed and the presence of intraventricular extension are correlated with increased mortality. Head CT is often diagnostic of SAH, but up to 15% of cases of aneurysmal SAH will have a normal study. If the head CT is normal but the suspicion for SAH is high, an emergent lumbar puncture should be performed to evaluate for blood or xanthrochromia in the spinal fluid, which is indicative of a sentinel bleed. Patients with sentinel bleeds have a >50% risk of rebleeding in the next 48–72 hours.

Initial management of SAH is focused on reducing the likelihood of rebleeding. Treating hypertension and maintaining blood pressure in a normal range has been shown to decrease the rate of rebleeding. After 4 days and for up to 2 weeks, patients are at increased risk for ischemic stroke from vasospasm and should receive nimodipine, which reduces long-term injury from vasospasm. The antifibrinolytic agent epsilon aminocaproic acid (AMICAR) has been shown to decrease mortality associated with rebleeding, but its benefits were offset by the increased risk for ischemic stroke. Surgical or endovascular interventions to secure ruptured aneurysms should be performed once patients are stabilized. Patients with extensive bleeding or intraventricular extension may develop obstructive hydrocephalus, and a ventricular drain may be necessary to treat elevated ICP. Anticonvulsants are often administered as prophylaxis against seizure.

Diseases associated with ischemic strokes

Hereditary and acquired hypercoagulable states

A number of factors have been implicated in the development of ischemic stroke.

Table 20.1 lists a variety of hypercoagulable states and the strength of their correlation with stroke. Notably, sickle cell disease, antiphospholipid antibody syndrome, and hyperhomocystinemia have the strongest association with arterial stroke.

Table 20.1 Strength of association of coagulopathy with arterial stroke.

Coagulopathy	Arterial stroke risk
Sickle cell disease	Strong
Antiphospholipid antibody syndrome	Strong
Hyperhomocystinemia	Moderate
Activated protein C resistance	Mild
Prothrombin gene mutation	Mild
Protein S deficiency	Mild
Protein C deficiency	Rare
Antithrombin III deficiency	Rare

Adapted from Moster ML. Coagulopathies and arterial stroke. *J Neuroophthalmol* 2003;23:63–71.

Activated protein C resistance/ factor V Leiden

Congenital activated protein C resistance (APC-R) is the most common inherited risk factor for venous thrombosis. A total of 95% of patients with APC-R have the factor V Leiden mutation. The mutation is present in 2–7% of the Caucasian population [11].

With respect to neurological complications, APC-R correlates almost exclusively with venous thrombosis, with only a few reported cases of arterial strokes in young patients. Symptoms of acute cerebral venous thrombosis include headache, seizure, somnolence, and cranial nerve palsies. Patients with suspected venous thrombosis should have neurological imaging with MRI/MRA and MRV. SAH can result from the rupture of congested cerebral veins. If cranial nerve palsies are present on examination (i.e. defects of cranial nerves III, IV, and VI associated with ptosis and facial pain), cavernous sinus thrombosis should be suspected. Treatment for stroke patients with cerebral venous thrombosis is low-molecular-weight heparin or warfarin.

Antiphospholipid antibody syndrome

Antiphospholipid syndrome (aPLs) is an acquired hypercoagulable state that is associated with venous as well as arterial thrombotic events. Arterial events occur most commonly in the cerebrovasculature. Stroke or TIA are the initial clinical manifestation in approximately 20% of patients subsequently diagnosed with aPLs. Involvement of the cerebral cortex and subadjacent white matter by platelet-fibrin microthrombi is most common [12]. The pathogenesis of thrombosis in aPLs is uncertain (see chapter 17).

Antiphospholipid antibodies are found in >10% of patients with acute ischemic stroke, and the vast majority of patients are young (<50 years) [11]. aPLs should be considered in the work-up of all young patients presenting with an ischemic arterial or venous stroke secondary to thrombosis. aPLs is suspected in patients with a history of multiple miscarriages, dementia, optic neuropathy, thrombocytopenia, SLE or SLE-like syndromes, or complicated migraine.

Testing for aPLs includes evaluation for IgG antiphospholipids on two separate occasions at least 12 weeks apart. Stroke risk is greatest with IgG antiphospholipids >40 GPL units and may not be clinically significant at lower levels [13]. Treatment is generally with warfarin to prevent recurrent systemic thrombosis. However, in patients with prior stroke and a single positive test result for antiphospholipid antibodies, aspirin (325 mg/day) appears to be as effective as moderate-intensity warfarin (PT 1.4–2.8) for preventing recurrent stroke [12].

Hyperhomocystinemia

Hyperhomocystinemia has a prevalence of 5–10% in the general population and is associated with accelerated premature atherosclerosis. Increased fasting levels of homocysteine have been related to the prevalence of extracranial common carotid artery stenosis of >25% in the Framingham cohort. Fasting homocysteine levels above 15.4 μmol/L significantly increase the patient's risk for stroke, with an odds ratio of 2.5–4.7. Elevated levels increase the odds of carotid intimal thickening more than three-fold. Proposed mechanisms of coagulopathy include increased platelet adhesion, activation of the coagulation cascade, conversion of LDL to a pro-atherogenic form, and endothelial damage.

Most often, hyperhomocystinemia is acquired due to a diet deficient in folate, B6, and/or B12. Folate and B12 levels should be checked in all patients, especially young patients with unexplained stroke and premature atherosclerosis [14]. Treatment includes vitamin supplementation with folic acid, B6, and B12. Elevated levels of homocysteine can also be seen with renal insufficiency and concurrent anti-epileptic drug use, especially phenytoin.

Hyperhomocystinemia needs to be distinguished from autosomal recessive homocystinuria. Patients who are homozygous for cystathionine beta synthase deficiency can have homocystine concentrations up to 400 μmol/L and present with a marfanoid body habitus, mental retardation, seizure, lenticular dislocations, skeletal abnormalities, and a 20-fold increase in urinary homocysteine excretion over other amino acids [11]. These patients are at high risk for myocardial infarction and ischemic stroke as well as premature death secondary to vascular disease. The incidence of stroke increases with increased homocysteine levels, and heterozygous patients have a milder course and clinical picture.

Sickle cell disease

Children with sickle cell disease (SCD) present with a wide variety of chronic neurological syndromes, including:

- ischemic and hemorrhagic stroke,
- dural VST,
- spinal cord infarction,
- transient ischemic attack,
- headache,
- seizure,
- altered mental status,
- cognitive difficulties, and
- covert "silent" infarction.

Up to 25% of children with HbSS will have covert or "silent" infarction by adolescence. Silent ischemia can be detected with diffusion-weighted MRI, which reveals ischemic regions, characteristically in the anterior or posterior watershed /border zones. One study enrolled and followed the neuroimaging of 213 HbSS children without a history of overt stroke. In this group, 160 children had normal baseline MRIs, and 53 children had MRIs showing silent infarcts. The patients were followed with serial MRIs, and the children with silent infarcts at baseline were significantly more likely to demonstrate new or progressive neurologically silent lesions compared with those whose baseline MRIs were normal. Only 2.5% children with normal baseline MRIs developed silent infarcts on follow-up MRI examination compared with 24.5% who had a baseline silent infarct [15]. These patients may have a normal T2-weighted MRI and a normal neurological examination. Seizure is common in patients with known cerebrovascular disease as well as in patients with covert infarction and should be treated with antiepileptic drug therapy as primary prevention. Interestingly, silent infarction is less common in patients with frequent sickle cell pain and more common in patients with a history of seizure [16].

SCD is the most common cause of pediatric ischemic stroke. The incidence of clinical stroke (i.e. a focal neurological deficit lasting >24 hours) is 250 times more common in a child with SCD than in the general pediatric population [17]. The peak incidence occurs between 2 and 5 years of age [18]. In the longitudinal Cooperative Study of Sickle Cell Disease, 25% of patients with HbSS and 10% of patients with HbSC disease had a stroke by the age of 45 years [17]. This study found that the risk of first ischemic stroke was increased by previous transient ischemic attacks, lower steady-state hemoglobin, previous acute chest syndrome, and systolic hypertension [19]. Neurological deficits are seen most often in the setting of acute infection triggering a sickle cell crisis, but it is not uncommon for overt stroke symptoms to present "out of the blue" in an otherwise well child. High white cell count, low hemoglobin, and oxyhemoglobin desaturation predict neurological complications. Ischemic stroke is often associated with stenosis or occlusion of moderate size vessels (i.e. distal internal carotid or proximal middle cerebral arteries). Sickle cell disease causes a vasculopathy in small arteries, "plugging of the microcirculation" with a resultant progressive segmental narrowing of medium size vessels in the cerebrovasculature (Fig. 20.3), leading to occlusion, disease, and eventually the classic "moyamoya" appearance on angiography.

In patients presenting with clinical signs of stroke, infarcts in the middle cerebral artery (MCA) territory, basal ganglia, or deep white matter usually predict proximal arterial stenosis or occlusion. Infarcts in the parietal–occipital lobes or thalamus associated with complaints of headache often predict VST. SAH and ICH may occur in the setting of acute hypertension or VST [17]. VST often goes undiagnosed, and whenever a sickle cell patient has moderate to severe headache, MRV or CT venography should be performed in addition to conventional neuroimaging.

Exchange transfusions to keep HbSS <30% are recommended along with adequate hydration, oxygenation, and blood pressure control. Transcranial doppler (TCD) is a useful screening tool to follow cerebral

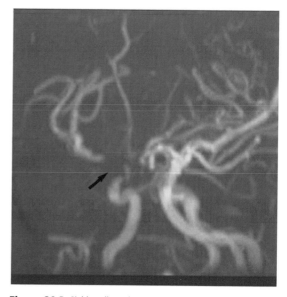

Figure 20.3 Sickle cell can lead to vascular occlusion as seen in this sickle cell patient who has total or near total occlusion of the right supraclinoid internal carotid artery, and M1 segment of the middle cerebral artery with possible reconstitution via the middle meningeal artery. This disease can progress further to a "moya moya" pattern and strokes without transfusion therapy.

blood flow in the internal carotid or MCA. TCD velocities over 200 cm/second are associated with a 40% increased stroke risk over the next 3 years [20]. The Stroke Prevention in Sickle Cell Disease Study demonstrated that regular exchange transfusion therapy in patients with transcranial doppler velocities >200 cm/second led to a 90% reduction in the incidence of stroke for the duration of the study [21]. Unfortunately, widespread patient access to TCD has been limited by both geographical and economic factors. The development of TCD screening programs is patchy in the United States and Europe with only a minority of patients (45% of children ages 2–12 with SCD or thalassemia) being screened annually, primarily due to barriers to care such as long travel distances to the nearest vascular laboratory [22]. Identifying children early on in the disease process and selecting for those who have potential for increased TCD velocities would allow them to be prioritized for routine TCD monitoring, exchange transfusion, and neuroimaging. Rees and colleagues developed a simple index using age and routine blood work (hemoglobin and aspartate transaminase) in order to predict which children are likely to have TCD readings >170 cm/second, placing them at higher risk of developing cerebrovascular disease and resultant ischemic infarcts. This index has been shown to have 100% sensitivity and between 60% and 70% specificity for predicting increased arterial velocities [19].

In addition to the standard therapies (exchange transfusions, hydroxyurea, and blood pressure management), antiplatelet therapy with aspirin has been shown to reduce ischemic stroke risk, as well as prevent silent ischemia and cognitive impairment. A pilot trial using aspirin therapy in sickle cell patients is underway. In the meantime, aspirin therapy should be used with caution in patients with a history of large territory ischemic stroke, subdural, or SAH because of the unknown risk of hemorrhage [1].

Diseases associated with hemorrhagic strokes

Hemophilia A

The most devastating and common neurological complication of hemophilia A is ICH. The incidence of ICH in the general population is around 2%. In contrast, the incidence of ICH in patients with hemophilia A can be as high as 12%. ICH can occur spontaneously or as a result of a minor/trivial trauma. A review of 170 patients with hemophilia A documented 42 episodes of ICH or spinal hemorrhage in 32 patients. Of those patients presenting with ICH or spinal hemorrhage, 36% were associated with a minor or obvious head trauma, whereas 64% occurred spontaneously. All of the patients presenting with an acute bleed where known to have severe hemophilia A, and 9 of the 32 patients (17.6%) presented with recurrent ICH [23].

Sudden onset of headache is the most common presenting symptom of ICH (97.5%) [23]. Other associated symptoms, including nausea, vomiting, and progressive neurologic deterioration, are strongly suggestive of intraparenchymal brain hemorrhage and warrant immediate neurological imaging with a CT of the head to assess for intra- or extraparenchymal blood. Patients with brain herniation at presentation have the worst prognosis, as concurrent herniation is near 100% fatal.

Acquired hemophilia A is a rare bleeding disorder caused by the development of autoantibodies that inhibit the action of naturally occurring factor VIII. Patients classically present with prominent extensive subcutaneous hematomas. Unlike classic hemophilia, ICH and hemarthroses are rare with hemophilia A.

In addition to standard management of ICH, treatment of bleeding in a patient with hemophilia consists of administration of coagulation factor concentrates in order to correct the deficiency. If FVIII concentrate is not available, one should not wait for concentrate but should begin treatment with cryoprecipitate, each unit of which generally contains 80–100 IU of FVIII, or FFP, which contains all clotting factors.

References

1 Zaidat OO, Lerner AJ. *The Little Black Book of Neurology (4th edition)*. St. Louis: Mosby, 2002.

2 Adams HP Jr., Adams RJ, Brott T, et al. Guidelines for the early management of patients with ischemic stroke. *Stroke* 2003;34:1056–83.

3 Goske-Bierska I, Wysokinski W, Brown RD Jr., et al. Cerebral venous sinus thrombosis: Incidence of venous thrombosis recurrence and survival. *Neurology* 2006;67:814–19.

4 Mohr JP, Choi D, Grotter J, Weir B, Wolf PA. *Stroke: Pathophysiology, Diagnosis, and Management* (4th edition). New York: Churchill Livingstone, 2004.

5 Ferro JM, Canhao P, Stam J, et al. Prognosis of cerebral vein and dural sinus thrombosis: results of the International Study on Cerebral Vein and Dural Sinus Thrombosis (ISCVT). *Stroke* 2004;35:664–70.

6 Broderick JP, Connolly S, Feldmann E, et al. Guidelines for the management of spontaneous intracerebral hemorrhage in adults: 2007 update: a guideline from the American Heart Association/American Stroke Association Stroke Council, High Blood Pressure Research Council, and the Quality of Care and Outcomes in Research Interdisciplinary Working Group. *Stroke* 2007;38:2001–23.

7 Ohwaki K, Yano E, Nagushima H, et al. Blood pressure management in acute intracerebral hemorrhage: relationship between elevated blood pressure and hematoma enlargement. *Stroke* 2004;35:1364–7.

8 Broderick JP, Adams HP, Barsan W, et al. Guidelines for the management of spontaneous intracerebral hemorrhage: a statement for healthcare professionals from a

special writing group of the Stroke Council, American Heart Association. *Stroke* 1999;30:905–15.

9 Mendelow AD, Gregson BA, Fernandes HM, et al. Early surgery versus initial conservative treatment in patients with spontaneous supratentorial intracerebral haematomas in the International Surgical Trial in Intracerebral Haemorrhage (STICH): a randomised trial. *Lancet* 2005;365:387–97.

10 Mayer SA, Brun NC, Begtrup K, et al. Efficacy and safety of recombinant activated factor VII for acute intracerebral hemorrhage. *N Engl J Med* 2008;358:2127–37.

11 Moster ML. Coagulopathies and arterial stroke. *J Neuroophthalmol* 2003;23:63–71.

12 Lim W, Crowther MA, Eikelboom JW. Management of antiphospholipid antibody syndrome: a systematic review. *J Am Med Assoc* 2006;295:1050–7.

13 Rand JH. The antiphospholipid syndrome. *Annu Rev Med* 2003;54:409–424.

14 Caplan LR. *Caplan's Stroke: A Clinical Approach* (3rd edition). Boston: Butterworth Heinemann, 2000.

15 Pegelow CH, Macklin EA, Moser FG, et al. Longitudinal changes in brain magnetic resonance imaging findings in children with sickle cell disease. *Blood* 2002;99:3014–18.

16 Kinney TR, Sleeper LA, Wang WC, et al. Silent cerebral infarcts in sickle cell anemia: a risk factor analysis. *Pediatrics* 1999;103:640–5.

17 Kirkham F. Therapy Insight: stroke risk and its management in patients with sickle cell disease. *Nat Clin Pract Neurol* 2007;3:264–78.

18 Ohene-Frempong K, Weiner SJ, Sleeper LA, et al. Cooperative study of sickle cell disease: cerebrovascular accidents in sickle cell disease: rates and risk factors. *Blood* 1998;91:288–94.

19 Rees DC, Dick MC, Height SE, et al. A simple index using age, hemoglobin, and aspartate transaminase predicts increased intracerebral blood velocity as measured by transcranial doppler scanning in children with sickle cell anemia. *Pediatrics* 2008;121:1628–32.

20 Adams RJ, McKie VC, Carl EM, et al. Long-term stroke risk in children with sickle cell disease screened with transcranial doppler. *Ann Neurol* 1997;42:699–704.

21 Adams RJ, McKie VC, Hsu L, et al. Prevention of a first stroke by transfusions in children with sickle cell anemia and abnormal results on transcranial doppler ultrasonography. *N Engl J Med* 1998;339:5–11.

22 Fullerton HJ, Gardner M, Adams RJ, Lo LC, Johnson SC. Obstacles to primary stroke prevention in children with sickle cell disease. *Neurology* 2006;67:1098–9.

23 Chinthamitr Y, Ruchutrakool T, Suwanawiboon B, Nakkinkun Y, Ayprasert N, Issaragrisil S. Intracranial and spinal hemorrhage in adult hemophelia A in siriraj hospital, Thiland. *J Thromb Haemost* 2007;5(Suppl 2):P-S150.

Hepatology

Raj K. Patel and Roopen Arya

Introduction

Hepatic diseases are associated with a variety of defects affecting both primary and secondary hemostasis (Table 21.1). It is therefore not surprising that advanced hepatic disease is associated with bleeding [1,2]. Chronic liver disease frequently causes portal hypertension with resultant hypersplenism and thrombocytopenia. This leads to formation of fragile vascular anomalies (varices) that may bleed profusely on a background of hemostatic failure. Not all patients with liver disease have bleeding manifestations, but these tend to be unpredictable when they occur. Common clinical manifestations include petechiae, ecchymoses, recurrent epistaxes, and gingival bleeding. Invasive procedures, such as liver biopsy and ascitic shunts, are particularly high risk in chronic liver disease as they may precipitate bleeding in previously stable patients.

Liver disease may be classified into two broad categories:

1 *Acute liver disease* (e.g. fulminant hepatic failure secondary to paracetamol overdose); or
2 *Chronic liver disease* (e.g. alcohol-induced cirrhosis, primary biliary cirrhosis).

Most advanced cases of liver disease are associated with at least one and frequently multiple hemostatic defects. Orthotopic liver transplantation corrects hepatic function and coagulopathy in long term but is associated with a substantial perioperative increase in bleeding risk.

A delicate balance exists between the procoagulant and anticoagulant defects associated with liver disease. Although bleeding episodes are more common, thrombotic events may occur despite a coexisting hemorrhagic tendency. These include symptomatic lower limb deep vein thrombosis, pulmonary embolism, thrombosis of the abdominal veins, and thrombosis in central venous catheters or extra-corporeal circuits. It is also possible that the prothrombotic state contributes to other hepatic disease processes, including portopulmonary hypertension, parenchymal extinction, and accelerated hepatic fibrosis [3]. Thrombosis may also occur as a result of local endothelial dysfunction. There is as yet no universally available laboratory test with which to accurately characterize the prothrombotic state in hepatic disease.

Pathophysiology of coagulopathy

Impaired coagulation factor synthesis

The liver is the major synthetic site for:
• Coagulation factors of both intrinsic and extrinsic pathways, including factors II, V, VII, VIII, IX, X, XI, and XII and fibrinogen;
• Anticoagulant proteins (antithrombin, protein C, protein S); and
• Fibrinolytic regulators (plasminogen, α_1-antiplasmin).

Coagulation proteins

Loss of hepatocyte function in disease states leads to a reduction in the levels of most coagulation proteins (except factor VIII) and therefore predisposes to bleeding. Reduced levels of these proteins broadly reflect the extent of liver damage but are poor predictors of bleeding risk in individual patients.

• In acute liver injury (e.g. following paracetamol overdose), prothrombin time (PT) has been shown to be an accurate predictor of hepatocellular damage,

Table 21.1 Hemostatic defects in hepatic disease.

Hemostatic abnormality
Reduced biosynthesis of hepatic coagulation factors
Reduced biosynthesis of anticoagulant and fibrinolytic proteins
Reduced clearance of coagulation proteins and inhibitors
Dysfibrinogenemia
Systemic fibrinolysis
Disseminated intravascular coagulation
Thrombocytopenia
Platelet dysfunction

bleeding risk, and likelihood of progression to fulminant liver failure.
• Factor V concentration is a particularly sensitive and specific indicator of hepatic synthetic function and plasma levels fall with increasing disease severity.
• Malabsorption of fat-soluble vitamins may lead to low levels of circulating vitamin K-dependent coagulation factors.

Whereas the majority of circulating coagulation factors decrease in liver disease, the reverse is true of factor VIII, von Willebrand factor (VWF), and fibrinogen. Fibrinogen and most of factor VIII are synthesized in hepatocytes, whereas VWF is synthesized by platelets and vascular endothelium. Circulating levels of these proteins increase in the acute phase response associated with hepatic disease, although low levels of fibrinogen in late disease may herald the onset of acute liver failure.

The formation of abnormal forms of vitamin K-dependent coagulation factors (e.g. des-γ-carboxyl prothrombin) may be seen in both acute and chronic liver disease. These proteins, raised in the absence of vitamin K (PIVKAs), form as a result of an acquired carboxylation defect but do not reach high enough concentrations to cause bleeding.

Thrombocytopenia and platelet dysfunction

Mild to moderate thrombocytopenia is common in hepatic disease, affecting up to 30% of all cases of chronic liver disease and 90% of subjects with end-stage disease.

Chronic liver disease is associated with:
• Portal hypertension and congestive splenomegaly. The resultant increase in platelet pooling by splenic

sequestration is the principal mechanism by which thrombocytopenia occurs in these patients.
• Increasing portal venous pressures, blood is shunted into the systemic circulation via portosystemic collaterals (varices) from which blood loss may occur, particularly on a background of thrombocytopenia.
• Ineffective production of platelets secondary to a decrease in liver thrombopoietin synthesis has been reported.

Alcohol-associated liver disease may cause thrombocytopenia by a variety of mechanisms:
• Alcohol is directly toxic to megakaryocytes, leading to inhibition of megakaryopoiesis and decreased platelet production.
• Folate deficiency resulting from poor dietary intake or ineffective hepatic metabolism may result in ineffective megakaryopoiesis.
• Alcohol ingestion is itself associated with decreased platelet survival.

In fulminant viral hepatitis, the marked thrombocytopenia often encountered is caused by both suppression of megakaryopoiesis by virus and increased platelet destruction.

The increase in bleeding time seen in many subjects with severe liver disease is often out of proportion to the associated degree of thrombocytopenia, suggesting the presence of platelet dysfunction. The results of platelet function testing in these patients are inconsistent. Whereas some studies have demonstrated abnormalities in primary and secondary aggregation to adenosine diphosphate (ADP), adrenaline, thrombin and ristocetin, others have failed to show any functional defect.

The cause of platelet dysfunction in liver disease is unclear. There is an increase in levels of circulating platelet-inhibitors, including fibrin degradation products. Ethanol or abnormal high-density lipoproteins may contribute to aggregatory abnormalities in some cases. In others, intrinsic platelet abnormalities have been demonstrated, including acquired storage pool deficiency (platelet nucleotide deficiency), reduced platelet arachidonic acid, and abnormalities of platelet membrane composition and signaling.

Disseminated intravascular coagulation

It is generally accepted that many patients with advanced liver disease have activated coagulation and chronic low-grade disseminated intravascular coagulation (DIC). The diagnosis of DIC in subjects with chronic liver disease is complicated by the fact that many of the laboratory abnormalities present are common to both conditions.

Bleeding or thrombosis is usually present in DIC but is not a frequent finding in patients with liver disease coagulopathy alone. Evidence of increased thrombin generation has been demonstrated in chronic liver disease. These effects are at least partially reversible by heparin and include reduced fibrinogen survival and increased markers of thrombin generation (D-dimer, thrombin–antithrombin complexes, fibrinopeptide A, and plasmin–antiplasmin complexes). It may be that liver disease confers a state of increased intravascular coagulation, whereas additional factors such as sepsis or bleeding trigger DIC.

A number of possible causes of chronic DIC in liver disease have been suggested:
• Procoagulant factors released from damaged hepatocytes.
• Release of intestinal endotoxins into the portal circulation.
• Impaired clearance of activated coagulation factors by the damaged failing liver.
• In addition, levels of naturally occurring anticoagulants, including antithrombin, protein C, protein S, and heparin cofactor II, are reduced in proportion to the degree of hepatic dysfunction.

Vitamin K deficiency

Vitamin K is a fat-soluble vitamin required for the production of a variety of coagulation proteins, including factors II, VII, IX, and X and proteins C and S. Vitamin K deficiency may occur in liver disease as a result of:
• poor dietary intake;
• destruction of vitamin K_2-producing intestinal bacteria by antibiotic therapy;
• bile salts are required for the absorption of vitamin K in the small intestine, so biliary obstruction may therefore lead to vitamin K deficiency; and
• prolonged cholestasis secondary to calculi or neoplasia leads to deficiencies in the vitamin K-dependent coagulation proteins and prolongation of the PT.

Dysfibrinogenemia

One of the earliest coagulation abnormalities seen in chronic liver disease is the production of a dysfibrino-

gen. This molecule is rich in sialic acid residues and results in abnormal fibrin polymerization. The reduced efficiency in fibrin clot production prolongs both the thrombin time and reptilase time, but has not been shown to contribute to clinical bleeding. Dysfibrinogenemia is most commonly seen in chronic hepatitis and cirrhosis but has also been reported in hepatocellular carcinoma.

Hyperfibrinolysis

Accelerated fibrinolysis is well recognized in hepatic cirrhosis. Forty percent of patients awaiting liver transplant show laboratory evidence of hyperfibrinolysis with short euglobulin lysis times and elevated serum fibrin degradation product concentrations. In addition, low plasminogen levels and elevated fibrinopeptide B, D-dimerm and plasmin–α_2-antiplasmin complex concentrations may be demonstrated in subjects with chronic liver disease. Possible mechanisms behind this include decreased hepatic clearance of plasminogen activators (e.g. tissue plasminogen activator, tPA) and a decrease in circulating the fibrinolytic inhibitors plasminogen activator inhibitor type 1 (PAI-1), α_2-antiplasmin, and histidine-rich glycoprotein.

Clinical manifestations of liver disease coagulopathy

Hemorrhage

Bleeding is a common manifestation of chronic liver disease (Table 21.2) and is associated with substantial

Table 21.2 Clinical manifestations of liver disease coagulopathy.

Ecchymoses
Purpura
Oozing from venipuncture or intravenous cannula sites
Dental bleeding
Hematuria
Gastrointestinal and variceal hemorrhage
Epistaxis
Postoperative hemorrhage

morbidity and mortality. Patients may present with both:

- *Mucosal bleeding:* resulting from thrombocytopenia and platelet dysfunction leading to failure of primary hemostasis; and
- *Soft tissue bleeding:* resulting from the reduction in coagulation proteins with failure of secondary hemostasis.

Once liver disease is diagnosed, it is important to remember that laboratory tests of hemostasis are poorly predictive of bleeding events. This is partly because liver disease bleeding is not only caused by defects in primary and secondary hemostasis, but also is frequently associated with anatomical abnormalities, such as portosystemic varices on a background of raised portal pressure.

Bleeding episodes may also be triggered by operative procedures in previously stable patients. Some patients with advanced chronic liver disease are identified for the first time prior to elective surgery when a coagulation screen is checked. At least 50% of patients with cirrhosis will have varices secondary to portal hypertension at diagnosis, and some will be diagnosed for the first time with liver disease following a variceal bleed.

Thrombosis (Table 21.3)

Abdominal vein thrombosis

Thrombosis of the hepatic veins (Budd-Chiari syndrome, BCS), portal, and/or mesenteric veins are infrequent but significant diseases that frequently occur in younger patients.

- *Hepatic vein thrombosis:* BCS due to hepatic venous thrombosis has a varied clinical presentation ranging from asymptomatic to fulminant liver failure [4]. A cause can be identified in 75% of these cases

Table 21.3 Hypercoaguability and liver disease.

Abdominal vein thrombosis
Deep vein thrombosis and pulmonary embolism
Thrombosis in central venous catheters and extracorporeal circuits
Parenchymal extinction and progressive hepatic fibrosis

Table 21.4 Causes of Budd-Chiari syndrome.

Hereditary prothrombotic disorders:
Factor V Leiden
PT 20210 G/A
Antithrombin deficiency
Protein C deficiency
Protein S deficiency

Acquired prothrombotic disorders:
Myeloproliferative disorders
Antiphospholipid syndrome
Paroxsysmal nocturnal hemoglobinuria
Malignancy
Pregnancy
Exogenous estrogen

Other:
Bechet's syndrome
Caval web
Dacarbazine
Aspergillosis
Inflammatory bowel disease
Hepatocellular/renal/adrenal carcinoma

(Table 21.4). These include hereditary and acquired prothrombotic states, trauma, and infection. The presence of multiple predisposing factors in BCS is well recognized. Myeloproliferative disorders (MPD) are the most common cause of BCS, with polychthemia vera implicated in 10–40% of cases [5–7]. In 25% of cases, the cause of BCS is not apparent ("idiopathic BCS"), although the presence of an underlying "latent" MPD is often suspected [8]. The diagnosis of MPD has been greatly improved by the discovery of a point mutation in the Janus kinase 2 (JAK2) gene on the short arm of chromosome 9. JAK2 is a tyrosine kinase that transduces signals triggered by hemopoeitic growth factors. In 2005, an acquired mutation in JAK2 (V617F) was reported in MPDs [9–12]. The presence of JAK2V617F in 90% of subjects with PV and 50% of those with primary thrombocythemia and myelofibrosis provides us with a new diagnostic test of clonality in these diseases. JAK2V617F has been shown to be present in up to 58.5% of cases of "idiopathic" BCS, indicating the presence of an underlying latent MPD [13].

• *Portal vein thrombosis:* Portal vein thrombosis (PVT) is often silent and may not be discovered until variceal hemorrhage occurs. Clinical features include abdominal pain, ascites, and rectal bleeding. Thrombosis extending to the mesenteric vessels may lead to mesenteric infarction. Common causes of PVT include hepatic cirrhosis, abdominal sepsis, tumors, and pancreatitis. As in BCS, the role of multiple etiological factors is well recognized, including hereditary and acquired prothrombotic disorders and estrogen therapy. JAK2V617F has been reported to occur in 17–36% of patients with PVT [14–17]. Anticoagulation therapy with vitamin K antagonists may be hazardous in patients with esophageal varices, and consequently, decisions on treatment are based on extent/age of thrombosis, presence of varices, history of bleeding, and the presence of an underlying prothrombotic disorder. In acute PVT, anticoagulation is frequently given for a period of 6 months; a longer duration of anticoagulation may be beneficial in chronic PVT or in patients with underlying prothrombotic disorders [18].

Venous thromboembolism (VTE)

Deep vein thrombosis and pulmonary embolism occur frequently in hospitalized medical patients, and routine risk assessment and thromboprophylaxis with heparin is now widely recommended [19]. Despite the hemorrhagic tendency of chronic liver disease, VTE occurs not infrequently in these patients. Prothrombotic coagulation disturbances in liver disease include reduced levels of anticoagulant proteins (antithrombin, protein C, protein S), antiphospholipid antibodies, and hyperfibrinolysis. The incidence of VTE in chronic liver disease may well be underestimated, as lower limb edema and dyspnea are nonspecific and commonly present in these patients. In one retrospective case-control study of patients with cirrhosis, new VTE was present in 0.5% of inpatients with cirrhosis [20].

Progression of fibrosis due to parenchymal extinction

It is clear that, in patients with chronic liver disease (particularly cirrhosis), the prothrombotic state can lead to further hepatic injury ("parenchymal extinction") and progression of fibrosis. This may be due to thrombosis in small intrahepatic vessels. There is some evidence that the prothrombotic state predisposes to accelerated fibrogenesis, for example, the observed association between factor V Leiden mutation and accelerated fibrosis in patients with hepatitis C infection. There is no good evidence to support the use of standard anticoagulation to prevent progression of hepatic fibrosis, but the advent of newer antithrombotics may kindle new interest in this area.

Extracorporeal circuits

Continuous venovenous hemodialysis (CVVH) and artificial liver support machines both require the exposure of blood to artificial surfaces, inevitably leading to coagulation activation and clotting in the extracorporeal circuit. A variety of anticoagulant strategies have been advocated, often depending on local expertise and the perceived bleeding risk in individual cases.

Laboratory investigation of hemostasis in liver disease

Clotting screen

The PT and activated partial thromboplastin time (APTT) are commonly prolonged in chronic liver disease, reflecting a reduction in coagulation factor production by the failing liver (Table 21.5). Patients with abnormal laboratory tests only require treatment to correct coagulopathy when there is evidence of active bleeding or prior to surgery.

Chronic liver disease

No single coagulation test is predictive of hemorrhage or thrombosis in patients with chronic liver disease:
• Factor VII has a short half-life and levels fall early in subjects with hepatic impairment. An isolated prolongation of the PT may be the only demonstrable laboratory abnormality in those with mild disease.
• A prolonged PT or international normalized ratio (INR) is a key indicator of hepatic dysfunction and commonly used as a trigger for liver transplantation; however, it is vitamin K-dependent. Although a prolonged PT is often used as a marker of hepatic dysfunction, it is most sensitive to low coagulation FVII levels

Table 21.5 Laboratory abnormalities in liver disease.

Laboratory abnormality	Likely etiology
Isolated ↑ PT	FVII deficiency
	Vitamin K deficiency (cholestasis, dietary)
↑ PT + ↑ APTT	Coagulation factor deficiencies
↑ Thrombin time + ↑ Reptilase time	Dysfibrinogenemia, hypofibringenemia
Thrombocytopenia	Hypersplenism, DIC
	Suppressed megakaryopoeisis
Abnormal platelet aggregometry	Acquired platelet function defect
↓ Euglobulin clot lysis time	Hyperfibrinolysis: ↓PAI ↓ α_2-antiplasmin

Abbreviations: APTT, activated partial thromboplastin time; DIC, disseminated intravascular coagulation; PAI, plasminogen activator inhibitor; PT, prothrombin time.

and does not accurately reflect the levels of other coagulation factors (e.g. FII, FVIII, FX, VWF).

• Factor V concentration is a sensitive indicator of hepatic disease as this protein is predominantly synthesized by hepatocytes and is not vitamin K-dependent.

• Thrombophilia tests: levels of the naturally occurring anticoagulants (antithrombin, protein C, protein S) may all be reduced as a consequence of liver disease. Combined antithrombin and protein C deficiency are usually due to liver disease rather than due to combined inheritance.

Cholestasis

Patients with early vitamin K deficiency secondary to cholestasis have isolated prolongation of the PT, which is correctable by administration of intravenous vitamin K.

Factor VII has the shortest half-life of all the vitamin K-dependent factors and is therefore the first coagulation factor to decrease, hence isolated prolonged PT. With severe prolonged vitamin K deficiency there is reduction in factors II, IX, and X with prolongation of both PT and APTT.

Advanced hepatocellular disease

These patients tend to have a more severe derangement of laboratory tests reflecting:

• high incidence of multiple coagulation factor deficiencies;
• hyperfibrinolysis; and
• DIC.

Fibrinogen level

Fibrinogen levels vary according to the type and severity of liver dysfunction. When measuring fibrinogen concentration, results may vary markedly depending on the methods used. Assays based on the rate of clot formation (e.g. Clauss fibrinogen) result in low levels of fibrinogen more often than assays based on final clot weight. This is because dysfibrinogens and circulating proteins that impair fibrin clot formation may (e.g. fibrinogen degradation products, FDPs) influence rate-dependent assays.

Dysfibrinogenemia

This may prolong thrombin time and reptilase time but is not usually associated with bleeding.

Hyperfibrinolysis

This may lead to hypofibrinogenemia with prolongation of the PT, APTT, thrombin time, and reptilase times. Other laboratory findings include a prolongation of the euglobulin clot lysis time, raised FDP levels, and decreased plasminogen concentration.

Thromboelastography (TEG®) is an investigation measuring the dynamics of clot formation and has been shown to be a more superior predictor of intraoperative bleeding in liver transplantation than standard coagulation tests.

Invasive procedures and liver disease

Liver biopsy

The risk of bleeding after liver biopsy is a small but significant one and has been estimated to occur in 0.4% of cases. In view of this risk, each case should be carefully reviewed to ensure that the procedure is only performed when absolutely necessary.

Percutaneous liver biopsy is relatively safe when the INR is below 1.5 and the platelet count is above

50×10^9/L. In subjects who do not fulfill these criteria, administration of vitamin K, plasma, and platelets should be considered prior to the procedure. Subjects with prolonged bleeding time and history of bleeding may be given desmopressin (DDAVP). Alternative strategies include laparoscopic liver biopsy and biopsy via the transjugular approach.

A high mortality rate has been reported in patients with sickle cell disease undergoing percutaneous liver biopsy and extreme caution is recommended, particularly in the setting of acute liver failure.

Shunt insertion in liver disease

Portocaval and mesocaval shunts may be inserted to alleviate portal hypertension in decompensated liver disease. These procedures are frequently associated with increased fibrinolysis and DIC. Peritoneal–venous shunt insertion in patients with chronic ascites may trigger significant bleeding. This is thought to be because of the flow of procoagulant and platelet-activating molecules from ascitic fluid into the systemic circulation triggering DIC. Clinically significant bleeding may be avoided by draining ascites prior to opening the shunt or by short-term occlusion of the shunt.

Liver transplantation

Liver transplantation is being increasingly offered to patients with end-stage decompensated liver disease. Marked hemostatic failure with substantial blood loss is frequently seen during liver transplant [21,22], with a strong association between blood loss and mortality rate. Research into the causes of liver transplant coagulopathy have led to improved intraoperative management strategies and decreased mortality rates.

The first operative (preimplantation) stage

There is mild deterioration in the baseline liver disease coagulopathy. This coincides with surgical dissection and mobilization of the diseased liver and is not usually associated with major blood loss.

The next three operative stages

The coagulation disturbance increases (Table 21.6) and is maximal during the anhepatic stage (because of loss of coagulation factor turnover) and early reimplantation (hyperfibrinolytic) stage. Consumptive thrombocytopenia with DIC often occurs, requiring

Table 21.6 Coagulation abnormalities during liver transplantation.

Stage of transplant	Hemostatic abnormality
Stage 1: Preimplantation	Mild deterioration of baseline liver disease coagulopathy
Stage 2: Anhepatic	Loss of coagulation factor synthesis and clearance Accelerated fibrinolysis and DIC Consumptive thrombocytopenia tPA released from graft on reperfusion
Stage 3: Reimplantation	Restoration of coagulation factor synthesis and clearance Resolution of hyperfibrinolysis

Abbreviations: DIC, disseminated intravascular coagulation; tPA, tissue plasminogen activator.

massive blood product replacement. This is followed by gradual resolution of hemostatic dysfunction in the third (reimplantation) stage and postoperative period.

Treatment of liver transplant coagulopathy

This varies according to stage of operation:
• Stage 1 is associated with mild surgical bleeding, not usually requiring aggressive hemostatic support.
• In the anhepatic and reperfusion stages, transfusion with blood, platelets, plasma, and cryoprecipitate is required to correct profound coagulopathy and inevitable major blood losses.
• The reperfusion stage is associated with tPA and endogenous heparin-like substance release from the graft, and antifibrinolytic therapy with aprotinin or tranexamic acid has been shown to be effective in reducing transfusion requirements in this setting.
• Stage 3 is usually associated with resolution of coagulopathy. However, if successful engraftment of the donor liver does not occur, tissue ischemia and necrosis may trigger DIC and further bleeding.

Treatment of liver disease coagulopathy

Treatment of coagulopathy in liver disease is required during episodes of bleeding or prior to invasive procedures. The type of treatment required will depend on the specific hemostatic abnormalities present and the nature of the bleeding event. It is important to remember that most patients with coagulopathy are stable and do not require specific therapy. When bleeding does occur, the associated triggers (e.g. esophageal varices secondary to portal hypertension) need to be addressed in conjunction with strategies to correct coagulopathy.

Vitamin K

Deficiency of vitamin K may occur in liver disease, resulting from poor diet or secondary to malabsorption. Administration of 10 mg vitamin K_1 will correct the PT, at least partially, in most patients within 48 hours. The PT will not fully correct if there is a coexisting defect in hepatic synthetic function.

Plasma

Fresh frozen plasma (FFP) or solvent detergent plasma (SDP) contains all the coagulation factors synthesized by the healthy liver. It may be used to correct multiple coagulation factor deficiencies in bleeding patients or prior to invasive procedures. A significant problem with FFP is the large volume of transfusion required to correct the PT and APTT in severe liver disease, particularly in volume-overloaded patients with ascites and peripheral edema. In addition, repeated transfusions are required to maintain circulating coagulation factor levels. Prothrombin complex concentrates should be used with caution in liver disease, as their use has been associated with thromboembolism and DIC. Cryoprecipitate or fibrinogen concentrate should be used to correct hypofibrinogenemia associated with hyperfibrinolysis or DIC.

Platelets

Platelet transfusions are indicated in bleeding patients with platelet counts of $<10 \times 10^9/L$, or in patients undergoing invasive procedures. Platelet increments are generally poor in subjects with portal hypertension because of sequestration of transfused platelets in the spleen. DDAVP ($0.3\mu g/kg$) may be of value in patients with acquired platelet dysfunction and prolonged bleeding time, but its value in bleeding patients is uncertain.

Antifibrinolytics

Aprotinin, tranexamic acid, and ε-aminocaproic acid have all been shown to reduce operative blood loss and transfusion requirements in liver transplantation. The use of these agents to reduce fibrinolysis associated with chronic liver disease is of uncertain value, and their use in DIC is not recommended.

Other agents

Heparin and antithrombin

Their use in DIC has not led to significant improvements in blood loss or mortality and is therefore not recommended.

Estrogens

There are some reports on efficacy in bleeding related to chronic liver disease, but further data from clinical trials are required before their use can be recommended.

Fibrin glue

Local endoscopic applications have been shown to be effective in the treatment of bleeding gastric varices.

Recombinant factor VIIa

Small studies have demonstrated reduced clotting times in chronic liver disease and a reduction in transfusion requirements in liver transplantation. The optimal role for recombinant factor VIIa in the treatment of liver coagulopathy has yet to be defined.

References

1 Amirano L, Guardascione MA, Brancaccio V, et al. Coagulation disorders in liver disease. *Semin Liver Dis* 2002;22:83–96.

2 Ratnoff OD. Hemostatic defects in liver and biliary tract disease. In: Ratoff OD, Forbes CD, eds. *Disorders of Hemostasis*. Philadelphia: WB Saunders, 1996:422.

3 Northup PG, Sundaram V, Fallon MB, et al. Hypercoagulation and thrombophilia in liver disease. *J Thromb Haemost* 2007;6:2–9.

4 Narayanan KV, Shah V, Kamath PS. The Budd–Chiari syndrome. *N Eng J Med* 2004;350:578–85.

5 Denninger MH, Chait Y, Casadevall N, et al. Cause of portal or hepatic vein thrombosis in adults: the role

of multiple concurrent factors. *Hepatology* 2000;31:587–91.

6 Valla D, Casadevall N, Lacombe C, et al. Primary myeloproliferative disorder and hepatic vein thrombosis: a prospective study of erythroid colony formation in vitro in 20 patients with Budd-Chiari Syndrome. *Ann Intern Med* 1985;103:329–34.

7 Primignani M, Martinelli I, Bucciarelli P. Risk factors for thrombophilia in extrahepatic portal vein obstruction. *Hepatology* 2005;41:603–8.

8 Pagliuca A, Mufti GJ, Janossa-Tahernia M, et al. In vitro colony culture and chromosomal studies in hepatic and portal vein thrombosis: possible evidence of an occult myeloproliferative state. *Q J Med* 1990;76: 981–9.

9 Baxter EJ, Scott LM, Campbell PJ, et al. Acquired mutation of the tyrosine kinase *JAK2* in human myeloproliferative diseases. *Lancet* 2005;365:1054–61.

10 Levine RL, Wadleigh M, Cools J, et al. Activating mutation in the tyrosine kinase *JAK2* in polycythemia vera, essential thrombocythemia, and myeloid metaplasia with myelofibrosis. *Cancer Cell* 2005;7:387–97.

11 James C, Ugo V, Le Couedic JP, et al. A unique clonal *JAK2* mutation leading to constitutive signaling causes polycythemia vera. *Nature* 2005;434:1144–8.

12 Kralovics R, Passamonti F, Buser AS, et al. A gain-of-function mutation of *JAK2* in myeloproliferative disorders. *N Engl J Med* 2005;352:1779–90.

13 Patel RK, Lea NC, Heneghan MA, et al. Prevalence of the activating JAK2 tyrosine kinase mutation V617F in the Budd-Chiari Syndrome. *Gastroenterology* 2006;130:2031–8.

14 Primigani M, Barosi G, Bergamaschi G, et al. Role of the JAK2 mutation in the diagnosis of chronic myeloproliferative disorders in splanchnic vein thrombosis. *Hepatology* 2006;44(6):1528–34.

15 Kiladjian J, Cervantes F, Leebeek F, et al. Role of JAK2 mutation detection in Budd-Chiari Syndrome (BCS) and portal vein thrombosis (PVT) associated to MPD. *Blood* 2006;108:Abstract 377.

16 Colaizzo D, Amitrano L, Tiscia GL, et al. The JAK2 V617F mutation frequently occurs in patients with portal and mesenteric venous thrombosis. *J Thromb Haemost* 2006;5:55–61.

17 Regina S, Herault O, D'Iteroche L, et al. The JAK2 mutation V617F is specifically associated with idiopathic splanchnic vein thrombosis. *J Thromb Haemost* 2007;5(4):859–61.

18 Condat B, Pessione F, Helene Denninger M, et al. Recent portal or mesenteric venous thrombosis: increased recognition and frequent recanalization on anticoagulant therapy. *Hepatology* 2000;32:466–70.

19 Hirsh J, Dalen JE, Master MPM, et al. American College of Chest Physicians The Sixth (2000) ACCP Guidelines for Antithrombotic Therapy for Prevention and Treatment of Thrombosis. *Chest* 2001;119:1S–2S.

20 Northup PG, McMahon MM, Ruhl AP, et al. Coagulopathy does not fully protect hospitalized cirrhosis patients from peripheral venous thromboembolism. *Am J Gastroenterol* 2006;101:1524–8.

21 Porte RJ, Knot EA, Bontempo FA. Hemostasis in liver transplantation. *Gastroenterology* 1989;97:488–501.

22 Starzl TE, Demertris A, van Thiel DH. Liver transplantation. *N Engl J Med* 1989;321:1014–22, 1092–99.

Stephanie Perry and Thomas L. Ortel

Bleeding in renal disease

Clinical presentation

In 1764, the association between bleeding and renal disease was first entertained in Morgagni's "Opera Omnia" [1,2]. Signs of bleeding may appear as easy bruising, petechia, gingival bleeding, epistaxis, or prolonged bleeding or hematomas from venipuncture or catheter sites [1,3,4]. Life-threatening bleeding can occur from pericardial tamponade, retroperitoneal bleeding, intracranial bleeding, and gastrointestinal bleeding [1,3]. Retroperitoneal bleeding can be spontaneous or postprocedure. For example, bleeding rates postrenal biopsy are reported to range from 11% to 22% [4]. Patients with uncontrolled hypertension and undergoing hemodialysis treatments are at risk of intracranial bleeds. Gastrointestinal bleeding has been reported to be the second leading cause of death in patients with acute renal failure [3].

Etiology

There are many factors that may contribute to bleeding in renal disease as can occur in other disease states. Factors such as anemia or use of antiplatelet or anticoagulant drugs may increase the risk of bleeding in patients. The mechanisms behind anemia contributing to risk of bleeding include the following:
- decreased laminar flow effect of red cell facilitating platelet interaction with the endothelial lining [3,5];
- red cells release ADP and thromboxane A2, which enhances platelet aggregation [3,5]; and
- hemoglobin scavenges nitric oxide (NO) [3,5].

Drugs that may reach higher levels in patients with renal disease, such as penicillin G, carbenicillin, ticarcillin, ampicillin, and moxalactam, can increase the risk of bleeding by binding to platelets and blocking platelet-membrane agonist receptors.

Even more specific to patients with renal disease is bleeding due to uremia, which disrupts normal platelet–platelet and platelet–vessel wall interactions [2,3]. These disruptions in platelet function due to uremia may be multifactorial. Mechanisms to explain uremia-induced platelet dysfunction have included the following:
- altered arachidonic acid metabolism [2,6];
- deficient platelet stores of adenosine diphosphate and serotonin [2,3,5,6]; and
- impaired binding of fibrinogen [2,3] and von Willebrand factor (vWF) [2,5,6].

One area of great interest in explaining the "uremia effect" on platelets is the role of guanidinosuccinic acid [2,5]. Guanidinosuccinic acid accumulates during ammonia detoxification when an amidine is transferred to aspartic acid from L-arginine. L-arginine has been found to be a major substrate for NO as well. NO is known to modulate vascular tone and interferes with platelet adhesion to endothelium and platelet–platelet interaction. NO has been found to be higher in uremic patients on hemodialysis when compared with healthy subjects. Similarly, guanidinosuccinic acid appears to have vasodilation effects on intact endothelium. In addition to having similar biological activities of NO, high guanidinosuccinic concentrations appear to cause formation of NO by uremic vessels [2].

Prevention and treatment

The site, extent, and acuity of bleeding will dictate the treatment. For external bleeding, mechanical maneuvers such as applying pressure over the area of bleeding and, if an extremity is involved, elevating the area above the level of the heart can help control or

Table 22.1 Prevention of bleeding in patients with renal failure.

Correction of anemia
Avoidance of antiplatelet drugs
Dialysis
Use of:
    Desmopressin
    Conjugated estrogens
    Antifibrinolytics
    Cryoprecipitate

alleviate bleeding [6]. Topical administration of hemostatic agents such as adsorbable collagen hemostat (bovine collagen) may be used. These agents work by interaction with platelets at the injury site. A fibrillar structure provides a mesh in which platelets are trapped and interact with the collagen fibrils to trigger further aggregation [4,5].

To prevent a bleeding complication (Table 22.1), patients should avoid antiplatelet drugs, such as aspirin and NSAIDs, for at least 1 week prior to invasive procedures or surgery [6]. Dialysis is useful in prevention and in the actively bleeding uremic patient. This is postulated to be due to the removal of urea and guanidiosuccinic acid [4]. During dialysis, heparin can be held for patients with risk for continued bleeding [5,6]. Although dialysis can be helpful in decreasing uremic bleeding, platelet dysfunction can occur due to the repeated mechanical stress [5,6].

Correcting severe anemia is another strategy for prevention and treatment of bleeding. Transfusions of packed red blood cells and platelets may be needed in the acutely bleeding patient [5,6]. For patients with less severe anemia and with normal iron stores, recombinant human erythropoietin 35–50 U/kg body weight three times a week can be given to achieve a hematocrit >30% [4,5]. Increases in reticulated platelets may occur in 7 days, so in short term, erythropoietin may improve platelet adhesion and aggregation [3]. However, the use of erythropoietin is not without risks, which include poorly controlled blood pressure, arteriovenous access thrombosis, and all-cause mortality in patients with target hemoglobin concentration of 12–16 g/dL [7].

Prior to invasive procedures, desmopressin (1-deamino-8-D-arginine vasopressin; DDAVP) can be used [3,6]. DDAVP increases vWF and factor VIII levels within 30 minutes to an hour of administration [3,5]. Intravenous doses of DDAVP at 0.3–0.4 µg/kg administered over 20–30 minutes can be used. Subcutaneous (0.3 µg/kg) and intranasal (2 µg/kg) routes are also effective, although less so than the intravenous route [4]. Adverse reactions to DDAVP include headache, facial flushing, rare thrombotic events, hypotension, and hyponatremia [4,6]. Tachyphylaxis can develop with repeated doses if given within a 24-hour interval [4,6]. Conjugated estrogen at 0.6 mg/kg daily, infused over 30 minutes, for 5 days has also been used with maximum effect in 5–7 days and duration of effect as long as 14–21 days. Side effects of conjugated estrogen include hot flashes [4–6].

Antifibrinolytic agents such as aminocaproic acid and tranexamic acid have been used for tooth extractions and minor oral surgery. However, systemic dosing of aminocaproic acid has been known to cause thrombosis in the glomerular capillaries of the renal pelvis and ureters of patients with upper urinary tract bleeding. Therefore, it is recommended not to treat hematuria in patients with upper urinary tract bleeding with aminocaproic acid [6].

Cryoprecipitate has been used in cases of nonresponsiveness to DDAVP in patients who are actively bleeding [5]. Cryoprecipitate is rich in factor VIII, vWF, fibrinogen, fibronectin, and factor XIII, begins to work within the hour, and has a duration of 18–24 hours [4,6]. Severe reactions to cryoprecipitate include rarely anaphylaxis, pulmonary edema, and intravascular hemolysis and the possible risk of post-transfusion hepatitis, HIV, fever, and allergic reactions [6].

Renal vein thrombosis

Clinical presentation

Renal vein occlusion caused by thrombosis was first described by Rayer in 1840 [8–10]. Patients may have an acute or gradual clinical presentation. Patients who develop an acute main renal vein thrombosis present with sudden onset of flank pain and tenderness to percussion, pleuritic chest pain, macroscopic hematuria, unilateral radiographic abnormalities by intravenous pyelogram, and worsening renal function. Patients with nephrotic syndrome may present with no symptoms except peripheral edema [11]. Neonates and infants more often have an acute presentation and are found to have abdominal distension, a flank mass from increase in kidney size, hematuria, and proteinuria and may also present with bilateral renal vein thrombosis. Neonates and infants are often diagnosed in the setting of severe dehydration and present with dry mouth, decreased urine output, and decreased skin turgidity. In cases of gradual onset, patients may have no symptoms or nonspecific chronic complaints of nausea, apathy, weakness, and generalized edema and may have symptoms of upper abdominal or flank pain [11].

Etiology

In adults, renal vessel occlusion is usually from vein thrombosis [8]. Renal vein thrombosis is a complication of nephrotic syndrome and has been found in patients with primary glomerular diseases, such as membranous glomerulopathy, minimal change disease, membranoproliferative glomerulonephritis, focal glomerulosclerosis, and rapidly progressive glomerulonephritis, and in other diseases with nephrosis, such as lupus erythematosus, diabetes mellitus, primary amyloidosis, familial Mediterranean fever with amyloidosis, sickle cell disease, sarcoidosis, and vasculiltis. Various studies have reported the incidence of renal vein thrombosis in nephrotic syndrome ranging from 5% to 62% with a high incidence among patients with membranous glomerulopathy with reports of 50–60% of patients evaluated [8,9,11].

Renal vein thrombosis is more common in primary glomerular disease but also occurs in other renal diseases, such as acute pyelonephritis, lupus nephritis, or amyloidosis in the setting of nephrotic syndrome. Other mechanisms associated with renal vein thrombosis include the following:
• thrombosis of the inferior vena cava with secondary renal vein involvement;
• direct extension of tumor into the lumen of the renal veins causing occlusion with thrombosis proximal to the tumor;
• alteration in renal blood flow (i.e. volume loss, diarrhea, sepsis, adrenal hemorrhage, hypoglycemia,

seizure disorders or hypoxia in cyanotic congenital heart disease, tricuspid insufficiency, constrictive pericarditis);
• systemic diseases with hypercoagulable states, such as sickle cell disease, primary antiphospholipid syndrome, advanced malignancy; and
• surgically induced renal vein occlusion with thrombosis beyond the ligature [8].

Diagnosis, treatment, and prognosis

In cases of acute onset with complete occlusion, kidney size increases within the first week with subsequent decrease in size over a couple of weeks and later renal atrophy. In the early phase, therefore, an ultrasound will show an enlarged kidney and hyperechogenic kidney in about 90% of cases [12]. Color Doppler ultrasound improves the ability to detect flow in the renal artery and the renal vein and has a high degree of sensitivity in detecting renal vein thrombosis in post-renal transplant patients. In chronic renal vein thrombosis, renal venous occlusion causes the development of varicosities, which shows a notching appearance in the ureter and collateral venous drainage around the kidney by intravenous urography [12].

The imaging method of choice is CT [12]. Screening with spiral CT has a sensitivity and specificity for covert renal vein thrombosis of 90–100% compared with the gold standard of renal venous angiography [10]. CT also has the advantage of detecting renal tumors and other renal diseases [12]. Doppler ultrasonography has high false-positive and false-negative rates for renal vein thrombosis (40% and 15%, respectively) [10].

Magnetic resonance angiography (MRA) has the advantage of avoiding nephrotoxic intravenous contrast agents. MRA is better at showing anatomic variants, vessel displacement, collateral circulation, and neoplastic vessel infiltration [10].

Treatment consists of correcting the underlying problem when due to secondary reasons for decreased renal blood flow. Dialysis may be needed in causes of renal failure from renal vein thrombosis [8]. The mortality rate can be high, and often patients with renal vein thrombosis are at risk of death from other thromboembolic events, such as pulmonary emboli. For patients with nephrotic syndrome and renal vein thrombosis, chronic anticoagulation therapy is warranted to prevent further extension of the thrombus and to prevent other thromboembolic events [9–11].

Thrombolytic agents have been given; however, this has been associated with high frequency of death due to bleeding complications [9]. Surgical thrombectomy has also been tried but is only rarely indicated for patients not responding to medical therapy [9]. Percutaneous mechanical thrombectomy has also been used with success [9].

Outcomes in a retrospective study from the Mayo Clinic from 1980 to 2000 found a high incidence of underlying renal malignancy (66%) and nephritic syndrome (20%) as the most common causes of renal vein thrombosis. In this cohort, the overall survival was poor with predictors of mortality including cancer and infection [13]. In patients with untreated renal vein thrombosis, the incidence of pulmonary embolus has been found to range from 20% to 40% [15].

In a retrospective review of neonatal renal vein thrombosis from 1992 to 2006, 70.6% of neonates, regardless of the treatment [about 40% with unfractionated heparin (UFH)/low-molecular-weight heparin (LMWH) and about 40% with supportive treatment] received, had irreversible damage. In this study, the mortality rate was observed to be 3.3% [14]. It is reported that approximately 20% of neonates may develop persistent hypertension and about 3% may need chronic dialysis or kidney transplantation [14].

Nephrotic syndrome/hypercoagulability

Incidence and prevalence of thromboembolic events

Addis in 1948 noted the frequent occurrence of thromboembolic events in patients with nephrotic syndrome. The increase in incidence that clinicians have noted since described by Addis could in part be due to longer survival of patients with improvements in care, especially with the introduction of antibiotics [11].

Certain renal diseases are associated with thrombophilia, notably primary and secondary nephrotic syndrome, systemic lupus erythematosus with lupus anticoagulant, granulamatous vasculitis (Wegener's granulomatosis), and Behçet syndrome. Consistently associated with thromboembolic events are membranous nephropathy (primary and secondary), membranoproliferative glomerulonephritis, minimal change disease, and possible amyloidosis [10].

Thromboembolic complications are one of the most serious outcomes for patients with nephrotic syndrome. Sites involved include pulmonary arteries, axillary and subclavian veins, femoral veins, coronary arteries, and mesenteric arteries. The most common presentation is for deep vein thrombosis (DVT) of the extremities [11]. Various studies have found that the prevalence for thromboembolic events other than renal vein thrombosis ranges from 8.5% to 44% [11]. About 15% of patients with nephrotic syndrome are reported to develop DVT, with or without renal vein thrombosis. Renal vein thrombosis, unilateral or bilateral, has been reported to develop in about 25–30% of patients with nephrotic syndrome from primary renal disease. The highest risks are reported with membranous glomerulonephritis at 37%, membranoproliferative glomeruonephritis at 26%, and minimal change disease at 24% [10]. The combined rates of DVT and renal vein thrombosis in patients with membranous nephropathy have been reported to be as high as 45% [10]. Others have reported that 40% of patients with membranous nephropathy and serum albumin <2.5g/dL had venous thromboembolism versus only 2.7% of patients with albumin >2.5g/dL [10]. The prevalence of thromboembolic events in children with nephrotic syndrome has been reported to range from 2% to 25% [16]. In patients older than 60 years with membranous nephropathy, it was found that the majority of deaths were caused by thromboembolic events [17].

Etiology

The thrombophilia associated in patients with nephrotic syndrome may be mulifactorial. Environmental risk shared by patients with medical illnesses include immobilization, obesity, need for surgeries and procedures, and co-morbidity such as congestive heart failure. Environmental factors that may be more specific for patients with nephrotic syndrome include volume depletion and the use of diuretic and/or steroid therapy [10].

The hypercoagulability state observed in patients with nephrotic syndrome may also be multifactorial [17,18] and include:

- increased levels of clotting factors,
- decreased levels of anticoagulant proteins,
- increased platelet activity,
- increase in vWF, and
- abnormal finbrinolysis.

Prothrombotic factors have been reported to include increased fibrinogen levels, factor VIII levels, and platelet adhesiveness; whereas, the antithrombotic factors that have been found to be decreased include antithrombin levels and proteins C and S activity. It has been reported that decreased plasminogen levels, elevated plasminogen activator inhibitor levels, or albumin deficiency-related impairment of the interaction of plasminogen–fibrin may account for the impaired thrombolytic activity [10]. Also reports of increases in platelet count and aggregation to ADP and collagen and increased β-thromboglobulin levels, a marker for platelet aggregation, have been noted [11]. Hypoalbuminemia may play a role in increasing free arachidonic acid and subsequent increase in thromboxane [18]. LDL cholesterol, which is usually elevated in patients with nephrotic syndrome, is toxic to the endothelium, which leads to impaired NO production and may increase platelet–vessel wall interactions [18]. Most likely, an increase in thrombin activity accelerates fibrinogen-induced fibrin formation and contributes to the thrombotic risk. This in part may be due to increases in clotting factors V and VIII and decreases in the inhibition of the coagulation cascade due to decreased levels of proteins C and S and antithrombin [18]. Antithrombin may be one of the most important coagulation inhibitors and inhibits activated factors XII, IX, X, and XI and plasmin. Antithrombin increases after steroid therapy [11]. Also, decreased fibrinolytic activity may be due to several mechanisms:

- increased α2-antiplasmin;
- decreased albumin may lead to decreased binding of plasminogen to fibrin; and
- elevated Lp (a) competes for the binding to fibrinogen or fibrin [18].

More specific to patients with membranous nephropathy is the association of anti-enolase autoantibodies. These autoantibodies may interfere with fibrinolysis [10].

Treatment

Treatment for thromboembolic events in patients with nephrotic syndrome is anticoagulation for the duration of the nephrotic state [10]. Given the high incidence of thromboembolic events in patients with nephrotic syndrome and membranous glomerulopathy, Bellomo and Atkins have recommended prophylactic anticoagulation [19].

Graft loss due to thromobosis/thrombophilias

Incidence and clinical presentation of thromboembolic events

Renovascular thrombosis was found to be the cause of graft loss posttransplant in approximately 8% of recipients, with thrombosis accounting for 25% of graft loss in <1 year posttransplant, as reported by Matas and colleagues [20]. Bakir and colleagues found thrombosis to be the cause of graft loss in 45% of recipients in <90 days posttransplant and 37% in <1 year [21]. Thrombosis of the renal vein graft is more common, causes pain and swelling of the graft, and can frequently lead to allograft rupture [20,21]. Thrombosis of the renal artery does not cause pain, swelling, or rupture. Also, thrombosis of both renal vein and artery can occur at the same time.

Etiology

Proposed mechanisms for renovascular thrombosis have included problems associated with the surgical procedure such as donor vessel abnormalities, including difference in diameter of vessels, multiple renal arteries, stenosis of the renal artery of the donor, atherosclerosis of the donor or recipient vessel, excessive surgical trauma of the vessels due to repeated re-anastomosis, lymphocele posttransplant, and prolonged ischemia with resulting reperfusion damage [21]. However, these technical problems or concerns for immunosuppressive drugs have not been able to explain the often unexpected graft thrombosis spurring the interest in thromphilia, inherited or acquired, as possible risk factors for renovascular thrombosis and subsequent graft loss [20,21].

Posttransplantation, the coagulation system is activated due to tissue trauma causing inflammation and expression of tissue factor, and fibrinolysis may be impaired due to overexpression of plasminogen activator inhibitor-I in the endothelium [20,21]. Inherited thrombophilia has been associated with allograft thrombosis. Irish reported a 6% prevalence of Factor V Leiden in 300 transplant recipients who had a four-fold increase in allograft thrombosis, which represented 20% of graft loss in this cohort [22]. One study found that the presence of prothrombin gene G20210A polymorphism was associated with a shorter median allograft survival of 65.9 months versus 149 months. Acquired thrombophilias have also been associated with allograft thrombosis. Another study evaluated 502 patients, of which 11 of 23 identified with antiphospholipid antibody syndrome underwent transplant. Of the 11 patients, 7 who did not receive anticoagulation had a graft thrombosis within 1 week, whereas 3 of the 4 patients who received anticoagulation maintained long-term graft function [19,22,23]. Allograft recipients with SLE and antiphospholipid antibodies were found to have a 40% risk of thrombosis, graft loss, or death caused by thromboembolism versus 8% of SLE patients without antiphospholipid antibodies [23].

Diagnosis and prevention

The diagnosis of allograft thrombosis can be made by performing angiography or by histology [21]. Color Doppler ultrasonography has become a standard procedure for evaluating renal allografts and can reliably detect complete allograft vein thrombosis if the pathognomonic reversed diastolic flow exists in the arteries [24]. Whether or not patients should be screened prior to transplant has been debated. Some have advocated thrombophilia screening for high-risk patients, such as patients with personal or family history of thrombosis and in children and adolescents who appear to be at higher risk of allograft thrombosis [19,21].

Using anticoagulation at prophylactic or treatment dosing to decrease allograft thrombosis needs to be weighed against the risk of bleeding. One study used dalteparin 2500 U daily just during the period of hospitalization for low-risk patients and dalteparin 5000 U daily for at least 1 month for high-risk patients. In 120 allograft recipients, the high-risk group included patients with hypercoagulable state (15%) or grafts with multiple vessels (31%) [25]. There were no reports of allograft thrombosis or major hemorrhagic

events; however, there was also no control group for comparison.

Dose adjustment of anticoagulants in renal insufficiency

Anticoagulants

As discussed in the previous sections, patients with renal disease may have problems with bleeding as well as thrombosis. Additionally, most of the anticoagulants that are used in practice are excreted by the kidneys. Therefore treating patients with anticoagulants offers a greater challenge with dosing and requires closer monitoring for signs of bleeding.

UFH is principally metabolized by the reticulendothelial system with approximately <10% excreted in the urine unchanged and, for this reason, is the anticoagulant of choice for patients with severe renal impairment. However, Thorevska and coworkers performed a retrospective cohort study which concluded that full-dose enoxaparin and UFH had similar major hemorrhagic events in patients with renal insufficiency [26]. In their cohort of 620 patients, there were a total of 149 hemorrhagic events of which 60 were major hemorrhages. Of interest is the timing of the hemorrhagic events between enoxaparin and UFH. A higher percentage of major hemorrhagic events in the enoxaparin group occurred after 3 days of therapy, whereas approximately half of the major hemorrhagic events in the UFH group occurred within the first 3 days of therapy. Also of interest is that patients with severe renal insufficiency (GFR ≤20 mL/min) had 20% more major hemorrhagic events and 150% more minor hemorrhagic events in the enoxaparin group. Although the increase in major hemorrhagic events in the enoxaparin group was not statistically significant, the number of patients receiving clopidrogel or glycoprotein IIB/IIIA drugs was statistically higher in the group receiving UFH and therefore there may have been a bias toward using UFH in patients who were more at risk of bleeding.

Guidelines for mild to moderate renal insufficiency

For the LMWHs, including enoxaparin, dalteparin, and tinzaparin, there are no dosage adjustments given for mild renal insufficiency (CL$_{cr}$ of 50–80 mL/min) and moderate renal insufficiency (CL_{cr} of 30–50 mL/min) [27]. For enoxaparin, it has been reported that the clearance is reduced by 30% in patients with moderate renal insufficiency. Because of concern for drug accumulation, it may be advisable to reduce the dose and perhaps follow anti-factor Xa levels to help guide therapy in patients with moderate renal insufficiency. Data are even more limited for dalteparin and tinzaparin. Also, for the factor Xa inhibitor fondaparinux, there are no dosage adjustments given for mild and moderate renal insufficiency. Therefore, patients need to be monitored closely for any signs of hemorrhage and consideration of following anti-factor Xa levels, especially if therapy is anticipated to be prolonged.

In the direct thrombin inhibitor (DTI) class of agents, only argatroban can be used without dosage adjustments for renal insufficiency. For acute coronary syndrome (ACS) patients undergoing percutaneous intervention, bivalirudin is not dose-reduced. However, for use in patients with heparin-induced thrombocytopenia (HIT), we would recommend reducing the dose from 0.15 mg/kg/hour to 0.05 mg/kg/hour. Patients should be monitored closely with checking activated partial thromboplastin time (APTT) 2–3 hours after initiation of drug and after dosage changes. For lepirudin, the manufacturer recommends dosage reduction for patients with CL_{cr} <60. For CL_{cr} between 30 mL/minute and 60 mL/minute, a reduced bolus dose of 0.2 mg/kg is recommended. For Cl_{cr} 45–60 mL/minute, the infusion rate should be reduced to 0.075 mg/kg/hour, and for Cl_{cr} 30–44 mL/minute, the infusion rate should be reduced to 0.045 mg/kg/hour. Others have advocated even lower doses of lepirudin infusion as follows: (1) normal renal function, 0.1 mg/kg/hour; (2) CL_{cr} 45–60 mL/minute, 0.05 mg/kg/hour; and (3) CL_{cr} 30–44 mL/minute, 0.03 mg/kg/hour [27]. When treating HIT with thrombosis a bolus dose is usually given; however, for isolated HIT, a bolus dose is not recommended. Also, some clinicians will not use a bolus dose in elderly patients and in patients with renal insufficiency. It is also recommended to monitor APTT 4 hours after initiating the infusion and after any dosage changes.

Guidelines for severe renal insufficiency

For severe renal insufficiency, defined as a Cl_{cr} <30 mL/minute, dose reductions are recommended for LMWHs. For DVT prophylaxis, enoxaparin is reduced to 30 mg once daily for the following: abdominal surgery, hip replacement, knee replacement, and in medical patients. For DVT treatment, enoxaparin is reduced to 1 mg/kg once daily. For dalteparin, the manufacturing guidelines only comment that, for cancer patients being treated for a venous thromboembolic event, anti-Xa levels should be monitored and the dose adjusted accordingly. For tinzaparin, there is a 24% decrease in clearance, and therefore it should be used with caution. Fondaparinux is contraindicated for patients with severe renal insufficiency.

As for mild and moderate renal insufficiency, argatroban is the only DTI that does not require a dose adjustment. For ACS patients undergoing percutaneous intervention, bivalirudin should be reduced to 1 mg/kg/hour. For dialysis-dependent patients on nondialysis days, the dose should be reduced to 0.25 mg/kg/hour. For use in patients with HIT, we would recommend reducing the dose to 0.03 mg/kg/hour. Patients should be monitored closely with checking APTT 2–3 hours after initiation of drug and after dosage changes. For lepirudin, the manufacturer recommends reducing the bolus dose to 0.2 mg/kg and to reduce the infusion rate to 0.0225 mg/kg/hour for Cl_{cr} 15–29 mL/minute and to not use lepirudin for Cl_{cr} <15 mL/minute. It is also recommended to monitor APTT after 4 hours of initiating the infusion and after any dosage changes.

Acknowledgment

Grant support: NIH K23-HL084233 (SLP); CDC UO1-DD000014 (TLO); NIH UO1-HL072289 (TLO); NIH U54-HL077878 (TLO).

References

1 Sohal AS, Gangji AS, Crowther MA, Treleavan D. Uremic bleeding: pathophysiology and clinical risk factors. *Thromb Res* 2006;118:417–22.

2 Salmaon S. Uremic bleeding: pathophysiology, diagnosis, and management. *Hosp Physician* 2001;76:45–50.

3 Hedges SJ, Dehoney SB, Hooper JS, Amanzadeh J, Busti AJ. Evidence-based treatment recommendations

for uremic bleeding. *Nat Clin Pract Nephrol* 2007;3: 138–53.

4 Kaw D, Malhaotra D. Platelet dysfunction and end-stage renal disease. *Semin Dial* 2006;19:317–22.

5 Noris M, Remuzzi G. Uremic bleeding: closing the circle after 30 years of controversies? *Blood* 1999;94:2569–74.

6 Gangji AS, Sohal AS, Treleaven D, Crowther MA. Bleeding in patients with renal insufficiency: a practical guide to clinical management. *Thromb Res* 2006;118:423–8.

7 Phrommintikul A, Haas SJ, Elsik M, Krum H. Mortality and target haemoglobin concentrations in anaemic patients with chronic kidney disease treated with erythropoietin: a meta-analysis. *Lancet* 2007;369:381–8.

8 Witz M, Kantarovsky A, Morag B, Shifrin EG. Renal vein occlusion: a review. *J Urol* 1996;155:1173–9.

9 Jaar BG, Kim HS, Samaniego, Lund GB, Atta MG. Percutaneous mechanical thrombectomy: a new approach in the treatment of acute renal-vein thrombosis. *Nephrol Dial Transplant* 2002;17:1122–5.

10 Wagoner RD, Stanson AW, Holley KE, Winter CS. Renal vein thrombosis in idiopathic membranous glomerulpathy and nephrotic syndrome: incidence and significance. *Kidney Int* 1983;23:368–74.

11 Llach F. Hypercoagulability, renal vein thrombosis, and other thrombotic complications of nephrotic syndrome. *Kidney Int* 1985;28:429–39.

12 Asgher M, Ahmed K, Shah SS, Siddique MK, Dasgupta P, Khan MS. Renal vein thrombosis. *Eur J Vasc Endovasc Surg* 2007;34:217–23.

13 Wysokinski WE, Gosk-Bierska I, Greene EL, Grill D, Wiste H, McBane RD. Clinical characteristics and long-term follow-up of patients with renal vein thrombosis. *Am J Kidney Dis* 2008;51:224–32.

14 Lau KK, Stoffman JM, Williams S, et al. Neonatal renal vein thrombosis: review of the English-language literature between 1992 and 2006. *Pediatrics* 2007;120:e1278–84.

15 Glassock RJ. Prophylactic anticoagulation in nephrotic syndrome: a clinical conundrum. *J Am Soc Nephrol* 2007;18:2221–5.

16 Fabri D, Belangero MS, Annichino-Bizzacchi JM, Arruda VR. Inherited risk factors for thombophilia in children with nephrotic syndrome. *Eur J Pediatr* 1998;157: 939–42.

17 O'Callaghan CA, Hicks J, Doll H, Sacks SH, Cameron JS. Characteristics and outcome of membranous nephropathy in older patients. *Int Urol Nephrol* 2002;33: 157–65.

18 Rabelink TJ, Zwaninga JJ, Koomans HA, Sixma JJ. Thrombosis and hemostasis in renal disease. *Kidney Int* 1994;46:287–96.

19 Bellomo R, Atkins RC. Membranous nephropathy and thromboembolism: is prophylactic anticoagulation warranted? *Nephron* 1993;63:249–54.

20 Matas AJ, Humar A, Gillingham KJ, et al. Five preventable cause of kidney graft loss in the 1990s: a single-center analysis. *Kidney Int* 2002;62:704–14.

21 Bakir N, Sluiter WJ, Ploeg RJ, van Son WJ, Tegzess AM. Primary renal graft thrombosis. *Nephrol Dial Transplant* 1996;11:140–7.

22 Irish A. Renal allograft thrombosis: can thrombophilia explain the inexplicable? *Nephrol Dial Transplant* 1999;14:2297–303.

23 Andrassy J, Zeier M, Anrassy K. Do we need screening for thrombophilia prior to kidney transplantation? *Nephrol Dial Transplant* 2004;19;iv64–8.

24 Schwenger V, Hinkel UP, Nahm A, Morath C, Zeier M. Color doppler ultrasonography in the diagnostic evaluation of renal allografts. *Nephron Clin Pract* 2006;104:c107–12.

25 Alkunaizi AM, Olyaei AJ, Barry JM, et al. Efficacy and safety of low molecular weight heparin in renal transplantation. *Transplantation* 1998;66:533–4.

26 Thorevska N, Amoateng-Adjepong Y, Sabahi R, et al. Anticoagulation in hospitalized patients with renal insufficiency: a comparison of bleeding rates with unfractionated heparin vs enoxaparin. *Chest* 2004;125:856–63.

27 Lobo BL. Use of newer anticoagulants in patients with chronic kidney disease. *Am J Health-Syst Pharm* 2007;64: 2017–6.

23 Oncology

Anna Falanga and Marina Marchetti

Introduction

The association between cancer and thrombosis has been known for more than a century. The occurrence of venous thromboembolism is a common complication of cancer. It can also precede the onset of an occult neoplasia, as first reported by Armand Trousseau in 1865. Almost at the same time, the possibility that a relation between the clotting mechanisms and the development of metastasis may occur was postulated by Billroth in 1878.

In the last three decades, remarkable progress has been made in this field, both by basic research and clinical studies. It is now clear that there is a two-way connection between coagulation and cancer [1]:
• malignant disease results in a prothrombotic imbalance of the host hemostatic system; and
• prothrombotic mechanisms may promote tumor growth and dissemination.

Recently, molecular studies have demonstrated that oncogenes responsible for neoplastic transformation also drive programs for hemostatic protein expression and clotting system activation [2–4]. Specifically,
• Targeting activated human mesenchymal–epithelial transition factor (MET) to the mouse liver with lentiviral vector determined progressive hepatocarcinogenesis, which is preceded and accompanied by a thrombohemorrhagic syndrome (i.e. venous thrombosis in tail vein and fatal internal hemorrhage) and laboratory signs of disseminated intravascular coagulation (DIC). Genome-wide expression profiling of hepatocytes expressing MET showed up-regulation of PAI-1 and COX-2 genes with a two- to three-fold increase in circulating protein levels [2].
• In an in vitro model of human glioma cells, the loss of the tumor suppressor gene *PTEN* up-regulated the expression of tissue factor (TF) and increased the levels of plasma clotting proteins [3].
• In a model of human colorectal cancer cells, TF expression was shown to be under the control of two major transforming events driving disease progression: the activation of *K-ras* oncogene and the inactivation of the *p*53 tumor suppressor [4].

Patients with cancer are exposed to a significant risk of thrombosis [5]. This situation is aggravated by antitumor therapies [6]. Data derived from large, randomized, controlled trials have been used to determine the true incidence of this complication and to define the major risk factors for thrombosis in cancer [7].

Very commonly, cancer patients present with abnormalities of laboratory tests of blood coagulation, even without clinical manifestations of thromboembolism and/or hemorrhage. These abnormalities reveal different degrees of blood clotting activation and characterize the hypercoagulable state of these subjects [8]. The results of laboratory tests in these patients demonstrate that a process of fibrin formation and removal is continuously ongoing during the development of malignancy.

The pathogenesis of thrombophilia in cancer is multifactorial; however, an important role is attributed to the tumor cell capacity to interact with and activate the host hemostatic system. Among other factors that contribute to the increased thrombotic diathesis in patients with cancer are the antitumor therapies.

Experimental studies show that fibrin and other coagulation proteins are involved in multiple steps of tumor growth and dissemination. Therefore, pharmacological interventions to prevent thrombotic phenomena in malignancy may possibly contribute to the control of the malignant disease progression.

The aim of this chapter is to summarize the most recent advances in our knowledge on the thrombophilic

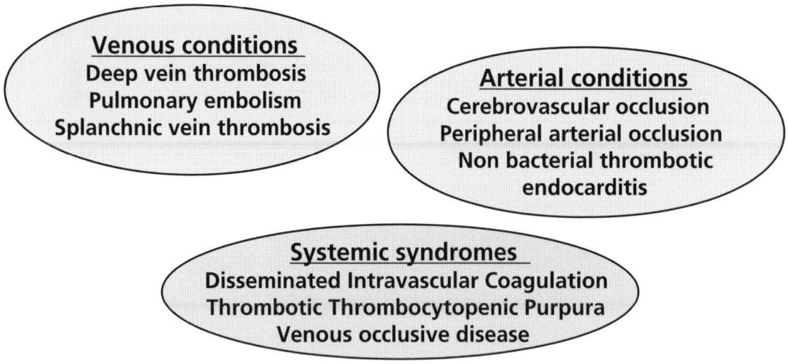

Figure 23.1 Thrombotic disorders associated with cancer. Clinical manifestations of thrombosis in patients with cancer can vary from localized DVT, more frequent in solid tumors, to systemic syndrome, such as DIC with consumption of coagulation factors and platelets, which is generally associated with leukemias or widespread metastatic cancer.

state of cancer patients and the pathophysiological mechanisms of blood clotting activation in this condition, giving also an overview of the current approaches to the prevention and treatment of venous thromboembolism (VTE) in cancer.

Clinical aspects

Although clinical manifestations of thrombosis in patients with cancer can involve both the venous and arterial systems (Plate 23.1), the thrombotic occlusions of the venous site have been more extensively studied (Fig. 23.1).

• VTE represents an important cause of morbidity and mortality in these patients [9].

• Epidemiological data clearly show that patients with cancer have a significantly increased risk of having clinical overt thrombosis (secondary deep vein thrombosis, DVT) upon triggering conditions (e.g. long-term bed rest, trauma, surgery), as compared with patients without malignancy.

• Medical treatments to cure cancer can worsen the patient's thrombophilic state and increase the thrombotic risk associated with this disease.

Recently, our understanding of the epidemiology of VTE in cancer has improved with the advent of large population-based studies and data from prospective series describing outcome with regard to VTE.

• DVT of the lower limbs is the most common clinical manifestation in these patients.

• The next most common manifestations are DVT of upper limbs, pulmonary embolism, central sinus thrombosis, and migratory superficial thrombophlebitis.

• Syndromes of more systemic involvement of the clotting system, such as DIC or thrombotic microangiopathy, have been described mainly in acute leukemia [10].

Occult malignancy

Thrombosis may be the earliest clinical manifestation of an occult malignancy. Initially, this observation was shown by anecdotal reports and retrospective clinical studies, but in more recent years, this concept has become well documented. Particularly important is the trial of Prandoni and coworkers [11], which evaluated the occurrence of cancer after a first episode of VTE among 250 patients without cancer at diagnosis. This study clearly showed that patients with an "idiopathic" VTE episode have a four- to seven-fold increased risk of being diagnosed with cancer in the first year after thrombosis when compared with patients with VTE secondary to known causes (e.g. surgery, congenital thrombophilia, oral contraceptives, pregnancy, and immobilization). In the case of recurrent VTE, this risk is further raised by up to ten-fold. A recent large population-based study has identified the type of cancers most commonly preceded by VTE in the year before diagnosis [12].

In spite of this evidence, the question as to whether aggressive diagnostic screening for cancer in patients with idiopathic DVT may lead to improved management of the malignant disease is still unanswered.

In the prospective Italian multicenter study, "Screening for Occult Malignancy in patients with venous Thromboembolism" (SOMIT), extensive screening was found to be effective in identifying precociously an occult malignancy [13]. Computerized tomography (CT) scanning of the abdomen and pelvis was the most effective diagnostic test, and CT scan and a gastro-intestinal investigation (such as hemoccult) was the best diagnostic combination. Based on the data from the SOMIT study, an analysis of costs of different screening strategies (in relation to the expected live years gained with each of them) shows that some of these strategies may be cost-effective. Finally, a prospective cohort follow-up study of 864 consecutive patients with acute VTE [14] suggests that a limited diagnostic workup (i.e. abdominal and pelvic ultrasound and laboratory markers for malignancy) may have the capacity to identify approximately one-half of the malignancies present in patients who were negative on routine clinical evaluation. In most of the cases, the malignancies identified by extensive screening are in an early stage; therefore, larger clinical trials to establish the impact of this finding on cancer prognosis are warranted.

The hypercoagulable state of malignancy

Even without thrombosis and before any therapy, patients with cancer present with multiple laboratory abnormalities of hemostasis showing a hypercoagulable condition [8].

Routine laboratory tests

Coagulation profiles performed in the past have revealed that the most frequent routine abnormalities reported are:
• Elevated levels of plasma coagulation factor (i.e. fibrinogen, factors V, VIII, IX, and X);
• Increased plasma levels of fibrin(ogen) degradation products (FDP or D-dimers); and
• Thrombocytosis.
  In two large prospective clinical trials evaluating routine coagulation tests in cancer patients:
• FDP levels and thrombin times were increased only in 8% and 14% of cases, respectively;
• Fibrinogen and platelet count were found more frequently elevated (48% and 36% of the cases, respectively);

• The increase in the levels of these two markers over time directly correlated with the disease progression; and
• Activation of the clotting system occurs in the absence of DIC or manifest thrombosis.

Specialized tests

Recently, the development of novel, more sensitive laboratory tests for the detection of the hypercoagulable state or subclinical DIC (which are listed in Table 23.1) has enabled the detection of ongoing activation of blood coagulation in vivo. These tests measure the final products of clotting reactions in plasma and include:
• Peptides released during the proteolytic activation of pro-enzymes into active clotting enzymes, i.e.:
  ○ prothrombin fragment 1 + 2 [F1+2],
  ○ protein C activation fragment,
  ○ factor IX and X activation fragments, and
  ○ fibrinopeptide A.
• Enzyme–inhibitor complexes produced during the activation of the coagulation and fibrinolytic systems, i.e.:
  ○ thrombin–antithrombin complexes [TAT] and
  ○ plasmin–antiplasmin complexes [PAP].
• Cross-linked fibrin degradation product, i.e.:
  ○ D-dimer.
• Cell membrane-associated markers to study the activation of cellular components of the hemostatic system, including platelets and leukocytes, i.e.:
  ○ P-selectin (or CD62P), and CD63 on platelet surface, and
  ○ Mac1 (or CD11b) and leukocyte alkaline phosphatase (LAP) on leukocyte surface.

Predictors of thrombosis
Studies on the plasma levels of these markers have provided a biochemical definition of the hypercoagulable state in humans. However, no studies of sound methodological design have been performed to indicate whether any of these tests of blood coagulation can serve as an adequate predictor of thrombosis in cancer patients. No studies have prospectively compared, in the same subjects, the levels of the plasma markers with the thrombotic events (confirmed by objective tests). Large studies are still required to answer

Table 23.1 Circulating markers of hemostatic system activation.

Coagulation
- Activated factor VII (FVIIa)
- Thrombin–antithrombin complex (TAT)
- Prothrombin fragment 1+2 (F1+2)
- Fibrinopeptide A and B

Fibrinolysis
- Tissue plasminogen activator (t-PA)
- Plasminogen activator inhibitor-1 (PAI-1)
- Plasminogen
- Plasmin–antiplasmin complex (PAP)
- Fibrin degradation products (FDPs)
- Soluble fibrin
- D-Dimer

Platelets
- β-Thromboglobulin
- Platelet factor 4 (PF4)
- Thromboxane A2 (TxA2)
- soluble P-selectin
- Membrane P-selectin, CD63

Leukocytes
- *Monocytes*
  - membrane tissue factor
  - soluble tissue factor
- *Neutrophils*
  - membrane CD11b
  - elastase
  - myeloperoxidase

Endothelium
- Thrombomodulin
- von Willebrand Factor (vWF)
- t-PA
- PAI-1
- s-E-Selectin
- s-VCAM-1 and s-ICAM-1
- Tissue factor pathway inhibitor (TFPI)

the question as to whether the measurement of any of these laboratory markers may be useful in assessing the risk level in the individual patient.

Predictors of survival

A number of studies have been conducted with the aim of defining the prognostic significance of some

thrombotic markers in patients with cancer [8]. The principal results of these studies have demonstrated a significant predictive value for shorter survival of high plasma levels of:

- TAT, fibrin monomer, and D-dimer, in patients with various different types of cancer;
- TAT and PAP, in a cohort of subjects with lung cancer;
- presurgical PAP, in patients operated for esophageal carcinoma; and
- presurgical D-dimer, in patients operated for colorectal cancer.

In contrast, plasma s-uPAR and other fibrinolytic parameters had no significant prognostic value in studies of breast cancer or gastric cancer patients.

Interestingly, a study of 3052 healthy men from the UK National Health Service Central Registry investigated whether the presence of a persistent hypercoagulable state may be predictive of death from cancer. The results found that healthy subjects with persistent hypercoagulability (defined as persistently elevated F1+2 and FPA levels) indeed have a significant risk of dying from cancer, particularly of the gastrointestinal tract, compared with subjects without persistent hypercoagulability [15].

Pathogenetic mechanisms

The activation of blood coagulation and thrombotic diathesis in patients with cancer is a complex and multifactorial phenomenon, which reflects the participation of different mechanisms [1,8].

General mechanisms related to the host response to the tumor include the acute-phase reaction, paraprotein production, inflammation, necrosis, and hemodynamic disorders, whereas tumor-specific clot promoting mechanisms include a series of prothrombotic properties expressed by tumor cells.

In addition, an important part in cancer-related thrombosis is played by the procoagulant effects triggered by anticancer therapies (Fig. 23.2).

Tumor cell prothrombotic mechanisms

There are several ways in which tumor cells can interact with and activate the hemostatic system [8].

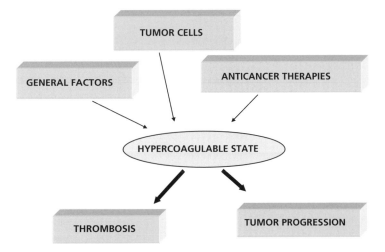

Figure 23.2 Mechanisms for activation of blood coagulation and thrombotic diathesis in patients with cancer. Even in the absence of overt clinical symptoms, almost all patients present with laboratory coagulation abnormalities, demonstrating a subclinical activation of blood coagulation, which characterizes a "hypercoagulable state." Multiple factors (i.e. general, tumor-specific, and antitumor therapy-related) concur to the activation of blood coagulation and to thrombotic manifestation in cancer patients.

The principal mechanisms can be summarized as follows:
- Production of tumor cell procoagulant activities, fibrinolytic proteins, and proinflammatory and proangiogenic cytokines.
- Direct interaction of tumor cell with host vascular and blood cells (i.e. endothelial cells, leukocytes, and platelets) by means of adhesion molecules. All these properties are listed in Table 23.2.

Procoagulant activities

Tumor cells may express different types of procoagulants, the best characterized of which are:
- Tissue factor (TF) and
- Cancer procoagulant (CP).

Table 23.2 Tumor cell prothrombotic properties.

– **Expression of procoagulants that directly activate coagulation:**
  - Tissue factor
  - Cancer procoagulant
– **Release of proinflammatory and proangiogenic cytokines that stimulate the prothrombotic potential of endothelial cells:**
  - IL-1β, TNF-α, VEGF, FGF
– **Expression of fibrinolyitc proteins**
  - t-PA, u-PA, PAI-1 and -2, uPAR
– **Expression of adhesion molecules for host vascular cells**
  - Integrins, selectins, immunoglobulin family

Other tumor cell procoagulant activities described are:
- Factor V receptor associated with vesicles shed from tumor cell plasma membranes, which facilitates the assembly of prothrombinase complex; and
- a Factor XIII-like activity that promotes the cross-linking of fibrin.

TF is a transmembrane glycoprotein that, in complex with factor VII (FVII)/FVIIa, triggers blood coagulation by proteolytically activating FIX and FX. TF is the procoagulant expressed by normal cells. Endothelial cells and monocyte–macrophages do not express TF in resting conditions, but expose this procoagulant in response to proinflammatory stimuli [i.e. interleukin 1β (IL-1β), tumor necrosis factor α (TNF-α), bacterial endotoxin]. TF expression by vascular cells induces intravascular thrombosis. Malignant cells are different in that they constitutively express TF in the absence of stimuli.

CP is a 68-kDa cysteine proteinase that, differently from TF, activates FX independently of FVII. CP has been found in extracts of neoplastic cells or in amnion–chorion tissues but not in extracts of normally differentiated cells. CP antigen has been found to be elevated in 85% of the sera of cancer patients. TF and CP have been identified in several human and animal tumor tissues. In recent years, a number of studies have characterized the procoagulant activities expressed by leukemic cells:
- Several authors have identified TF in leukemic cells.

- CP has been found in blasts of various acute myelogenous leukemia phenotypes, with the greatest expression in acute promyelocytic leukemia (APL) subtype.
- The differentiating treatment with all-*trans* retinoic acid (ATRA) of APL blasts in vitro reduces the expression of both TF and CP.
- In patients with APL, the remission induction with ATRA treatment induces the rapid resolution of the severe coagulopathy of this disease and significantly affects the procoagulant activities expressed by the bone marrow cells in vivo.
- Similar observations have been reported for breast cancer.

Recent studies suggest a new role for TF in the tumor growth and metastasis, which is not entirely mediated via clotting activation, but may be dependent on signaling through the cytoplasmic domain, suggesting a "non-coagulation" role for TF in cancer disease.

Fibrinolytic activities

Tumor cells can express all the proteins of the fibrinolytic system, including the urokinase-type (u-PA) and the tissue-type (t-PA) plasminogen activators, and their inhibitors, i.e. plasminogen activator inhibitor 1 and 2 (PAI-1 and PAI-2). Cancer cells also carry on their membranes the specific plasminogen activator receptor u-PAR, which favors the assembly of all the fibrinolytic components, facilitating the activation of the fibrinolytic cascade. It has been suggested that, in leukemia patients, the expression of these activities by blast cells may have a role in the pathogenesis of the bleeding symptoms. An impaired plasma fibrinolytic activity has been found in patients with solid tumors, which represents per se another tumor-associated prothrombotic mechanism.

Fibrinolysis is also a key component in tumor biology, as it is essential in releasing tumor cells from their primary site of origin, in neo-angiogenesis, and in promoting cell mobility and motility. Fibrinolytic proteins are under evaluation as potentially valuable predictors of disease-free interval and long-term survival in malignant disease. In breast cancer, patients with low levels of u-PA and PAI-1 have a significantly better survival than patients with high levels of either factor, particularly in node-negative breast cancer [16].

Cytokine activity

Down-regulation of anticoagulant activity
Tumor cells synthesize and release a variety of pro-inflammatory cytokines (i.e. TNF-α, IL-1β) and proangiogenic factors (VEGF, bFGF), which can act on the different hemostatic cells and affect their antithrombotic status.

These cytokines can induce the expression of TF procoagulant activity by endothelial cells and monocytes, and in parallel down-regulate the expression of thrombomodulin (TM), a potent anticoagulant, expressed by endothelial cells. The up-regulation of TF, together with the down-regulation of TM, leads to a prothrombotic condition of the vascular wall.

Increased fibrinolysis
The same cytokines stimulate endothelial cells to increase the production of the fibrinolysis inhibitor PAI-1, resulting in a subsequent inhibition of fibrinolysis, which further contributes to the prothrombotic state. Cytokines also contribute to enhance the adhesion potential of the vascular wall, by increasing the expression of cell adhesion molecules of endothelial cells, which become more capable to attract tumor cells and support their extravasation.

Procoagulant properties
Further, tumor cells and/or tumor cell cytokines can induce the expression of monocyte TF. Monocyte activation has been described to occur both in vitro and in vivo. Indeed, tumor-associated macrophages harvested from experimental and human tumors express significantly more TF than control cells. In addition, circulating monocytes from patient with different types of cancer have been shown to express increased TF activity. The generation of procoagulant activity by monocyte–macrophages in vivo is conceivably one mechanism for clotting activation in malignancy.

Recruitment of white cells
The cytokines and chemokines produced by malignant cells are also mitogenic and/or chemoattractants for polymorphonuclear leukocytes. These cells, upon activation, secrete proteolytic enzymes, which

can damage the endothelial monolayer, and produce additional cytokines and chemokines, which support tumor growth, stimulate angiogenesis, and enable metastatic spread via engagement with either venous or lymphatic networks. They also synthetize VEGF which is chemotactic for macrophages and can induce TF procoagulant activity by monocytes and endothelial cells.

Cell adhesion molecules

During the hematogenous spread, tumor cells directly interact with endothelial cells, platelets, and leukocytes. These interactions occur through surface cell-adhesion molecules (i.e. integrins, selectins, and immunoglobulin superfamily).

• The integrin family of cell-adhesion proteins promotes the attachment and migration of cells to the surrounding extracellular matrix (ECM). Through signals transduced upon integrin ligation by ECM proteins or immunoglobulin superfamily molecules, this family of proteins has key roles in regulating tumor growth and metastasis as well as tumor angiogenesis.

• Selectins are multifunctional cell-adhesion molecules that mediate the initial interactions between circulating leukocytes and activated endothelium as well as the adhesion of tumor cells during the metastatic process.

The tumor cell capacity to adhere to the endothelium and the underlying matrix is well described, and adhesion molecule pathways specific to different tumor cell types have been identified. The relevance of the tight interaction of tumor cells with endothelial cells in the pathogenesis of thrombosis in cancer is related to the localized promotion of clotting activation and thrombus formation. The tumor cell attached to endothelium can release its cytokine content into a protected milieu that favors their prothrombotic and proangiogenic activities. In addition, the adhesion of tumor cells to leukocytes or vascular cells represents the first step for cell migration and extravasation.

Experimental and in vitro studies have shown that polymorphonuclear leukocytes may function to promote tumor growth and metastasis. Tumor cell-derived factors can regulate the expression of various adhesion molecules (i.e. the β2-integrin CD11b/CD18) by leukocytes, which in turn attach to

tumor cells and facilitate tumor cell migration through the endothelium.

Platelets

Similarly to leukocytes, clinical and experimental evidence suggests the importance of platelets in tumor cell dissemination via the bloodstream. Platelets can facilitate tumor cell adhesion and migration through the vessel wall by a variety of mechanisms, including bridging between tumor cells and endothelial cells, and allowing migration of tumor cells through the endothelial cell matrix by heparanase activity. Tumor cells can activate platelets directly or through the release of proaggregatory mediators, including ADP, thrombin, and a cathepsin-like cysteine protease. Upon activation, platelets aggregate and release their granule contents, as shown by the detection of elevated plasma levels of β-thromboglobulin and PF4 (which are both localized in alpha-granules of platelets), and of increased expression of platelet membrane activation markers, such as P-selectin (or CD62P) and CD63, in patients with malignancy.

In addition, activated platelets release VEGF and PDGF, which play an important part in tumor neo-angiogenesis.

Antitumor therapy prothrombotic mechanisms

The pathogenesis of thrombosis during antitumor therapies is not entirely understood, but a number of mechanisms have been identified (Table 23.3) [17].

Table 23.3 Antitumor therapy prothrombotic mechanisms.

a. Release of procoagulant activities and cytokines from damaged cells
b. Direct drug toxicity on vascular endothelium
c. Induction of monocyte tissue factor
d. Decrease of physiological anticoagulants (i.e. protein C, proteins S, antithrombin)
e. Apoptosis

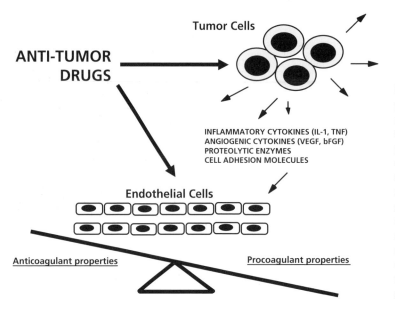

ANTI-TUMOR DRUGS

Tumor Cells

INFLAMMATORY CYTOKINES (IL-1, TNF)
ANGIOGENIC CYTOKINES (VEGF, bFGF)
PROTEOLYTIC ENZYMES
CELL ADHESION MOLECULES

Endothelial Cells

Anticoagulant properties   Procoagulant properties

Figure 23.3 Antitumor therapy prothrombotic mechanisms. Tumor cells perturbed by antitumor drugs release a series of soluble mediators (i.e. proinflammatoy and proangiogenic cytokines, proteolytic enzymes), which can act on endothelial cells by altering their normal antithrombotic and antiadhesive status or by damaging the endothelial monolayer, with the subsequent exposure of the highly procoagulant endothelial cell matrix. The same antitumor drugs can up-regulate the expression of adhesion molecules by tumor cells, which become adhesive toward the endothelium.

The possible role of cytokine released by damaged tumor cells in response to chemotherapy in increasing the thrombotic risk was suggested by experiments showing that plasma samples collected from women with breast cancer after chemotherapy contained higher levels of mediators (likely cytokines) able to increase the reactivity of endothelial cells to platelets. The direct damage exerted by chemotherapy on vascular endothelium represents another mechanism of drug-induced thrombosis (Fig. 23.3). Profound changes in plasma markers of endothelial damage have been reported in patients receiving different types of chemotherapy. Some chemotherapeutic agents can directly stimulate the expression of TF procoagulant activity by macrophages and monocytes, thus inducing a procoagulant response from host cells. In animal studies:

• Bleomycin determines morphologic damage to the vascular endothelium of the lung, resulting in pulmonary thrombosis and fibrosis.

• Adriamycin can directly affect glomerular cells, impairing their permeability and leading to a nephrotic syndrome, accompanied by hypercoagulation and increased thrombotic tendency.

Anti-angiogenic drugs, such as thalidomide and lenalidomide, and the anti-VEGF receptor SU5416, represent a new class of substances with endothelial toxic activity [18]. In cancer patients, during anti-angiogenic therapy with SU5416A, a significant increase in circulating markers of endothelial cell activation has been observed, particularly in those patients experiencing a thromboembolic event [19].

Radiation therapy can cause endothelial injury, as demonstrated by the release of von Willebrand protein from endothelial cells irradiated with doses up to 40 Gy.

Another prothrombotic mechanism of anti-tumor therapy is likely related to the direct hepatotoxicity of radio- and chemotherapy, which can cause a reduction in the plasma levels of natural anticoagulant proteins (antithrombin, protein C, and protein S), which is a well-known risk factor for thrombosis.

Prevention and treatment of thrombosis in cancer

Prophylaxis of VTE

Patients with diagnosed malignant disease are at an increased risk of developing "secondary" VTE in specific conditions (e.g. surgery, immobilization; Table 23.4). These patients have been stratified by the Consensus Conference of the American College of Chest Physicians (ACCP) in their highest risk category for developing "secondary" VTE. In addition, the risk of recurrences is significantly increased in cancer compared

Table 23.4 Risk of VTE in cancer patients undergoing surgery.*

Type of surgery	Risk (%)
General	29
Gynecologic	41
Orthopedic	50–60
Neurosurgery	28

*Adapted from Clagett et al. *Ann Surg* 1988;208:227.

with noncancer patients, even during treatments for VTE. There is no evidence that there is a benefit from giving antithrombotic prophylaxis to all cancer patients; however, there are selected conditions in which prophylaxis has to be considered, such as surgical interventions, acute medical illness, and administration of antitumor therapies [20].

Cancer surgery

Cancer surgery carries a two- to three-fold increased thrombotic risk compared with noncancer surgery of equal intensity. Perioperative prophylaxis with low doses of unfractionated heparin (UFH) or with fixed dose low-molecular-weight heparin (LMWH) is effective in significantly reducing the incidence of postoperative VTE. LMWH has a good safety profile also in this condition. Further, a higher dose of LMWH has been shown to be more effective than a lower dose in surgical cancer patients, without increasing the hemorrhagic risk [21]. This is of particular relevance as cancer patients are also at high risk of bleeding. A prolonged postoperative prophylaxis up to

1 month after surgery for cancer can add a benefit to reduce the rate of postoperative VTE. Two large clinical trials have shown the safety and efficacy of extended prophylaxis in cancer patients undergoing abdominal or pelvic surgery. In the ENOXACAN II study, a trial designed ad hoc for cancer patients, a 60% reduced rate of postoperative VTE was observed in the arm randomized to receive prolonged prophylaxis with LMWH. The FAME study confirmed the same results in a subgroup of patients with cancer (Table 23.5) [20].

Medical conditions

The advantages of thromboprophylaxis in nonsurgical conditions, such as in cancer patients with central venous catheters (CVC) or during chemotherapy, are still under evaluation. In recent prospective clinical studies, the incidence of CVC-related thrombotic complications in cancer patients appears to be lower than that reported by earlier studies, with a rate of about 4% for symptomatic VTE. These studies show no significant benefit of thromboprophylaxis with either LMWH or 1 mg/day fixed dose warfarin in preventing CVC-related thrombosis. Therefore, routine thromboprophylaxis has not been recommended so far [20,22].

The role of thromboprophylaxis in medical cancer patients receiving chemo- and/or hormone therapy is still undefined. In hospitalized cancer patients with an acute medical illness, thromboprophylaxis is recommended as for all other acute medical patients [20,22,23].

In ambulatory cancer patients receiving chemo- and/or hormone-therapy, there is no sufficient

Table 23.5 Prolonged prophylaxis with LMWH in surgical cancer patients.

Study	Cancer patients n %	Prophylaxis	Major bleeding %	VTE incidence %
ENOXACAN II *Bergqvist, NEJM 2002*	332 (100%)	Enoxaparin vs. placebo for:		
		19–21 days	0.4	4.8
		6–10 days	0	12
FAME	198 (58%)	Dalteparin vs. no prophylaxis for:		
Rasmussen, JTH 2006		4 weeks	0	8.8
		1 week	0	19.6

evidence to recommend routine thromboprophylaxis. A randomized, controlled trial demonstrated that prophylaxis with low-dose warfarin [international normalized ratio (INR) range 1.3–1.9] is effective and safe in reducing the incidence of thrombosis in women with stage IV metastatic breast cancer receiving chemotherapy. Recently, other clinical trials to test the efficacy of LMWH to prevent VTE in cancer patients receiving chemotherapies have been conducted. The preliminary results are presented in abstract form and do not demonstrate the efficacy of prophylaxis.

In two double-blind, placebo-controlled trials, patients with metastatic breast cancer (TOPIC I) or with non-small cell lung carcinoma stage III or IV (TOPIC II) were randomly assigned to receive or not a LMWH during chemotherapy.
• In the breast cancer trial, no differences in the rate of VTE were observed.
• In contrast, in the lung cancer trial, an effectiveness of LMWH prophylaxis was found in the subgroup with stage IV disease.

In the placebo-controlled, double-blind PRODIGE trial, patients with malignant glioma were assigned to receive LMWH prophylaxis or placebo in association with chemo- and radiotherapy.
• In this glioma trial, no statistically significant reduction in VTE rate was observed in the experimental arm, and there was a significant increase in bleeding complications.

A multicenter Italian study (acronym PROTECHT) has been recently conducted to test the efficacy of LMWH thromboprophylaxis in patients receiving chemotherapy for five types of solid tumors, including lung, breast, gastrointestinal, ovary, and head/neck cancers. The results are currently under evaluation.

Therefore, thromboprophylaxis in ambulatory cancer patients receiving pharmacological antitumor drugs cannot be recommended until more definite data will be produced by large randomized clinical trials. One exception is made for ambulatory patients with multiple myeloma receiving thalidomide and lenalidomide in combination with chemotherapy or steroids. Due to the unacceptably high thrombotic risk associated with this condition, an antithrombotic prophylaxis is recommended [20].

Treatment of VTE

The standard treatment for an acute episode of VTE consists of:
• The administration of LMWH at dose adjusted to body weight or UFH i.v. adjusted to achieve and maintain an activated partial thromboplastin time (APTT) prolongation of 1.5–2.5 times the basal value.
• Heparins are administered for 5 days concomitantly with vitamin K antagonists and suspended when full anticoagulation with vitamin K antagonists has been achieved (i.e. INR range 2–3) for at least two consecutive days.
• Thereafter, vitamin K antagonists are continued for at least 3–6 months.

In cancer patients with VTE, a new regimen exists:
• Initial treatment with weight-adjusted dose of LMWH for 1 month,
• Long-term treatment with 70–80% of initial dose LMWH from the 2nd to the 5th month.

This regimen was tested in the international randomized multicenter CLOT trial and demonstrated to be more effective than the conventional treatment in preventing recurrent VTE in cancer patients. The data are confirmed by two other randomized clinical trials [20,22,23].

However, vitamin K antagonists with a targeting INR of 2–3 are acceptable when LMWH is not available [20].

The duration of VTE treatment depends on the activity of the cancer.
• Indefinite anticoagulation is recommended for patients with active malignancy, i.e. those with metastatic disease or receiving continued chemotherapy, as cancer is a strong continuing risk factor for recurrent VTE [20].
• The role of the new oral anticoagulant drugs needs to be tested.

Anticoagulation and cancer survival

An antineoplastic effect of antithrombotic agents in various experimental models (i.e. tumor cell in culture, experimental animals, and cancer patients) has often been suggested. Anticoagulant drugs such as heparins and vitamin K antagonists have both been tested in this context. However, heparins have been more extensively studied.

Table 23.6 Randomized clinical trials testing the effect of LMWH on survival in cancer patients.

Study	Cancer	Control	LMWH
Altinbas M, et al. *J Thromb Haemost*, 2004	Small cell lung cancer	Nil	*Dalteparin* 5000 IU/day 18 weeks
Kakkar AK, et al. *J Clin Oncol*, 2004	Advanced cancer	Placebo	*Dalteparin* 5000 IU/day 1 year
Klerk CPW, et al. *J Clin Oncol*, 2004	Metastasized and advanced cancer	Placebo	*Nadroparin* Therapeutic dose 2 weeks + half dose 4 weeks
Sideras K, et al. *Mayo Clin Proc*, 2006	Advanced cancer	Nil	*Dalteparin* 5000 IU/day

Several reports in animal models and in vitro studies demonstrate that:

• heparin can reduce the primary tumor growth or its metastatic spread, and

• LMWH can inhibit neoangiogenesis induced by tumor cell environment [24,25].

Clinical studies of thrombosis in cancer patients show that, aside from their role as antithrombotics, heparins may have beneficial effects on survival in these patients, with a major role for LMWH compared with UFH. In recent years, a number of prospective randomized clinical trials of LMWH administration to improve survival (as a primary end-point) in cancer patients have been accomplished (Table 23.6). Altogether the results of these trials, although not conclusive, look promising in suggesting a benefit of cancer prognosis from LMWH administration, particularly in nonadvanced disease stage. However, the use of anticoagulants as adjuvant therapy for cancer cannot be recommended until additional clinical trials confirm these results [26].

References

1 Falanga A, Marchetti M, Vignoli A, Balducci D. Clotting mechanisms and cancer: implications in thrombus formation and tumor progression. *Clin Adv Hematol Oncol* 2003;1(11):673–8.

2 Boccaccio C, Sabatino G, Medico E, et al. The MET oncogene drives a genetic programme linking cancer to haemostasis. *Nature* 2005;434(7031):396–400.

3 Rong Y, Post DE, Pieper RO, Durden DL, Van Meir EG, Brat DJ. PTEN and hypoxia regulate tissue factor expression and plasma coagulation by glioblastoma. *Cancer Res* 2005;65(4):1406–13.

4 Yu JL, May L, Lhotak V, et al. Oncogenic events regulate tissue factor expression in colorectal cancer cells: implications for tumor progression and angiogenesis. *Blood* 2005;105(4):1734–41.

5 Blom JW, Vanderschoot JP, Oostindier MJ, Osanto S, van der Meer FJ, Rosendaal FR. Incidence of venous thrombosis in a large cohort of 66,329 cancer patients: results of a record linkage study. *J Thromb Haemost* 2006;4(3):529–35.

6 Khorana AA, Francis CW, Culakova E, Lyman GH. Risk factors for chemotherapy-associated venous thromboembolism in a prospective observational study. *Cancer* 2005;104(12):2822–9.

7 White RH, Chew H, Wun T. Targeting patients for anticoagulant prophylaxis trials in patients with cancer: who is at highest risk? *Thromb Res* 2007;120(2):S29–40.

8 Falanga A. Thrombophilia in cancer. *Semin Thromb Hemost* 2005;31(1):104–10.

9 Khorana AA, Francis CW, Culakova E, Kuderer NM, Lyman GH. Thromboembolism is a leading cause of death in cancer patients receiving outpatient chemotherapy. *J Thromb Haemost* 2007.

10 Falanga A, Barbui T, Rickles F. Hypercoagulability and tissue factor gene upregulation in hematologic malignancies. *Semin Thromb Hemost* 2008;34:204–10.

11 Prandoni P, Lensing AW, Buller HR, et al. Deep-vein thrombosis and the incidence of subsequent symptomatic cancer. *N Engl J Med* 1992;327(16):1128–33.

12 White RH, Chew HK, Zhou H, et al. Incidence of venous thromboembolism in the year before the diagnosis of cancer in 528,693 adults. *Arch Intern Med* 2005;165(15):1782–7.

13 Piccioli A, Lensing AW, Prins MH, et al. Extensive screening for occult malignant disease in idiopathic

venous thromboembolism: a prospective randomized clinical trial. *J Thromb Haemost* 2004;2(6):884–9.

14 Monreal M, Lensing AW, Prins MH, et al. Screening for occult cancer in patients with acute deep vein thrombosis or pulmonary embolism. *J Thromb Haemost* 2004;2(6):876–81.

15 Miller GJ, Bauer KA, Howarth DJ, Cooper JA, Humphries SE, Rosenberg RD. Increased incidence of neoplasia of the digestive tract in men with persistent activation of the coagulant pathway. *J Thromb Haemost* 2004;2(12):2107–14.

16 Annecke K, Schmitt M, Euler U, et al. uPA and PAI-1 in breast cancer: review of their clinical utility and current validation in the prospective NNBC-3 trial. *Adv Clin Chem* 2008;45:31–45.

17 Lee AY, Levine MN. The thrombophilic state induced by therapeutic agents in the cancer patient. *Semin Thromb Hemost* 1999;25(2):137–45.

18 Palumbo A, Rajkumar SV, Dimopoulos MA, et al. Prevention of thalidomide- and lenalidomide-associated thrombosis in myeloma. *Leukemia* 2008;22(2):414–23.

19 Kuenen BC, Levi M, Meijers JC, et al. Analysis of coagulation cascade and endothelial cell activation during inhibition of vascular endothelial growth factor/vascular endothelial growth factor receptor pathway in cancer patients. *Arterioscler Thromb Vasc Biol* 2002;22(9):1500–5.

20 Lyman GH, Khorana AA, Falanga A, et al. American Society of Clinical Oncology guideline: recommendations for venous thromboembolism prophylaxis and treatment in patients with cancer. *J Clin Oncol* 2007;25(34):5490–505.

21 Bergqvist D, Burmark US, Flordal PA, et al. Low molecular weight heparin started before surgery as prophylaxis against deep vein thrombosis: 2500 versus 5000 XaI units in 2070 patients. *Br J Surg* 1995;82(4):496–501.

22 Mandala M, Falanga A, Piccioli A, et al. Venous thromboembolism and cancer: guidelines of the Italian Association of Medical Oncology (AIOM). *Crit Rev Oncol Hematol* 2006;59(3):194–204.

23 National Comprehensive Cancer Network. NCCN Clinical Practice Guidelines in Oncology. Venous Thromboembolic Disease. 2008;vol 1:Available from: http://www.nccn.org/professionals/physician_gls/PDF/vte.pdf. Accessed June 2, 2008.

24 Marchetti M, Vignoli A, Russo L, et al. Endothelial capillary tube formation and cell proliferation induced by tumor cells are affected by low molecular weight heparins and unfractionated heparin. *Thromb Res* 2008;121(5):637–45.

25 Norrby K. Low-molecular-weight heparins and angiogenesis. *APMIS* 2006;114(2):79–102.

26 Kuderer NM, Khorana AA, Lyman GH, Francis CW. A meta-analysis and systematic review of the efficacy and safety of anticoagulants as cancer treatment: impact on survival and bleeding complications. *Cancer* 2007;110(5):1149–61.

24 Obstetrics, contraception, and estrogen replacement

Isobel D. Walker

Introduction

Thrombosis prevention and management has become the major focus for hematologists with an interest in women's health. Normal pregnancy is associated with increasing hypercoagulability as gestation progresses. In addition, the pregnant woman experiences increasing lower limb venous stasis due to compression of the venous flow by the gravid uterus and inevitably suffers endothelial damage due to the vascular trauma associated with delivery, particularly operative delivery. Thrombophilias may play a role in the etiology of not only venous thromboembolism (VTE) but a range of other vascular complications of pregnancy, and much debate has centered on the possibility of intervention to reduce the burden of these adverse pregnancy outcomes.

Advances in artificial reproductive technology and in the management of women with serious medical disorders, including valvular heart disease, have meant that increasingly women who would have been denied pregnancy in the past now have the opportunity to have a child of their own, but these women inevitably need specialist care, often involving a hematologist.

The risk of VTE associated with the use of female hormones for contraception or for estrogen replacement is now widely recognized, but much work remains to identify products that are as safe and effective as possible.

Hemostasis in normal pregnancy

Normal pregnancy is associated with major changes in all aspects of hemostasis: increasing concentrations of most clotting factors, including fibrinogen and factors VII, VIII, IX, X and XII; decreasing levels of some of the natural anticoagulants, such as protein S; increased resistance to activated protein C, and reducing fibrinolytic activity (see Table 24.1). As a result, as pregnancy progresses, and during the puerperium, the overall hemostatic balance is shifted toward hypercoagulability.

Choice of anticoagulation

Warfarin

Coumarins such as warfarin cross the placenta. Maternal coumarin ingestion between 6 and 12 weeks gestation may result in developmental abnormalities of fetal cartilage and bone, including stippling of the epiphyses and nasal hypoplasia. Different series have reported widely varying incidences of warfarin embryopathy, but a reasonable estimate of the incidence is around 5%. Warfarin use later in pregnancy is linked to abnormalities of the fetal central nervous system, including impaired brain growth due to repeated microhemorrhage and scarring. It has been suggested that the risks of fetal warfarin complications may be dose-dependent with an increased risk when the daily warfarin dose exceeds 5 mg [1]. It is generally recommended that coumarins should not be used for the prevention or treatment of VTE during pregnancy, but coumarins remain the anticoagulants of choice for the management of some pregnant women with mechanical heart valve prostheses. In all pregnant women, because of the hemorrhagic risk to both mother and fetus, warfarin should be avoided beyond 36 weeks gestation.

Table 24.1 Changes in levels of procoagulant factors and natural anticoagulants.

Procoagulant factors	Change in level by third trimester*
Fibrinogen	↑ 10%
Prothrombin	↑ 6%
Factor V	↑ 30%
Factor VIII	↑ 64%
Factor IX	↑ 14%
Factor X	↑ 22%
Factor XI	↓ 9%
Factor XII	↑ 31%
Von Willebrand factor antigen	↑ 87%
Ristocetin cofactor activity	↑ 105%
Natural anticoagulants	
Free protein S antigen	↓ 30%
Protein C activity	↓ 1%
Antithrombin activity	↑ 6%
Activated protein C resistance	Increased

*Percentage increase (↑) or decrease (↓) at 36 weeks gestation compared with level at 6–11 weeks gestation [25].

Heparins

Neither unfractionated heparins (UFH) nor low-molecular-weight heparins (LMWH) nor heparinoids (e.g. danaparoid) cross the placental barrier. Heparins are therefore devoid of any known teratogenic risk, and the fetus is not anticoagulated as a result of maternal heparin use. LMWH have a number of advantages over UFH, including better bioavailability with a more predictable dose response, an enhanced anti-Xa (antithrombotic) to anti-IIa (anticoagulant) ratio with a reduced risk of bleeding, and a longer plasma half-life. Compared with UFH, LMWHs are less likely to cause bone demineralization or heparin-induced thrombocytopenia. LMWHs are used increasingly in pregnant women requiring anticoagulation and are considered safe in general [2].

Gestational VTE

In the developed world, pulmonary embolism (PE) remains a leading cause of maternal death. Furthermore, gestational VTE is a major cause of morbidity not only during pregnancy but also in the longer term. Effective primary prevention of venous thrombosis and management of acute events when they occur are essential constituents of maternity care.

Incidence of gestational VTE

The incidence of objectively confirmed pregnancy-associated VTE is approximately 1 in 1000 deliveries [3]. Numerically, more VTE events occur during pregnancy than in the puerperium, but when the incidences of direct vein thrombosis (DVT) and PE are expressed as events per year at risk, the annual incidence of VTE (DVT + PE) in postpartum women is 4–5 times greater than the annual incidence in antepartum women. About 85% of pregnancy-associated DVTs are left-sided, compared with only 55% left-sided in non-pregnant women. Seventy-two percent of pregnancy-associated DVTs are ileofemoral, and only 9% are confined to distal calf veins. Almost two-thirds of women who have a gestational DVT develop objective signs of venous insufficiency.

Risk factors for gestational venous thrombosis

The etiology of venous thrombosis is multifactorial and, as in nonpregnant patients, women who develop a pregnancy-associated VTE frequently have more than a single identifiable risk. The common risk factors for gestational VTE are shown in Table 24.2.

Table 24.2 Risk factors for pregnancy-associated VTE.

Patient factors	Obstetric factors
Age over 35 years	Hyperemesis
Obesity; BMI ≥30	Preeclampsia
Dehydration	Operative vaginal delivery
Immobility >4 days	Cesarean section, particularly emergency section
Medical illness or infection	Extended surgery, e.g. cesarean hysterectomy
Gross varicose veins	
Intravenous drug use	
Long-distance travel	
Previous venous thrombosis	
Thrombophilia	

Thrombophilia and the risk of gestational venous thrombosis

By definition, thrombophilias are disorders of hemostasis that predispose to thrombosis. Included are heritable deficiencies of the natural anticoagulants antithrombin, protein C, and protein S and common mutations in the genes encoding clotting factors V and II, factor V Leiden, and the prothrombin G20210A and acquired thrombophilias such as antiphospholipid antibodies (Table 24.3).

Early studies suggested that, in the absence of anticoagulant prophylaxis, more than 40% of pregnancies in women with heritable thrombophilia might be complicated by VTE. Because these studies were retrospective reports of events occurring in women from already symptomatic kindred, the risk of gestational VTE may have been overestimated. However, a study of consecutive, unselected women with a history of gestational VTE suggested that, for women with the most severe type of antithrombin deficiency (type I quantitative defects), the risk of developing gestational VTE is indeed almost 40%, even in otherwise asymptomatic kindred [3]. In a systematic review of 9 studies that included a total of 2526 pregnancies [4], the risk of pregnancy-related VTE was greatest in factor V Leiden and prothrombin G20210A homozygotes, but significant also for women with heterozygous factor V Leiden, heterozygous prothrombin G20210A, or deficiency of antithrombin, protein C, or protein S (Table 24.4).

Although the results of studies indicate significantly increased relative risk, given that the incidence of pregnancy-associated VTE in an unselected population of women is around 1:1000, the absolute risk

Table 24.4 Odds ratios for pregnancy-associated VTE in women with heritable thrombophilias [4].

Defect		Odds ratio (95% CI)
Factor V Leiden	Homozygous	34.40 (9.86–120.05)
	Heterozygous	8.32 (5.44–12.70)
Prothrombin G20210A	Homozygous	26.36 (1.24–559.29)
	Heterozygous	6.80 (2.46–18.77)
Antithrombin deficiency		4.69 (1.30–16.96)
Protein C deficiency		4.76 (2.15–10.57)
Protein S deficiency		3.19 (0.48–6.88)

in women with a heritable thrombophilia usually remains modest. The risk of VTE in pregnancy with acquired thrombophilia remains unclear.

History of previous venous thrombosis

It has been suggested that, compared with the general obstetric population, women with a history of previous VTE may be at increased risk of a recurrence in pregnancy. Estimates of the risk of recurrence have varied widely. In a prospective study of women with a history of a previous objectively confirmed VTE in whom antenatal thromboprophylaxis was withheld, the overall rate of objectively confirmed recurrence during a subsequent pregnancy was 2.4% [5].

There were no recurrent events in women who did not have an identifiable thrombophilia and in whom the previous event was associated with a temporary acquired thrombotic risk factor. On the other hand, the recurrence rate in women who had an identifiable thrombophilia and/or in whom the previous event had occurred apparently spontaneously was 5.9%.

Prevention of gestational VTE

Using an assessment tool based on the known risk factors for gestational VTE, all pregnant women should be assessed for thrombotic risk at the time of booking, at each antenatal visit, on admission for delivery, and following delivery.

Routine screening of all women for thrombophilic defects is not justifiable, but screening of women who have a history of previous VTE is frequently

Table 24.3 Thrombophilias: prevalences in the general population of Caucasians.

Thrombophilia	Prevalence %
Antithrombin deficiency	0.25–0.55
Protein C deficiency	0.20–0.33
Protein S deficiency	0.03–0.13
Factor V Leiden (heterozygous)	2–7
Prothrombin G20210A (heterozygous)	2
Antiphospholipid antibodies	5

recommended, and many clinicians would also offer thrombophilia screening to women who give a family history of proven VTE [6].

All women assessed to be at increased risk of gestational VTE should be encouraged to wear graduated compression stockings throughout their pregnancy and puerperium. Given the evidence that the risk of VTE is greatest following delivery, many obstetricians would also offer women assessed to be at increased risk of pregnancy-associated VTE, who have no contraindication to anticoagulation or antithrombotics, pharmacological thromboprophylaxis following delivery—usually daily prophylactic doses of LMWH, self-administered subcutaneously, for 6 weeks following delivery [6,7].

Consideration may also be given to offering pharmacological thromboprophylaxis during pregnancy to women perceived to be at relatively higher risk of gestational VTE [6,7]. This group includes:
• Any woman who has a history of spontaneous (idiopathic) VTE, and
• Women who have had a thrombotic event in relation to a previous pregnancy or while using a combined oral contraceptive (COC), and any woman who has been found to have a thrombophilic defect because she has been investigated following a previous thrombotic event.

Also in this group are women who have no personal history of thrombosis, but who have been investigated because of a family history of VTE and have been found to have a thrombophilic defect associated with a relatively high risk of gestational VTE (e.g. type 1 antithrombin deficiency, homozygosity for factor V Leiden or prothrombin G20210A, or double heterozygosity for factor V Leiden and prothrombin G20210A).

Daily self-administered LMWH in prophylactic doses throughout pregnancy and for 6 weeks following delivery is usually considered adequate for most of these women at higher risk, but in some cases, the daily dose of LMWH may be increased to a level intermediate between that which is usually used for prophylaxis and the dose usually used for treatment of acute VTE [6,7].

The incidental finding of antiphospholipids in pregnancy should trigger increased clinical surveillance, but pharmacological intervention should be reserved for these women with antiphospholipids who are symptomatic. Women with antiphospholipids and a past history of VTE may usually be considered to be at highly increased risk of recurrent VTE associated with pregnancy and offered pharmacological thromboprophylaxis, using intermediate doses of LMWH as described above during pregnancy and the puerperium.

Diagnosis of gestational VTE

The general poor specificity of the clinical diagnosis of DVT and PE is compounded in pregnancy by the relative frequency of nonthrombotic leg swelling, breathlessness, and chest discomfort in pregnant women. Objective diagnosis is essential in all women presenting with suspected VTE in pregnancy or the puerperium. Failure to identify and treat thrombosis places mother's life at risk while unnecessary treatment exposes both her and her unborn child to risk.

In pregnant women presenting with suspected VTE, anticoagulation with heparin (usually LMWH) in full therapeutic doses should be commenced while awaiting confirmation of the diagnosis, except in the few cases where there is a contraindication to anticoagulation. D-dimer assays are generally unhelpful during pregnancy because normal pregnancy is associated with elevated D-dimer levels. In pregnant women, compression duplex ultrasound is the primary diagnostic tool for the confirmation of DVT.

Women in whom the presence of a DVT is confirmed should continue anticoagulation. Patients with a negative ultrasound and a low level of clinical suspicion do not require continuing anticoagulation. Patients with a negative ultrasound but a high level of clinical suspicion should continue on anticoagulation and either have a repeat ultrasound in a week or undergo alternative diagnostic testing. If this repeat or alternative testing is negative, anticoagulation may be discontinued. In patients with back pain and swelling of the entire leg in whom iliac vein thrombosis is suspected, magnetic resonance venography or conventional contrast venography may be considered [8].

Maternal chest x-ray exposes the fetus to a negligible dose of radiation, and although it is uninformative in over half of pregnant women who have an objectively proven PE, it may reveal PE-related abnormality or non-PE-related pulmonary disease, such as pneumonia. If the chest x-ray is normal, bilateral lower limb compression duplex ultrasound may be considered. A diagnosis of DVT will indirectly support a diagnosis of PE and, because the management is the same for DVT or PE, it may be possible to avoid further investigation that would expose the fetus to radiation [8]. Whatever the chest x-ray shows, if there is clinical suspicion of PE, definitive testing is essential. The choice of technique—ventilation perfusion (V/Q) scanning or computed tomographic pulmonary angiography (CTPA)—will depend on local availability and policy. During pregnancy, it is often possible to omit the ventilation component of the V/Q scan, thereby reducing the radiation dose to the fetus. Compared with V/Q scanning, maternal CTPA exposes the fetus to only about 10% of the radiation dose. However, there is a relatively high radiation dose to maternal breast tissue with a postulated associated increased lifetime risk of breast cancer. For this reason, some clinicians recommend lung perfusion scanning in young pregnant women, particularly if there is a family history of breast cancer. If iodinated contrast medium is administered to a mother having CTPA, thyroid function should be checked in the neonate.

Management of gestational VTE

The recommended treatment dose of LMWH varies according to manufacturer. Pregnancy alters the pharmacokinetics of some LMWHs (enoxaparin and dalteparin), and 12-hourly dosing with these products is recommended for the treatment of pregnant women with VTE. Because of the physiological hypercoagulability of pregnancy with its associated risk of recurrent VTE, most experts suggest continuation of full therapeutic doses of LMWH for the remainder of the pregnancy [8].

A modified regimen with intermediate LMWH doses after the first month at full doses may be useful in patients considered to be at increased risk of bleeding. The total duration of anticoagulation should usually be no less than 6 months, and anticoagulation should continue until at least 6–12 weeks after delivery.

Warfarin can be used after delivery, but many women find it more convenient to remain on a LMWH for this period. For women with a DVT, pain and swelling improve more rapidly and the risk of post-thrombotic syndrome is reduced if the patient is mobile and properly fitting compression hosiery is worn on the affected leg during the daytime. In women in whom a proximal DVT is diagnosed close to the time of expected delivery, there is evidence that (temporary) insertion of an inferior vena caval filter prior to labor or delivery reduces the risk of PE [8]. In general, delivery should be delayed if possible.

Management of delivery in women using anticoagulants during pregnancy

To avoid unwanted anticoagulation during delivery, pregnant women should be advised to discontinue their heparin injections as soon as they think they may be in labor.

Because the prolongation of the activated partial thromboplastin time (APTT) may persist longer than expected, in women using UFH, the APTT should be checked and protamine sulphate given if necessary. Epidural or spinal anesthesia is generally safe in women using UFH, providing their coagulation screen is within normal and their platelet count is $>80 \times 10^9$/L.

When the delivery date is planned, LMWH should be stopped 12–24 hours ahead of induction or cesarean section. In spite of considerable debate, it remains unclear what period of time should elapse between the last dose of LMWH and insertion or removal of an epidural or spinal catheter or how long the time interval should be until the next dose. For guidance, the Royal College of Obstetricians, London suggest that, in women on full treatment doses of LMWH, 24 hours should elapse after the last dose of LMWH before insertion of an epidural or spinal catheter, the cannula not be removed within 12 hours of the most recent injection, and no further dose of LMWH given for at least 4 hours after its removal [8]. For women on prophylactic doses of LMWH, regional anesthetic techniques should not be used until 12 hours have elapsed since the last injection. As above, the cannula should not be removed within 12 hours of the most recent injection, and no further dose of LMWH should be given for at least 4 hours after its removal. Local policies should be decided after discussion with the anesthetists providing the service.

Thrombophilia and vascular complications of pregnancy

Inadequate or abnormal placental vasculature may result in a number of complications that have potentially serious or even lethal consequences for the mother and her unborn child. These complications include:

- preeclampsia,
- placental abruption,
- intrauterine growth retardation, and
- miscarriage and stillbirth.

Pregnancy loss

Thrombi in the spiral arteries or fibrin deposition in the intervillous spaces on the maternal side of the placenta may result in inadequate placental perfusion. Microthrombi are frequently found in the vessels of the placentae from women who have experienced pregnancy loss, and placental infarction has been described in the placentae of some, but not all, women with thrombophilia who have a pregnancy loss. Placental thrombosis and infarction are, however, not uncommon in fetal loss cases in the absence of any identifiable thrombophilia. No placental lesion is specific for thrombophilia.

Recurrent fetal loss (RFL)

This is a well-documented finding in patients with antiphospholipids (APLs). The prevalence of persisting APL positivity among women who have a history of recurrent fetal loss is around 15%. In women with persistent APLs and a history of RCL, the prospective fetal loss rate (without intervention) has been put as high as 90%. The detection of positive APL tests in unselected women, however, is not predictive of poor pregnancy outcome.

Testing for the presence of APLs

After three or more consecutive early pregnancy losses or one unexplained late pregnancy loss, the recommended practice is to test for APLs, but it is possible that screening for APLs should be extended to include women who have had two consecutive miscarriages or three or more nonconsecutive events [9].

Treating RFLs associated with APL

Randomized trials have demonstrated improved fetal survival with aspirin plus heparin compared with only aspirin [10].

Link between heritable thrombophilias and RFL

There have been many studies examining possible associations between heritable thrombophilias and pregnancy loss, and two meta-analyses [4,11] have demonstrated associations between heritable thrombophilias, factor V Leiden, prothrombin G20210A and protein S deficiency, and recurrent first trimester pregnancy loss and single late-pregnancy loss (Table 24.5).

Treatment of RFL in heritable thrombophilias

It has been suggested that prophylactic doses of LMWH throughout pregnancy may improve pregnancy outcome in women with heritable thrombophilia and a history of recurrent fetal loss [12], but there is a lack of evidence of efficacy of thromboprophylaxis for this indication from randomized,

Table 24.5 Heritable thrombophilia and pregnancy loss.*

	Factor V Leiden Odds ratio (95% CI)		Prothrombin G20210A Odds ratio (95% CI)		Protein S deficiency Odds ratio (95% CI)	
	Rey [11]	**Robertson [4]**	**Rey**	**Robertson**	**Rey**	**Robertson**
Recurrent first trimester loss	2.01 (1.13–3.58)	1.91 (1.01–3.61)	2.56 (1.04–6.29)	2.70 (1.37–5.34)	14.7 (0.99–218)	–
Non-recurrent second trimester loss	–	4.12 (1.93–8.81)	–	8.60 (2.18–33.95)	–	–
Late-pregnancy loss	3.26 (1.82–5.83)	2.06 (1.10–3.86)	2.30 (1.09–4.87)	2.66 (1.28–5.53)	7.39 (1.28–42.6)	20.09 (3.70–109.15)

*Data from two meta-analyses [4,11].

controlled trials. This insufficient evidence on which to recommend antithrombotic intervention in women with a history of pregnancy loss with no other identified abnormality apart from a heritable thrombophilia has been recognized by the British Committee for Standards in Haematology [6] and by the authors of a recently published Cochrane Review [13].

However, some will extrapolate from the evidence in randomized, controlled trials, a benefit from intervention with heparin and low-dose aspirin in women with APL syndrome and recurrent pregnancy loss and judge that the prophylactic doses of LMWH in pregnancy are relatively safe, so an increasing number of clinicians are willing to prescribe antithrombotic agents to women with heritable thrombophilia and a history of two or more otherwise unexplained miscarriages or one unexplained later intrauterine fetal death.

Preeclampsia

The weight of evidence currently available would appear to support the conclusion that the prevalent types of inherited thrombophilia (factor V Leiden and prothrombin G20210A) are not strong independent risk factors for preeclampsia. They may, however, characterize a subpopulation of women in whom the risk is elevated or in whom the clinical presentation may be more severe. In particular, there is evidence that carriage of factor V Leiden may increase the risk of severe preeclampsia in women who are susceptible to preeclampsia [14,15].

Artificial reproductive technology

In artificial reproductive technology (ART), exogenous gonadotrophins and gonadotrophin-releasing hormone are given to induce ovulation. Between 1% and 25% of women undergoing ART develop ovarian hyperstimulation syndrome (OHSS), a condition associated with increased levels of coagulation factors and reduced levels of some natural anticoagulants. Venous thrombosis occurs with an incidence of around 1 in 1000 treatment cycles in women undergoing ART and is usually associated with severe forms of OHSS, but may occur in patients who do not display evidence of OHSS.

Many of the case reports describing VTE in association with OHSS report DVT in subclavian and internal jugular veins. VTE should be suspected in patients who have had ovarian stimulation who present with neck pain and/or swelling. The reason for localization of VTE in these sites in OHSS patients is not clear. In one review, 9 of 22 (41%) women who had an ART-associated upper extremity DVT had an identifiable thrombophilic defect [16].

Pregnant women with heart valves

Throughout the world each year, a large number of prosthetic heart valves are implanted, many of them in women of childbearing age. Maternal mortality in women with prosthetic heart valves is estimated to be between 1% and 4% and is mostly related to thromboembolism.

Choice of prosthetic valve: bioprosthetic

The choice of prosthesis is in itself difficult. In general, unless they have atrial fibrillation or an intracardiac thrombus, patients with bioprosthetic (tissue) heart valves do not need long-term anticoagulation, although some may take aspirin. Women with bioprosthetic valves may expect an uncomplicated pregnancy providing they have a normally functioning prosthesis, normal ventricular function, and no significant pulmonary hypertension. Tissue valves, however, undergo structural degeneration, and this appears to happen particularly with mitral tissue valves and more quickly in younger patients (under the age of 40 years). Some, but not all, studies have suggested that valve structural deterioration is accelerated by pregnancy.

Choice of prosthetic valve: mechanical

Patients with mechanical heart valve prostheses require lifelong anticoagulation, and this includes a requirement for continuing anticoagulation throughout pregnancy with the attendant risks to both mother and fetus. Women have a high thrombotic risk with:
• older type mechanical prostheses (e.g. Starr-Edwards or Bjork-Shiley),
• a prosthesis in the mitral position,
• multiple prosthetic valves,
• atrial fibrillation,
• a history of a previous thrombotic event.

On the other hand, women with newer less thrombogenic bileaflet valves, particularly if they are in the aortic position (and providing they are in normal sinus rhythm and have normal left ventricular function), may be regarded as being at lower thromboembolic risk.

Efficacy and safety of anticoagulants in pregnant women with prosthetic heart valves

In a review of six published cohort studies and twenty-two case series, three commonly used approaches to anticoagulation during pregnancy were identified:

1 oral anticoagulants throughout pregnancy;
2 replacing oral anticoagulants with UFH from weeks 6 to 12 and pre-delivery; and
3 use of UFH throughout pregnancy [17].

The incidences of maternal thromboembolic complications and maternal mortality were highest in the group of women using UFH throughout pregnancy and least in those using oral anticoagulation throughout their pregnancy, substituting heparin only in the last few weeks before their expected delivery (Table 24.6). Seventeen of the 25 reported maternal deaths were due to thrombosis of the prosthesis or related complications, and 2 were due to hemorrhage.

Warfarin

In pregnant women with mechanical heart valve prostheses, when warfarin is used the target international normalized ratio (INR) target is usually 3.0 (range 2.5–3.5). However, a lower INR target of 2.5 (range 2.0–3.0) may be acceptable for women with bileaflet valves in the aortic position, providing they are in sinus rhythm and do not have left ventricular dysfunction. Some clinicians advise women in the high thromboembolic risk category to use an INR target of 3.5. Warfarin should be avoided close to term and LMWH substituted.

LMWH

Only a few case reports of LMWH use in pregnant patients with prosthetic heart valves have been published [18]. Not all have had successful outcomes [19]. In nonpregnant patients with prosthetic heart valves, LMWH has been shown to be at least as safe as UFH for "bridging" of patients taken off their long-term coumarin anticoagulation periprocedure. However, in pregnancy, a randomized, open label study that planned to recruit 110 women comparing LMWH with UFH and warfarin was terminated after 2 of the first 12 recruits died (one with a prosthetic mitral valve and one with prostheses in both the mitral and aortic positions). Both were in the LMWH-treated group, and both had subtherapeutic levels of anticoagulation around the time of death.

Currently, both the European Society of Cardiology [20] and the American College of Cardiology/American Heart Association [21] caution against the use of LMWH because of the lack of published evidence on the use of LMWH in pregnant women with prosthetic heart valves.

The most appropriate choice

Decisions about the most appropriate anticoagulant regimen during pregnancy for women with mechanical heart valve prostheses must be made on an individual patient basis after careful counseling, and should be based as much as possible on the relative risks of the various thromboprophylaxis regimens and whether the patient is perceived to be at high or lower thromboembolic risk.

On the basis of one report that the risk of fetal complications with warfarin appears to be dose-related, providing their daily warfarin requirement does not exceed 5 mg [1], some women may feel reassured about the relatively low risk to their fetus if they use warfarin throughout pregnancy or with substitution of

Table 24.6 Efficacy of thromboprophylaxis in pregnant women with mechanical heart valve prostheses, comparing three different approaches to anticoagulation [17].

Treatment approach	Maternal thromboembolism	Maternal mortality
Warfarin throughout pregnancy with UFH from 35 weeks to delivery	3.9%	1.8%
Warfarin with UFH from 6–12 weeks gestation and from 35 weeks to delivery	9.2%	4.2%
UFH throughout pregnancy	33.3%	15.0%

LMWH from 6–12 weeks gestation. However, women whose daily warfarin requirement exceeds 5 mg, particularly if they are classified into the lower thromboembolic risk group, may wish to minimize the risk of fetal complication and may be prepared to rely on adjusted doses of LMWH. Women with mechanical heart valve prostheses who choose to use LMWH for anticoagulation during pregnancy must be made aware that both the European Society of Cardiology [20] and the American College of Cardiology/American Heart Association [21] recommend warfarin as the anticoagulant of choice for pregnant women with mechanical heart valve prostheses.

For patients with prosthetic valves on either UFH or LMWH, regular (at least weekly) monitoring is recommended. With UFH, the APTT should be maintained between 2.0 and 2.5 times the control APTT, and for LMWH, the peak anti-Xa level 4 hours postinjection should be between 1.0 and 1.2 U/mL [7].

Female hormone use and the risk of VTE

Oral contraceptives

Since their introduction in the 1960s, it has been evident that COCs are associated with an increased risk of VTE. Although it was originally assumed that the magnitude of this risk was related to the estrogen dose in the COC, more recently the role of the progestogen content has been examined. Oral contraceptives containing third-generation progestogens (desogestrel or gestodene) are associated with an approximately two-fold increased risk of VTE compared with COCs containing second-generation progestogens (levonorgestrel). COCs cause slight increases in some procoagulant factors, reduce the levels of some natural anticoagulants, and increase resistance to activated protein C. These effects are more marked with third-generation than with second-generation COCs.

Although there is a significantly increased risk of VTE for COC users, because these products are used by young women in whom VTE is uncommon, the overall absolute risk of VTE for COC users remains low at around 3–4 in 10,000 users per year. The relative risk of VTE for third-generation COC users is around six- to nine-fold that in non-COC users, and in a prospective study, the absolute risk of VTE associated with third-

generation COC use was around 1 in 1000 new users per year.

Thrombophilia and COC

A super-additive risk of VTE has been observed between the use of COCs and the presence of thrombophilia, with the odds of developing VTE substantially amplified in women with thrombophilia who use a COC. The most significant increased risk has been observed with factor V Leiden [22,23]. The interaction between the factor V Leiden mutation and COCs is enhanced for users of COCs containing third-generation progestogens. Prothrombin G20210A has also been shown to increase the risk of VTE in COC users, as has deficiency of antithrombin or protein C [23]. The increased risk of VTE associated with COC use in patients with heritable thrombophilias has led to the suggestion that women should be screened for these defects prior to prescription of a COC, but this is widely accepted as not cost effective [24].

Progestogen-only preparations

These are used to treat menstrual disorders and are associated with increased risk of VTE, but in the general population, progestogen-only pills used for contraception appear not to be associated with significantly increased VTE risk.

Hormone replacement therapy

Hormone (estrogen) replacement therapy (HRT) can be administered orally, transdermally, transvaginally, or subcutaneously.

Nonoral administration avoids the hepatic "first pass" effect and has minimal effects on blood coagulation. Oral preparations include unopposed estrogen and combined preparations, usually containing conjugate equine estrogens (CEEs) or micronized estradiol combined with a progestogen. Transdermal HRT may also contain both estrogen and progestogen or estrogen only. The changes in hemostasis associated with HRT use are similar in type and direction to those associated with COC use but lesser in magnitude. Nonoral HRT preparations provoke lesser changes in hemostasis than oral preparations.

Early studies suggested that HRT did not significantly increase the risk of VTE. Later, however, case control studies linking HRT use and VTE have been published, and the increased risk of VTE has been confirmed in randomized studies. The evidence is consistent in demonstrating a relative risk of VTE of the order of two to four in women using HRT compared with nonusers. The risk of VTE is greatest for orally administered preparations and is minimal for women using nonoral HRT. In observational studies, the risk appeared similar irrespective of the type of estrogen used, and no significant difference in risk was observed in users of opposed (with progestogen) versus unopposed estrogen. Recently, however, a lower risk of VTE was found in women using unopposed estrogen HRT compared with women using combined HRT.

As in COC users, the risk of VTE in HRT users seems to be higher near the start of therapy and in women with thrombophilia, in particular factor V Leiden. Although the relative risk of VTE is similarly increased in COC and HRT users, the absolute risk is higher in HRT than in COC users, due to their older age.

Others

There is limited information about the risk of VTE in users of Selective Estrogen Receptor Modulators, but in a randomized, placebo-controlled trial, the relative risk of VTE in users of Raloxifene was 3.1 (95% CI 1.5–6.2), suggesting that the risk is similar to that with estrogen-containing HRT. A similarly increased risk of venous thrombosis has been reported in women using tamoxifen for the prevention or treatment of breast cancer.

References

1 Vitale N, De Feo M, De Santo LS, Pollice A, Tedesco N, Cotrufo M. Dose-dependent fetal complications of warfarin in pregnant women with mechanical heart valves. *J Am Coll Cardiol* 1999;33(6):1637–41.

2 Greer IA, Nelson-Piercy C. Low-molecular-weight heparins for thromboprophylaxis and treatment of venous thromboembolism in pregnancy: a systematic review of safety and efficacy. *Blood* 2005;106(2):401–7.

3 McColl MD, Ramsay JE, Tait RC, et al. Risk factors for pregnancy associated venous thromboembolism. *Thromb Haemost* 1997;78(4):1183–8.

4 Robertson L, Wu O, Langhorne P, et al. Thrombophilia in pregnancy: a systematic review. *Br J Haematol* 2006;132(2):171–96.

5 Brill-Edwards P, Ginsberg JS, Gent M, et al. Safety of withholding heparin in pregnant women with a history of venous thromboembolism. *N Engl J Med* 2000; 343(20):1439–44.

6 Walker ID, Greaves M, Preston FE. Investigation and management of heritable thrombophilia. *Br J Haematol* 2001; 14(3):512–28.

7 Bates SM, Greer IA, Pabinger I, Sofaer S, Hirsh J. Venous thromboembolism, thrombophilia, antithrombotic therapy, and pregnancy: ACCP Evidenced based Clinical Practice guidelines (the Eighth edition). *Chest* 2008;133(6 Suppl):844S–86S.

8 Greer IA, Thomson AJ. Thromboembolic disease in pregnancy and the puerperium: acute management. Green Top Guideline. No 28. 2007. London, Royal College of Obstetricians. Available from: http://www.rcog.org.uk/resources/Public/pdf/green_top_28_thromboembolic_minorrevision.pdf.

9 Greaves M, Cohen H, Machin SJ, Mackie I. Guidelines on the investigation and management of the antiphospholipid syndrome. *Br J Haematol* 2000;109(4): 704–15.

10 Rai R, Cohen H, Dave M, Regan L. Randomised controlled trial of aspirin and aspirin plus heparin in pregnant women with recurrent miscarriage associated with phospholipid antibodies (or antiphospholipid antibodies). *Br Med J* 1997;314(7076):253–7.

11 Rey E, Kahn SR, David M, Shrier I. Thrombophilic disorders and fetal loss: a meta-analysis. *Lancet* 2003; 361(9361):901–8.

12 Brenner B, Hoffman R, Carp H, Dulitsky M, Younis J. Efficacy and safety of two doses of enoxaparin in women with thrombophilia and recurrent pregnancy loss: the LIVE-ENOX study. *J Thromb Haemost* 2005; 3(2):227–9.

13 Di Nisio M, Peters L, Middeldorp S, Di Nisio M, Peters L, Middeldorp S. Anticoagulants for the treatment of recurrent pregnancy loss in women without antiphospholipid syndrome. *Cochrane Database Syst Rev* 2005;(2):CD004734.

14 Morrison ER, Miedzybrodzka ZH, Campbell DM, et al. Prothrombotic genotypes are not associated with preeclampsia and gestational hypertension: results from a large population-based study and systematic review. *Thromb Haemost* 2002;87(5):779–85.

15 Lin J, August P, Lin J, August P. Genetic thrombophilias and preeclampsia: a meta-analysis. *Obstet Gynecol* 2005;105(1):182–92.

16 Chan WS, Ginsberg JS. A review of upper extremity deep vein thrombosis in pregnancy: unmasking the 'ART' behind the clot. *J Thromb Haemost* 2006;4(8): 1673–7.

17 Chan WS, Anand S, Ginsberg JS. Anticoagulation of pregnant women with mechanical heart valves: a

systematic review of the literature. *Arch Intern Med* 2000;160(2):191–6.

18 Ellison J, Thomson AJ, Walker ID, Greer IA. Use of enoxaparin in a pregnant woman with a mechanical heart valve prosthesis. *Br J Obstet Gynaecol* 2001;108(7): 757–9.

19 Lev-Ran O, Kramer A, Gurevitch J, Shapira I, Mohr R. Low-molecular-weight heparin for prosthetic heart valves: treatment failure. *Ann Thorac Surg* 2000;69(1): 264–5.

20 Vahanian A, Baumgartner H, Bax J, et al. Guidelines on the management of valvular heart disease: The Task Force on the Management of Valvular Heart Disease of the European Society of Cardiology. *Eur Heart J* 2007;28(2):230–68.

21 Bonow RO, Carabello B, de Leon AC Jr, et al. Guidelines for the management of patients with valvular heart disease: executive summary. A report of the American College of Cardiology/American Heart Association Task Force on Practice Guidelines (Committee on Management of Patients with Valvular Heart Disease). *Circulation* 1998;98(18):1949–84.

22 Vandenbroucke JP, Koster T, Briet E, Reitsma PH, Bertina RM, Rosendaal FR. Increased risk of venous thrombosis in oral-contraceptive users who are carriers of factor V Leiden mutation. *Lancet* 1994;344(8935): 1453–7.

23 Wu O, Robertson L, Langhorne P, et al. Oral contraceptives, hormone replacement therapy, thrombophilias and risk of venous thromboembolism: a systematic review. The Thrombosis: Risk and Economic Assessment of Thrombophilia Screening (TREATS) Study. *Thromb Haemost* 2005;94(1):17–25.

24 Wu O, Robertson L, Twaddle S, et al. Screening for thrombophilia in high-risk situations: a meta-analysis and cost-effectiveness analysis. *Br J Haematol* 2005; 131(1):80–90.

25 Clark P, Brennand J, Conkie JA, McCall F, Greer IA, Walker ID. Activated protein C sensitivity, protein C, protein S and coagulation in normal pregnancy. *Thromb Haemost* 1998;79(6):1166–70.

25 Pediatrics

Mary E. Bauman and M. Patricia Massicotte

Quaternary care pediatrics: trading one problem for another

The age of highly specialized pediatric care has resulted in many medical and surgical successes. However, new life-threatening challenges have resulted, which include thrombosis. Prior to this era, there were little data concerning the risk or occurrence of both venous and arterial thrombosis in infants and children. The studies over the last 15 years, although inferior in design, have begun to define a number of important areas in pediatric thrombosis:
- cohorts at high risk,
- the overall incidence,
- clinical presentation,
- diagnostic methods,
- treatment modalities, and
- long-term outcomes.

Many health professionals are now confronted with these surviving infants and children who require special care, which cannot be extrapolated from adult practice as a result of many differences compared with adults. These unique differences include nutrition sources and ongoing growth, developmental hemostasis, and drug metabolism.

(Note: For the purposes of this chapter, the term "children" will be used to describe infants and children, unless otherwise stated.)

Kids are not little adults: the differences

Normal growth and development
The differences in children compared with adults alter incidence and etiology of thrombosis, but also the type and dose of anticoagulant agent used.

- Full-term infants double their birth weight by 5 months of age and triple their birth weight by 1 year.
- Nutrition sources differ among infants; for example, breastfed infants receive almost no vitamin K, whereas bottle-fed infants receive varying amounts of vitamin K depending on the amount and type of formula taken.
- Young children will binge eat, then not eat for a period of time [1].
- Renal function (GFR) increases over time until adulthood.

Developmental hemostasis
Normal physiological hemostasis is dependent on maintaining a fine balance between thrombosis and hemorrhage. Coagulation and fibrinolysis, the two pathways responsible for hemostasis, have a number of protein components that, when activated by a stimulus, interact with red blood cells and platelets and result in thrombus formation (coagulation) and/or thrombus degradation (fibrinolysis). Historically, alterations in blood flow, composition, and vessel wall integrity have been recognized as the most important elements involved in thrombus formation, known as Virchow's Triad.

Normal hemostasis results in a fine balance between bleeding and clotting (Fig. 25.1).
- Procoagulant proteins present in the blood (factors XII, XI, HMWK, X, IX, VIII, VII, V, II, and fibrinogen).
- Procoagulant factors are activated by a stimulus (e.g. sepsis, trauma, surgery).
- Thrombin (FIIa) is then produced.
- Thrombin activates fibrinogen into fibrin, the precursor of a polymerized clot.
- The fibrinolytic system is subsequently activated to break down the clot.

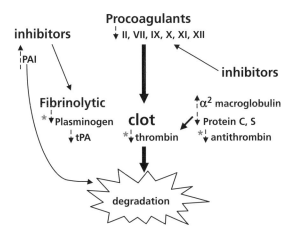

Figure 25.1 Coagulation/fibrinolytic system: the essence. Abbreviations: PAI, plasminogen activator inhibitor; tPA, tissue plasminogen activator. Dotted arrows demonstrate differences in children. Asterisks (*) indicate differences in children that influence therapy.

• Inhibitor proteins of hemostasis (antithrombin, protein C, protein S, α2-macroglobulin) and fibrinolysis (plasminogen activator inhibitor 1) are present to prevent massive clot formation or clot lysis, respectively (Fig. 25.1).

Compared with adults, children have a number of differences in hemostasis and fibrinolysis that affect the incidence, treatment, and long-term outcome of thrombosis (Fig. 25.1) [2,3].
• Contact factors XII, X, HMWK and the vitamin K-dependent factors II, VII, IS, and X are decreased until approximately 6 months of age [2–4].
• Thrombin generation is decreased 30–50% compared with adult levels [4].
• Inhibitors of hemostasis are present.
• The fibrinolytic system is downregulated [2].

Neonatal platelets are demonstrated to be hyporeactive to thrombin, adenosine diphosphate/epinephrine, and thromboxane A_2 due a a defect intrinsic to neonatal platelets [5].

The importance of antithrombotic therapy

Treatment of thrombosis is important due to resultant morbidity and mortality. Unlike adults, even asymptomatic clots result in serious sequelae in children.

• Many children have intracardiac blood shunts (right–left), thus venous thrombi may result in stroke [6].
• There is an association between sepsis and thrombosis [7].
• Pulmonary embolism is often asymptomatic in children due to large cardiopulmonary reserves and may be life-threatening [8].
• Loss of venous access, which may be required for future intervention in a patient population who will require life-long medical support [9].
• Post-thrombotic syndrome [10].

Difficulties in performing clinical trials in children

The practice of evidence-based medicine is based on the results of properly designed, conducted, and analyzed studies. Evidence for the safety and efficacy of therapies is established through clinical trials. However, there are a number of difficulties in the design and management of clinical trials in children. A significant challenge is that pediatric studies are largely underfunded due to the perception that adult knowledge may be applied to children [4].

Laboratory measures of hemostasis

Common surrogate measures of hemostasis
The most common surrogate measures of in vivo coagulation are the activated partial thromboplastin time (PTT also known as APTT) and the prothrombin time (PT) converted to the international normalized ratio (INR). PTT measures contact factors (XI, XII), factors II, VIII, and X, and the conversion of fibrinogen to fibrin. This part of the pathway is often referred to as the intrinsic system and the common pathway (Fig. 25.2).

The PT measures factors synthesized in the liver, including vitamin K-dependent factors (II, VII, IX, X) measuring the extrinsic and common pathways (Fig. 25.2). Developmental hemostasis alters age-related normal values of tests that measure hemostasis, especially for the PTT [2–4]. The INR is not a true value but is calculated using the patient PT value in seconds divided by the geometric mean of the reference PT range (for the respective reagent/analyzer

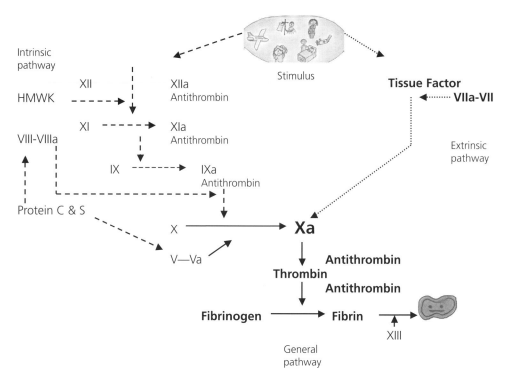

Figure 25.2 Simplified coagulation cascade. Dashed lines indicate intrinsic pathway. Dotted lines indicate extrinsic pathway. Solid lines indicate common pathway.

combination), taken to the power of the international sensitivity index. The use of the INR value is an attempt to account for different analyzers and thromboplastin reagents used in PT testing.

The INR and PTT measure interaction of coagulation factors in plasma (as compared to whole blood) in a test tube. The inability to measure the presence and interaction of red blood cells and platelets provides an incomplete measure of hemostasis.

Global measures of hemostasis

Activated clotting time (ACT)
The ACT uses activated whole blood and measures clotting time in seconds as a measure of global hemostasis, which more closely reflects in vivo coagulation. This point-of-care test is used in extracorporeal life support (cardiopulmonary bypass, extracorporeal membranous oxygenation) to monitor anticoagulation, specifically heparin. There are no well-designed studies evaluating safety and efficacy of

the use of ACTs to monitor anticoagulation in children. Although many health care professionals use the ACT to measure anticoagulation, the ACT does not solely reflect the effect of heparin but also reflects recent infusion of blood products.

Thromboelastogram
The thromboelastogram uses whole activated whole blood to measure hemostasis (formation of a clot) as well as fibrinolysis (clot degradation). The most common devices used to measure thromboelastography are the ROTEM® (Pentafarm, Munich, Germany) and the TEG® (Haemoscope, Niles IL,). Formal well-designed studies are required to evaluate the validity, accuracy, and application of the measure in children.

Therapeutic agents and metabolism
Evidence for the safety and efficacy of therapies is established through clinical trials. It is challenging to perform rigorous studies in children [4], and as a result, the agents that are commonly used for treatment

of thrombosis in children include heparin therapy and vitamin K antagonists. Current data in adults support the premise that, when patients are maintained within their defined therapeutic range, they will be adequately protected from the risk of thrombosis and minimize the risk of a serious adverse event [11,12]. Newer agents, such as direct thrombin inhibitors, are available, although there are limited data available to support their use. Despite this, there are clinical situations where these agents must be used, for example in confirmed heparin-induced thrombocytopenia (HIT).

In addition, there are multiple variables that make the use of antithrombotic drugs in children different from adults, which include:

• Epidemiology of thrombosis in children is different.
• Hemostatic system is dynamically evolving.
• Distribution, binding, and clearance of antithrombotic drugs are age-dependent.
• Many children requiring antithrombotic therapy have underlying conditions that often require concurrent medication.
• Frequency and type of intercurrent illnesses vary with age.
• Practical ability to deliver the drug is impacted by difficult venous access, needle phobias, etc.
• Pediatric formulations of antithrombotic drugs are not available, making accurate dose measurement difficult.
• Dietary differences that are inherent to normal growth and development particularly influence the use of vitamin K antagonist therapy.

Heparin is a term that encapsulates unfractionated heparin (UFH) and low-molecular-weight heparins (LMWH).

Unfractionated heparin (UFH)

UFH remains a commonly used anticoagulant agent used in hospital settings for children at potential increased risk of hemorrhage (i.e. postoperatively) or when rapid reversal of anticoagulant effect is required. Heparin is not absorbed orally, therefore must be administered intravenously or subcutaneously.

UFH: metabolism

UFH acts via antithrombin-mediated catabolism of thrombin and inhibition of factors IIa, IXa, Xa, XIa, and XIIa (Fig. 25.2). UFH is poorly bioavailable and binds with a number of plasma proteins, endothelial

cells, and macrophages, which results in variability in anticoagulant response.

• UFH binds with antithrombin to catabolize thrombin. Antithrombin is at decreased levels in infants and children compared with adults, further increasing the variable anticoagulant response.
• Antithrombin concentrate may be administered when patient levels are low to strengthen UFH response and reduce anticoagulant variability.
• UFH binds to von Willebrand factor and inhibits von Willebrand factor-dependent platelet function [13].

UFH therapy: dosing and monitoring

Dosing of UFH in children is age-dependent (Table 25.1). Dosing guidelines are provided in Table 25.2. Children will achieve therapeutic UFH (anti-factor Xa) levels more quickly if a UFH bolus dose of 75–100 U/k/hour is administered; however, it is important to consider the risk–benefit ratio with regards to hemorrhage. Heparin doses are then titrated based on laboratory measure of anti-factor Xa, or PTT if anti-factor Xa measures are unavailable.

The internationally accepted gold standard measure of UFH is an anti-factor Xa level, with a target range of 0.35–0.7 U/mL [12] to reflect a therapeutic heparin level. Recent data suggest that extrapolating the PTT from adults to pediatric patients is likely to be invalid, as normal PTTs in infants and children are increased secondary to developmental hemostasis [14]. Equally, there is a different response to heparin compared with adults; therefore, the use of the PTT to monitor heparin therapy may be invalid. In addition, in vitro and in vivo data support that the PTT that corresponds to an anti-factor Xa level of 0.35–0.7 U/mL varies significantly with age [14].

Some health professionals are using anti-factor Xa in children despite the absence of studies because of the lack of correlation between anti-factor Xa levels and PTT, as investigations have validated UFH dosing nomograms in children. Depending on the reagent and the machine used to measure the PTT, therapeutic PTTs can be anywhere from 1.5 to 6.2 times baseline [13].

UFH: benefits and limitations

• Short half-life,therefore clears within 4–6 hours of cessation.
• Fully reversible with protamine sulphate.

Table 25.1

Anticoagulant	Properties	Indications	Contraindications	Dose	Monitoring
UFH	Half-life dose dependent (max 150 minutes). Completely reversible with protamine sulphate. Poorly bioavailable, requires frequent blood monitoring. Antithrombin required to achieve heparin effect. If no heparin effect achieved with high doses of heparin, determine antithrombin level as antithrombin may be required.	Immediate post-op. Increased risk of bleeding. Frequent invasive procedures requiring reversal of anti-coagulation. Presence of intracardiac lines.	HIT. Poor venous access due to parenteral administration. Frequent monitoring is required.	Age-dependent dosing: <12 months of age = 28 U/kg/ hour; >12 months of age = 20 U/kg/ hour.	q24h at minimum. UFH level is gold standard (0.35–0.70 U/mL). If it is necessary to use a PTT to monitor therapy, the PTT range must be determined by each hospital to correspond to UFH 0.35–0.7 U/mL.
LMWH	Highly bioavailable, "stable drug." Not fully reversible. Antithrombin has less influence. Requires 24 hours to clear anticoagulant effect.	When bleeding risk considered stable. Bridge between heparin and warfarin post-op. Poor venous access.	High risk for bleeding. Reversal required frequently for interventions. Hold LMWH for 24 hours before procedure. Renal insufficiency.		LMWH level (anti-Xa) target 0.5–1.0 U/mL. Dose titrated to achieve level. Minimum monthly levels. INR or PTT will not be affected.
Enoxaparin q12h	Half-life is 3–6 hours.	Stable anticoagulant effect required.		Age-dependent dosing, <3 months of age = ~1.5 mg/kg/ dose; 3 months of age ~1.0 mg/kg/dose.	LMWH level 4–6 hours post dose.
Tinzaparin q24h	Half-life is 3–6 hours.	Needle-phobic children on long-term therapy.		200 mg/k/dose	Age-dependent LMWH levels. <5 years = 2 hours post dose; >5 years = 4 hours post dose.
VKA Warfarin	Half-life is 160 hours, oral administration.	Long-term anticoagulant therapy.	Relative: <1 years of age unless mechanical valve in situ.	Load: 0.1–0.2 mg/kg (see text) Maintenance: individualized dosing titrated to INR.	INR daily until therapeutic, then decreased frequency when stable with minimum monthly testing. Test INR with illness, medication, or diet change.

Table 25.2 UFH dosing nomogram.

PPT(s)	Anti-Xa (U/mL)	Hold UFH (minutes)	Rate Δ	Repeat PTT
<50	<0.1	0	↑20%	4 hours
50–59	0.1–0.34	0	↑10%	4 hours
60–85	0.35–0.70	0	0	24 hours
86–95	0.71–0.89	0	↓10%	4 hours
96–120	0.90–1.20	30	↓10%	4 hours
>120	>1.20	60	↓15%	4 hours

Table 25.3 UFH: reversal.

Time since end of infusion, or last UFH dose (minutes)	Protamine per 100 U UFH dose (maximum 50 mg/dose) (mg)
<30	1
30–60	0.5–0.75
61–120	0.375–0.5
>120	0.25–0.375

- Requires venous access for administration and monitoring.
- Poor bioavailability.
- Osteopenia (although may be reversible).
- HITHIT is an immune-mediated platelet reaction response to heparin. HIT is characterized by a sudden drop in platelets by more than 50% after 5 days of first-time heparin exposure or any time after a previous heparin exposure. The incidence among children is <0.1% [15].

The gold standard test to determine HIT is the serotonin release assay. This assay is performed in few laboratories. The ELISA is most commonly available; however, the sensitivity is variable compared with the serotonin release assay, as shown by Warkentin and coworkers [15]. If there is a strong suspicion or a positive diagnosis for HIT, all heparin and LMWH should be discontinued.

UFH: subcutaneous dosing

Therapeutic UFH may be administered subcutaneously. The daily dose in U/kg/hour is divided in two daily doses and is given subcutaneously every 12 hours. For subcutaneous UFH, the total daily dose in U/kg is divided into two doses given every 12 hours.

Dosing is calculated using the following formula:

Dose = Patient weight × age-dependent U/kg/hour

(i.e. 20/28) × the # of hours of coverage.

Subcutaneous (SC) UFH is monitored by using either the PTT or anti-factor Xa level measured at 4–6 hours after the SC dose. Dose is adjusted according to the UFH nomogram (Table 25.2).

UFH: reversal

Dosing instructions for protamine sulphate are shown in Table 25.3. Except for reversal of UFH following cardiopulmonary bypass, the maximum dose of protamine sulphate regardless of the amount of UFH received is 50 mg, and should be administered in a concentration of 10 mg/mL at a rate not to exceed 5 mg/minute. When administered too quickly, protamine sulphate may result in cardiovascular collapse. Patients with known hypersensitivity reactions to fish and those who have received protamine-containing insulin or previous protamine therapy may be at risk of hypersensitivity reactions to protamine sulphate. An APTT 15 minutes after administration will demonstrate the effect obtained through administration.

Low molecular weight heparin (LMWH)

LMWHs have rapidly become the anticoagulant of choice for pediatric patients in the absence of a high risk for bleeding [16]. LMWHs are reported among adults to have equal efficacy to the higher molecular weight UFH and are associated with a decreased risk for hemorrhage in adults. However, there are no well-designed studies evaluating safety and efficacy in children.

LMWH: metabolism

LMWHs inhibit the activation of the same activated factors as UFH; however, the greatest inhibition occurs on factor Xa (Fig. 25.2) [17]. LMWHs have an average molecular weight of 5000 and are synthesized from higher molecular weight heparins (molecular weight 15,000). LMWHs have increased bioavailability, resulting in a more stable anticoagulant effect. There are three commonly used LMWHs (Table 25.1):

1 Enoxaparin,
2 Tinzaparin, and
3 Dalteparin

LMWH: dosing and monitoring

Dosing of LMWHs is age-dependent (Table 25.1). Recent publications describing enoxaparin dosing have suggested that age-dependent dose requirements [18] may be higher than suggested in Table 25.1. Dosing guidelines are provided in Table 25.4.

• Enoxaparin doses <10 mg; when LMWH level is subtherapeutic, increasing the dose by 1 mg is suggested and repeat LMWH level.

• Tinzaparin doses <1000 units; when LMWH level is subtherapeutic, increasing the dose by 100 units is suggested and repeat LMWH level.

Dosing in this way allows for more precise measurement and accurate dosing. Enoxaparin may be administered using an insulin syringe as 1 U on an insulin syringe is equivalent to 1 mg Enoxaparin. This ease of measurement may assist in reducing dose measurement errors.

Monitoring LMWH effect can only be performed by using an anti-factor Xa level, as LMWH maximally inhibits the activation of procoagulant factor X.

Table 25.4 LMWH dosing nomogram.

Anti-Xa level (U/mL)	Hold dose?	Dose Δ	Next anti-factor Xa level?
<0.35	No	↑25%	4 hours post next morning dose
0.35–0.49	No	↑10%	4 hours post next morning dose
0.5–1.0	No	0	q1–4 weeks
<1.20	Consider	↓20%	Consider drawing a trough level 10 hours post. If trough <0.5, administer next dose at 20% of previous dose.

Note: For doses of Enoxaparin <10 mg and for Tinzaparin <1000 U, increase or decrease dose by 1 mg or 100 U, respectively.

The influence of LMWH on the activation of factor II is diminutive, and therefore a PTT will not measure LMWH effect. The target anti-factor Xa level on blood samples drawn 2–6 hours post LMWH dose is 0.5–1.0 U/mL.

It is recommended that anti-factor Xa levels be monitored on a monthly basis and dose adjustments be made to maintain an anti-factor Xa (LMWH) level (Table 25.4). This is necessary in the pediatric population, as children often outgrow their current dose or there may be some accumulation over time due to insufficient renal clearance.

LMWH: benefits and limitations

• 95% bioavailability making it a more stable agent.
• Requires less frequent blood monitoring.
• Subcutaneous administration.
• Decreased incidence of HIT.
• Does not interfere with platelet function.
• Caregivers may be taught administration of LMWH.

LMWH: reversal

If anticoagulation with LWMH needs to be terminated for clinical reasons, discontinuation of LMWH injections for 24 hours will usually suffice. If an immediate reversal of effect is required, protamine sulphate reverses 80% of the anti-factor Xa activity of LMWHs.

Oral vitamin K antagonists

The most commonly prescribed oral vitamin K antagonist (VKA) is warfarin with a half-life of 162 hours. Alternatively, in Europe and South America, phenprocoumon is frequently prescribed with a half-life of 140 hours [19].

VKA: metabolism

VKAs prevent gamma carboxylation of vitamin K-dependent procoagulant factors II, VII, IX, and X (Fig. 25.2) [12].

VKAs: dosing and monitoring

• Children have increased dose requirements compared with adults.
• Children with fontan procedures require a decreased loading dose of warfarin (0.1 mg/kg/day) compared with the usual loading dose of 0.2 mg/kg/day with a maximum loading dose of 5 mg [20]. If the INR

Table 25.5 Warfarin dosing nomogram: maintenance phase for target INR 2.5 (2.0–3.0).

INR*	Action
1.1–1.4	Increase dose by 20%.
1.5–1.9	Increase dose by 10%.
2.0–3.0	No change.
3.1–3.5	Decrease dose by 10%.
>3.5–4.0	Administer one dose at 50% less than maintenance dose. Then restart at 20% less than previous maintenance dose.
4.1–5.0	Hold 1 dose then restart at 20% less than previous maintenance dose.
>5.0	Consider reversal.

*This nomogram is intended for use once loading phase is completed. Prior to each dose adjustment, assess patient for medication change, illness (cold, flu), and adherence.

reaches 1.6 within the first 3 days of dosing, the loading dose should be decreased by 50%.
• Dosing nomogram is provided in Table 25.5.
• There are indication-related target INRs extrapolated from adult ranges.
  ○ Systemic thrombosis/pulmonary embolism INR 2.5 (2–3)
  ○ Fontan target INRs can vary upon individual practice between 1.5 and 3.0.
  ○ Mechanical heart valves
    ▪ Aortic valve: target INR 2.5 (2–3)
    ▪ Mitral valve: target INR 3.0 (2.5–3.5)
• Pharmacogenomics are currently ongoing to evaluate single nucleotide polymorphisms in cytochrome P450 2C9 (CYP2C9) and vitamin K epoxide reductase (VKORC1) and their effect on warfarin dose requirements.

Frequent INR monitoring is important as a result of the variability of INRs in children due to the above-mentioned challenges. The side effects associated with oral anticoagulant therapy (bleeding and new or extension of thrombus) increase with poor oral anticoagulant control as reflected by out-of-range INR. The event rate in children requiring oral antithrombotic therapy for varying etiologies is reported to range from 0% to 0.5% per patient year and 0% to 1.3% per patient year for bleeding and thrombosis, respectively [12].

Point-of-care (POC) INR monitoring: a solution to VKA therapy
The use of the POC INR meter represents a solution to effective management of VKA therapy in children. The ease of using a POC INR meter at home facilitates:
• More frequent testing and improved time in therapeutic range as compared with children who perform laboratory INR testing [21].
• The POC INR meter requires a minimal volume blood sample, produces an INR result within 1 minute, enables timely drug dosage adjustment, and allows prompt attention to critical values.
• The POC INR can be performed at the patients' convenience and eliminates the need for the patient to visit the laboratory.
• This convenience facilitates more frequent INR testing [22], a requirement for children when illness is present or when there is a change in diet or medication [12].
• POC INR monitoring provides a solution to the problem of pain associated with venipuncture, difficult venous access, and needle phobias.
• In addition, POC INR meter use is believed to improve quality of life.

For these reasons, POC INR meters are used for INR measurement in children as an option for improving VKA monitoring [21].

VKAs: benefits and limitations
VKAs are administered orally; however, VKA therapy in children is difficult [12] as there is no pediatric formulation available, and children requiring anticoagulant therapy often have:
• Complex underlying health problems that result in frequent reversal for invasive interventions, multiple medication changes, and require illness-associated dose requirements [12].
• Multiple simultaneous medications that interfere with VKA metabolism.
• Inconsistent nutritional intake, such as breast milk that contains little vitamin K, bottled formula with varying amounts of vitamin K, and normal age-appropriate fluctuations in daily intake.
• Increased susceptibility to the common cold and flu as part of normal growth and development.
• Poor venous access that limits monitoring VKAs, which is a narrow therapeutic index drug.

- Anxiety and needle phobias.
- The nonreported use of complementary alternative medications.

In addition, the care of children requiring long-term primary thromboprophylaxis, such as children with congential heart disease (CHD), presents increased challenges, including life-long monitoring (a child with a mechanical heart valve may initiate anticoagulation at age 5 years, whereas an adult may begin VKAs much later in life; this results in many more patient years of anticoagulation). In addition, there are data to strongly suggest that long-term VKA therapy in children may be associated with osteoporosis [23].

VKAs: the challenge of complementary alternative medicines

Complementary alternative medicines (CAMs) include nutritional and dietary supplements. The use of CAMs is highly underreported by children and their families [24]. When children receiving anticoagulation use CAMs, this may influence their level of anticoagulation, resulting in thrombosis or hemorrhage. It is necessary to educate families about CAM use and its potential influence on their child's level of anticoagulation increasing their risk of thrombosis and/or hemorrhage [25].

VKA: reversal

The antidote for warfarin is dependent on whether urgent or nonurgent reversal is necessary. For nonurgent reversal, vitamin K is administered at a dose of 0.5–1 mg orally, depending on the patient's size. The administration of vitamin K either intravenously or intramuscularly has been shown to be less efficacious than orally, as long as gut absorption is not severely compromised. For urgent reversal (major bleeding or interventional procedure), factor VIIa 50 U/kg IV or FFP 20 mL/kg IV is administered.

As described in adults, in children who are considered to be at high risk for thrombosis (i.e. mechanical valves), bridge anticoagulant therapy using heparin may be considered [26].

New agents

Direct thrombin inhibitors, such as argatroban, lepirudin, and bilvalirudin, are approved in many countries for use in adults with confirmed HIT. There are no well-designed studies published describing their use in children. However, there are a few case reports and small cohort studies describing their use.

Danaparoid, a factor Xa inhibitor, is available in many countries with the exception of the United States. Dosing guidelines for children are published elsewhere [12].

Thrombolytic therapy

In the presence of thrombosis that threatens the viability of organ, limb, or life, rapid clot lysis should be strongly considered in the absence of contraindications, such as an elevated PTT and INR, decreased fibrinogen, platelets <100,000, cerebral bleeding, early post-op, or massive bleeding.

The most common agent used is tissue plasminogen activator (tPa) (activase, alteplase; Genentech, San Francisco, CA).

- The doses in the literature range from 0.01 to 0.6 mg/kg/hour for varying amounts of time [12].
- It is important to ensure that plasminogen levels are sufficient to allow thrombolysis. For this reason, in the absence of clinical trials, the use of fresh frozen plasma (10–20 mL/kg IV every 8-12 hours with tPa infusion) as a plasminogen source is recommended prior to/during tPa infusion.

In children, the risk of major hemorrhage is as high as 68% with bleeding requiring transfusion in 39%.

- Serious discussion about the risk/benefit of thrombolytic therapy with other health care professionals and parents/caregivers followed by documentation of the discussion within the patients' medical records should occur prior to use.

Streptokinase, another thrombolytic agent, is not recommended in children due to the potential for anaphylactic reaction secondary to antibody development.

Factor VIIa

Factor VIIa is a recombinant activated blood product that has been used to manage bleeding. There are little data in nonhemophiliac children to support recommendations for its use.

The suggested dosing is 15–30 µg/kg body weight.

Antiplatelet therapy

Antiplatelet therapy is used for a number of indications, although there are no dose finding, safety, and efficacy studies. Common indications include:
• Cardiac (extracardiac palliative shunts, intravascular stents, mechanical aortic valves, kawasaki's disease, following heart transplantation, and others).
• Post organ transplant (heart, liver).

The most common antiplatelets used are aspirin and dipyridamole. There are other agents with some data appearing in the literature. These agents include clopidogrel and abciximab [12].

Antiplatelet therapy: metabolism

Each agent inhibits platelet function by interrupting different metabolic pathways that are important for optimal platelet shape change, adhesion, and aggregation.

Antiplatelet therapy: dosing and monitoring

• Aspirin 1–5 mg/kg/day
• Dipyridamole 2–5 mg/kg/day
• Clopidogrel 0.2 mg/kg/day

There have been various methods used to monitor antiplatelet effect (platelet aggregation, PFA100, accumetrics, TEG®); however, none has been demonstrated to be associated with safety and efficacy outcomes.

Antiplatelet therapy: benefits and limitations

• Monitoring not currently recommended.
• Oral administration.
• Aspirin is associated with gastrointestinal bleeding.

Antiplatelet therapy: reversal

• Discontinuation of therapy is sufficient to clear effect (may take up to 7 days).
• Special consideration should be given to withholding aspirin with fever or exposure to chicken pox due to the small risk of developing Reyes syndrome.
• Immunizations and injections may be administered; however, it is imperative to apply 5 minutes of firm pressure on the injection site to minimize bruising.
• The manufacturer of the varicella vaccine recommends withholding aspirin for 1 week before and 6 weeks following varicella immunization.

Cohorts of children at risk for thrombosis

There are a number of cohorts of children that are identified to be at high risk for venous or arterial thrombosis:
• Children with central lines
  ○ Central venous (CVL)
  ○ Central arterial lines
• Children with congenital heart disease
• Children who undergo organ transplantation

Children with central venous or arterial lines

Systemic venous thromboembolic events in children most often occur due to interaction of multiple risk factors with the presence of a CVL appearing to be one of the strongest risk factors.

Systemic arterial thromboembolic events in children most often occur as a result of the placement of an arterial line or following cardiac catheterization. Thromboprophylaxis during cardiac catheterization using UFH of 50–150 U/kg bolus has been demonstrated to be safe and efficacious in children in a randomized clinical trial [27].

Diagnosis of venous and arterial or intracardiac thrombosis

Clinical symptoms of thrombosis vary depending on the location of the thrombus. For example, a deep venous thrombosis in a limb may be associated with pain, swelling, skin discoloration, and altered perfusion, whereas an intracardiac thrombus may range from asymptomatic to congestive heart failure, pulmonary embolism, or sequelae secondary to an embolus, including stroke, and organ or limb compromise.

Both venous and arterial thromboses require rapid diagnosis and treatment to prevent thrombus extension or embolism, which could result in mortality or morbidity.

Clinical studies have determined that the most sensitive diagnostic methods for diagnosing upper system thrombosis are the ultrasound for jugular venous thrombosis and venography for intrathoracic vessels. For symptomatic thrombosis of both the upper and lower system, ultrasound may be used; however, if the clinical suspicion for thrombosis is high and ultrasound is negative, consideration should be given to further imaging, such as magnetic resonance imaging

(MRI), computed tomography (CT), and/or venography of the suspicious venous or arterial system. There are no studies determining the sensitivity and specificity of these newer imaging techniques in children; however, they are commonly used. The concern in children using diagnostic tests with high radiation doses has resulted in a move toward MRI [28].

Intracardiac thromboses are often incidental findings for children with comprised cardiac function and may be identified through echocardiogram, cardiac catheterization, angiogram, or cardiac MRI or CT.

Duration of antithrombotic therapy for systemic venous thrombosis

Duration and intensity of therapy is based on adult recommendations and may be in excess of what is required in children. Until studies are completed, it is reasonable to base therapy on adult recommendations.

Duration of treatment: systemic venous thrombosis

This depends on several factors:
- Risk factor resolved; 3 months duration.
- Continued risk factor; long-term therapy.
- Idiopathic; minimum 6–12 months of therapy.
- Life-threatening pulmonary embolus; consider thrombectomy or thrombolytic therapy.

There are no data to support the use of routine thromboprophylaxis of CVLs in children.

Some outcomes of systemic venous thrombosis

Postthrombotic syndrome is reported to be approximately 20%. Postthrombotic syndrome is characterized by pain, swelling, and alterations in perfusion that may result in skin ulceration. There is no treatment; however, palliation may include the use of compression stockings.

Frequently there are challenges associated with thrombosis-related loss of venous access that is often required for future procedures or treatment.

Duration of treatment: systemic arterial thrombosis

- Catheter related; immediate removal of the catheter with variable duration of therapy described. Thrombolysis and or thrombectomy may be considered.

- Idiopathic; if life threatening, thrombectomy or thrombolysis would be recommended as initial treatment. Anticoagulation following clot removal has been used in varying doses and duration.

Outcomes of systemic arterial thrombosis

- Loss of life, limb, or organ dependent on thrombus location.
- Alteration of organ function.
- Limb length discrepancy.
- Intermittent claudication secondary to decreased perfusion.

Pulmonary embolism

Pulmonary embolism (PE) is rare in children, and most commonly occur as a result of deep venous thrombosis [29]. The following radiographic tests may be used to diagnose PE in children: ventilation perfusion scan, spiral CT, MRI, MRV, or pulmonary angiogram.

Altered quality of life associated with long-term anticoagulation

Quality of life (QOL) is an abstract entity that can be measured by a questionnaire developed specific to the patient condition. There are a number of characteristics of long-term anticoagulation that may induce treatment dissatisfaction and reduce QOL for children. A validated pediatric QOL inventory for children requiring long-term anticoagulation would assess general constructs that are most salient for this patient population. Identification and systematic evaluation of these constructs is critical to recognizing influences on patient adherence to improve patient care. Once confounders are identified, the "best" management (best QOL associated with best safety and efficacy) for children requiring long-term anticoagulation can be established.

Children with congenital heart disease

CHD is one of the most common inborn defects occurring in 0.8% of newborn infants. Many children with CHD have extracardiac shunts surgically placed as palliation for their condition, including Blalock Taussig shunts, Norwood Sano, Central Right Ventricle to Pulmonary Artery shunts, Glenn shunts, and Fontan shunts. These shunts vary in diameter and flow characteristics and are often considered at increased risk for thrombosis. Although there are no well-designed studies evaluating the use of anticoagulant or antiplatelet agents in this patient population, they are commonly used as thromboprophylaxis [12]. There are a number of other cardiac indications where anticoagulants and/or antiplatelets are used as thromboprophylaxis; however, there are no well-designed studies to provide safety and efficacy data for any therapeutic agent.

Children with mechanical heart valves placed are prescribed long-term VKAs as thromboprophylaxis as per adult guidelines [12].

Children with CHD: duration of antithrombotic therapy

There are no evidence-based guidelines for duration of therapy with the exception of mechanical heart valves (life-long as per adult guidelines). Discussion of duration of therapy based on the available literature may be found in *Chest* 2008 [12].

Children with organ transplantation: liver transplant

Vascular complications at the site of vessel anastamosis are more common in pediatric patients and are demonstrated to be a significant cause of graft loss and patient morbidity. These complications have decreased in recent years due to the use of microsurgical techniques; however:

• Hepatic artery thrombosis is reported as 5–17% [30]. One-third of the patients who develop hepatic artery thrombosis will develop hepatic gangrene and liver failure requiring further high-risk interventions.

• Portal vein thrombosis is reported as high as 33% [30].

There are no properly designed studies investigating the use of antithrombotics or antiplatelet agents for thromboprophylaxis post liver transplant.

Future perspectives

Thrombosis in children occurs as sequelae secondary to quaternary care pediatrics. Currently, there are few properly designed clinical studies to determine the best prevention and treatment in children with or at risk for thrombosis. The complications of thrombosis in children may be catastrophic, and thus therapy is indicated. The incidence of thrombotic complications continues to increase as a result of continued advances in medical and surgical therapy. It is imperative that internationally collaborative clinical studies be performed to determine the best diagnostic, treatment, and preventative measures for thrombosis in children. New agents have significant potential due to ease of administration and stable metabolism, resulting in the lack of the need for monitoring. Studies evaluating the use of new agents in children are in the early phases and may provide new options for therapy.

References

1 Satter E. *How to Get Your Kid to Eat - But Not Too Much*. Boulder, CO: Bull Publishing Company, 1987.

2 Andrew M, Vegh P, Johnston M, Bowker J, Ofosu F, Mitchell L. Maturation of the hemostatic system during childhood. *Blood* 1992;80(8):1998–2005.

3 Kuhle S, Massicotte PM. Maturation of the coagulation system during childhood. *Prog Pediatr Cardiol* 2005;21(1):3–7.

4 Massicotte MP, Sofronas M, deVeber G. Difficulties in performing clinical trials of antithrombotic therapy in neonates and children. *Thromb Res* 2006;118(1):153–63.

5 Rajasekhar D, Barnard MR, Bednarek FJ, Michelson AD. Platelet hyporeactivity in very low birth weight neonates. *Thromb Haemost* 1997;77(5):1002–7.

6 Barnes C, Newall F, Furmedge J, Mackay M, Monagle P. Arterial ischaemic stroke in children. *J Paediatr Child Health* 2004;40(7):384–7.

7 Randolph AG, Cook DJ, Gonzalez CA, Andrew M. Benefit of heparin in central venous and pulmonary artery catheters: a meta-analysis of randomized controlled trials. *Chest* 1998;113(1):165–71.

8 Biss TT, Brandaao LR, Kahr WH, Chan AK, Williams S. Clinical features and outcome of pulmonary embolism in children. *Br J Haematol* 2008;142(5):808–18.

9 Monreal M, Davant E. Thrombotic complications of central venous catheters in cancer patients. *Acta Haematol* 2001;106(1–2):69–72.

10 Goldenberg NA. Long-term outcomes of venous thrombosis in children. *Curr Opin Hematol* 2005;12(5):370–6.

11 Ansell J, Hirsh J, Hylek E, Jacobson A, Crowther M, Palareti G. Pharmacology and management of the vitamin K antagonists: American College of Chest

Physicians Evidence-Based Clinical Practice Guidelines (8th Edition). *Chest* 2008;133(6 Suppl):160S–98S.

12 Monagle P, Chan A, Massicotte P, Chalmers E, Michelson AD. Antithrombotic therapy in neonates and children: the Eighth ACCP Conference on Antithrombotic and Thrombolytic Therapy. *Chest* 2008;133(6 Suppl): 645S–87S.

13 Hirsh J, Bauer KA, Donati MB, Gould M, Samama MM, Weitz JI. Parenteral anticoagulants: American College of Chest Physicians Evidence-Based Clinical Practice Guidelines (8th Edition). *Chest* 2008;133(6 Suppl); 141S–59S) [Published erratum in *Chest* 2008;134(2): 473.]

14 Ignjatovic V, Summerhayes R, Gan A, et al. Monitoring unfractionated heparin (UFH) therapy: which anti factor Xa assay is appropriate? Thromb Res 2007;120(3): 347–51.

15 Warkentin TE, Sheppard JI, Moore JC, Sigouin CS, Kelton JG. Quantitative interpretation of optical density measurements using PF4-dependent enzyme-immunoassays. *J Thromb Haemost* 2008;6(8):1304–12.

16 Kuhle S, Massicotte P, Dinyari M, et al. Dose-finding and pharmacokinetics of therapeutic doses of tinzaparin in pediatric patients with thromboembolic events. *Thromb Haemost* 2005;94(6):1164–71.

17 Hirsch J, Warkenton T, Shaughnessy S. Heparin and low molecular weight heparin. Mechanism of action, pharmacokinetics, dosing, monitoring, efficacy, and safety. *Chest* 2001;119:64S–94S.

18 Malowany J, Knoppert D, Chan A, Pepelassis D, Lee D. Enoxaparin use in the neonatal intesnive care unit: experience over 8 years. *Pharmacotherapy* 2007;27(9): 1263–71.

19 Hirsh J, Dalen J, Anderson DR, et al. Oral anticoagulants: mechanism of action, clinical effectiveness, and optimal therapeutic range. *Chest* 2001;119(1 Suppl):8S–21S.

20 Crowther MA, Ginsberg JB, Kearon C, et al. A random-ized trial comparing 5-mg and 10-mg warfarin loading doses. *Arch Intern Med* 1999;159(1):46–8.

21 Newall F, Monagle P, Johnston L. Home INR monitoring of oral anticoagulant therapy in children using the CoaguChek trademark S point-of-care monitor and a robust education program. *Thromb Res* 2006;118(5): 587–93.

22 Bauman ME, Conroy S, Massicotte MP. Point-of-care INR measurement in children requiring warfarin: what has been evaluated and future directions. *Pediatr Health* 2008;2(5):651–9.

23 Barnes C, Newall F, Ignjatovic V, et al. Reduced bone density in children on long-term warfarin. *Pediatr Res* 2005;57(4):578–81.

24 McCann LJ, Newell SJ. Survey of paediatric complementary and alternative medicine use in health and chronic illness. Arch Dis Child 2006;91(2):173–4.

25 Smith LFP, Ernst E, Ewings P, Myers P, Smith C. Co-ingestion of herbal medicines and warfarin. *Br J Gen Pract* 2004;54(503):439–41.

26 Douketis JD, Berger PB, Dunn AS, et al. The perioperative management of antithrombotic therapy: American College of Chest Physicians evidence-based clinical practice guidelines (8th edition). *Chest* 2008;133(6 Suppl):299S–339S.

27 Freed MD, Keane JF, Rosenthal A. The use of heparinization to prevent arterial thrombosis after percutaneous cardiac catheterization in children. *Circulation* 1974;50(3):565–9.

28 Frush DP, Goske MJ, Hernanz-Schulman M. Computed tomography and radiation exposure [5]. *N Engl J Med* 2008;358(8):851.

29 Babyn PS, Gahunia HK, Massicotte P. Pulmonary thromboembolism in children. *Pediatr Radiol* 2005; 35(3):258–74.

30 Aw MM, Phua KB, Ooi BC, et al. Outcome of liver transplantation for children with liver disease. *Singapore Med J* 2006;47(7):595–8.

Introduction

Thrombotic and bleeding problems are common problems in the intensive care unit (ICU). The management of bleeding, massive blood loss, and disseminated intravascular coagulation are covered elsewhere in this book, whereas this chapter covers the prevention and acute management of venous thromboembolism, the thrombotic microangiopathies, heparin-induced thrombocytopenia, thrombocytopenia and thrombocytosis, sepsis, and SERS.

Thrombocytosis

Thrombocytosis is defined, as a platelet count of greater than $450 \times 10^9/L$. Reactive thrombocytosis is common in ICU patients, particularly in association with surgery or trauma, hemorrhage, acute and chronic infection, malignancy, iron deficiency anemia, inflammatory disease, and post splenectomy. The platelet count does not usually exceed $1000 \times 10^9/L$ in reactive thrombocytosis. Differential diagnoses include myeloproliferative disorders, such as essential thrombocythemia, chronic idiopathic myelofibrosis, and polycythemia vera. A blood film and even assessment of JAK-2 status may be helpful in discriminating an underlying malignancy in difficult cases. If a patient is not actively bleeding, thromboprophylaxis with aspirin 75 mg daily is appropriate as there is an increased risk of thrombosis with thrombocytosis [1].

Thrombocytopenia

Patients with thrombocytopenia may have petechiae, purpura, and bruising or frank hemorrhage. A full blood count and blood film will confirm a low platelet count and the presence or absence of other diagnostic features, such as red cell fragmentation, platelet morphological abnormalities, or evidence of dysplasia or hematinic deficiency.

Thrombocytopenia may arise because of:
- decreased platelet production,
- increased platelet destruction, and/or
- sequestration in the spleen.

It occurs in up to 20% of medical and 35% of surgical admissions to ICU and may be multifactorial. Table 26.1 lists the differential diagnoses of thrombocytopenia in the ICU setting. There is an inverse relationship between severity of sepsis and platelet count.

Platelet clumping

Patients with sepsis may develop ethylene diaminetetraacetic acid (EDTA)-dependent antibodies, which cause platelet clumping ex vivo, resulting in pseudothrombocytopenia. If platelet clumping is seen on a blood film, a fresh sample should be taken into an alternative anticoagulant, such as citrate.

Patients with sepsis

Immune mechanisms
Nonimmune destruction of platelets occurs in sepsis. Immune mechanisms may also contribute, with nonspecific platelet-associated antibodies detected in up to 30% of ICU patients. It is thought that IgG binds to bacterial products on the platelet surface or to an altered platelet surface. A subset of patients with platelet-associated antibodies also have autoantibodies directed against glycoprotein IIb/IIIa [i.e. they have

Table 26.1 Differential diagnosis of thrombocytopenia in the ICU setting.

Pseudothrombocytopenia
    Clotted blood sample
    EDTA-dependent antibodies

Drugs
    Heparin, including HAT and HITT
    IIb/IIIa inhibitors (abciximab, eptifibatide, tirofiban)
    Adenosine diphosphate (ADP) receptor antagonists
        (clopidogrel)
    Acute alcohol toxicity

Sepsis
Disseminated intravascular coagulation
Massive blood loss—a dilutional thrombocytopenia

Post cardiopulmonary bypass
    Intra-aortic balloon pump

Renal dialysis
    Immune thrombocytopenic purpura (ITP)

Antiphospholipid syndrome
    Thrombotic thrombocytopenic purpura (TTP)
    Hemolytic uremic syndrome (HUS)
    Hypersplenism
    Hematinic deficiency, particularly acute folate deficiency

Pregnancy-associated thrombocytopenia
    Benign gestational thrombocytopenia
    Postpartum HUS
    HELLP
    Preeclampsia

Myelodysplastic syndrome
Carcinoma
Post-transfusion purpura
Hereditary thrombocytopenia

idiopathic thrombocytopenic purpura (ITP)]. Unfortunately tests for platelet-specific IgG are nonspecific and do not help in the management of septic patients. Bone marrow hemophagocytosis is a common finding in septic thrombocytopenic patients. The marrow is often hypocellular with reduced megakaryocyte numbers.

Nonimmune mechanisms

Other causes of thrombocytopenia should be sought in a critically ill patient. Thrombocytopenia may occur as:

• a complication of heparin treatment. A mild thrombocytopenia of no clinical significance may be seen in the first few days of heparin therapy—heparin associated thrombocytopenia (HAT).
• This should be differentiated from heparin-induced thrombocytopenic thrombosis (HIT; see below).
• Dilutional thrombocytopenia may occur after trauma or complex surgery.
• Acute folate deficiency has been described in ICU patients.
• Preexisting disease, such as ITP, cancer, hypersplenism, and myelodysplastic syndrome, may contribute to a low platelet count.

Consumptive coagulopathy is associated with an elevated INR, APTT, thrombin time, D-dimer, and a reduced fibrinogen.

Thresholds for therapy

British Society for Haematology [2] and other guidelines suggest a platelet threshold of $10 \times 10^9/L$ for platelet transfusion in thrombocytopenic patients without additional risk factors, such as sepsis, concurrent antibiotic use, or other abnormalities of hemostasis.

Patients with chronic sustained failure of platelet production, such as myelodysplasia or aplastic anemia, may remain free from serious hemorrhage with platelet counts below $5–10 \times 10^9/L$.

As standard platelet counts are produced by cell counters that categorize by size, an immunoplatelet count is occasionally helpful in providing a "true" platelet count by labeling platelet antigens [3]. Long-term prophylactic platelet transfusions may lead to alloimmunization, platelet refractoriness, and other complications of transfusion.

Procedures

For procedures such as lumbar puncture, epidural anesthesia, gastroscopy and biopsy, insertion of indwelling lines, trans-bronchial biopsy, liver biopsy, and laparotomy, the platelet count should be raised to at least 50×10^9/L. For operations on critical sites, such as the brain or eyes, recommendations are for a platelet count of 75–100 $\times 10^9$/L.

Antiplatelet therapy

Drugs known to have antiplatelet activity should be withdrawn. Any underlying disorder associated with platelet dysfunction, such as uremia, should be treated if possible. The hematocrit should be corrected to >0.30 in those with renal failure. The use of DDAVP can be considered.

Massive transfusion

In massive blood loss, the platelet count is preserved until relatively late. A platelet count of around 50 $\times$ 10^9/L is expected when red cell concentrates equivalent to two blood volumes have been transfused. The platelet count should be maintained above 50×10^9/L in patients with acute bleeding. A higher target of 100×10^9/L is recommended for those with multiple trauma or central nervous system injury.

Disseminated intravascular coagulopathy (DIC)

Platelet transfusions are indicated in acute DIC when there is bleeding associated with thrombocytopenia. Management of the underlying disorder and coagulation factor replacement are also required. Frequent full blood count and coagulation screening tests should be carried out, and the platelet count maintained above 50×10^9/L. Platelet transfusions should not be given simply to correct a low platelet count in chronic DIC in the absence of bleeding.

Immune thrombocytopenia

In patients with ITP, platelet transfusions are reserved for patients with life-threatening gastrointestinal, genitourinary, or central nervous system bleeding or other bleeding associated with severe thrombocytopenia. In ITP, the residual platelets tend to be young and have good hemostatic effect, so patients tend not to bleed unless the platelet count is very low. Platelet transfusions may not produce an incremental rise in patients with ITP due to the effect of the platelet antibodies on the donor platelets. IV methylprednisolone, IVIg or anti-D (only to be used in the Rhesus-positive patients

who have a spleen) can be given to produce platelet increments [4]. The emerging thrombopoeitic agents may gain a place in the future management of acute ITP.

Post-transfusion purpura

Post-transfusion purpura is due to the presence of a platelet specific allo-antibody [usually anti-human platelet antigen-1a (HPA-1a)] in the recipient, which reacts with donor platelets, destroying them and also the recipient's own platelets. High dose IVIg (2g/kg given over 2 or 5 days) is used in the treatment of post-transfusion purpura, with responses in about 85% of patients. Large doses of platelet transfusions may be required to control severe bleeding before there is a response to IVIg. There is limited evidence that HPA-1a-negative platelets are more effective than those from random donors [5].

The thrombotic microangiopathies

Profound thrombocytopenia and microangiopathic hemolytic anemia characterize thrombotic microangiopathy, which includes three major disorders: thrombotic thrombocytopenic purpura (TTP), hemolytic uremic syndrome (HUS), and HELLP syndrome (Haemolysis, Elevated Liver function tests and Low Platelets). The hemolysis is due to the breakdown of red cells as they pass over areas of thrombosis.

Thrombotic thrombocytopenic purpura (TTP)

TTP is a clinical diagnosis characterized by:
• thrombocytopenia,
• microangiopathic hemolytic anemia,
• fluctuating neurological signs,
• renal impairment, and
• fever.

Excessive platelet aggregation results in platelet microvascular thrombi, which particularly affect the cerebral circulation. This is mediated by ultra-large von Willebrand factor (vWF) multimers due to a deficiency of vWF cleaving protease (vWF-CP), also known as ADAMTS13. Deficiency of vWF-CP activity may be genetic due to absence of the enzyme or acquired due to the presence of an autoantibody to vWF-CP. Cirrhosis, acute inflammation, DIC, and malignancy have all been associated with reduced VWF-CP activity but do not cause TTP.

TTP is characterized by:
• severe thrombocytopenia.
• Red cell fragments may be absent from the peripheral blood in the first 24–48 hours following clinical presentation.
• Coagulation profiles are usually normal.

Secondary DIC due to prolonged tissue ischemia is an ominous prognostic indicator.

Many specialized units now measure levels of vWF-CP and its inhibitor to confirm the diagnosis of TTP, but results are not available quickly. Thus, if a case of TTP is suspected, they must be treated immediately and the diagnosis must be confirmed or refuted retrospectively. Renal or skin biopsy performed after recovery of the thrombocytopenia may also aid retrospective diagnosis. There is a prominent arteriolar and capillary thrombosis with thrombi, largely composed of platelets, which stain strongly for VWF. This contrasts with HUS, where the primary histological changes are glomerular, and arteriolar fibrin thrombi and subendothelial widening of the glomerular capillary wall.

Factors that may precipitate TTP

These include drugs, autoimmune disease, malignancy, and infection and are listed in Table 26.2. In some series, up to 14% of TTP episodes have been associated increasingly with HIV infection, with the greatest risk at CD4 counts of less than 250×10^9/L. E. coli O157:H7 is more closely linked with HUS, but there have been cases with typical TTP features.

A panel of investigations required in a suspected case of TTP includes:
• FBC and film (Plate 26.1),
• Reticulocyte count,
• Clotting screen including fibrinogen and D-dimers,
• Urea and electrolytes,
• Liver function tests,
• Lactate dehydrogenase,
• Urinalysis,
• Direct antiglobulin test, and
• HIV and hepatitis serology.

Table 26.2 TTP precipitating factors.

Drugs	Autoimmune disease
Oral contraceptives	Systemic lupus erythematosis
Ticlopidine	
Ciclosporin	Malignancy
Mitomycin C	Pregnancy
Infection	Post–bone marrow transplantation
HIV	

Immediate treatment (plasma exchange)

If a patient presents with signs suggestive of TTP (i.e. those with neurological signs and a microangiopathic haemolytic anemia and thrombocytopenia in the absence of any other identifiable cause), it is increasingly being recognized that delay in treatment may result in sudden death due to thrombotic occlusion of the coronary arteries [6].

Single volume daily plasma exchange should be commenced within 24 hours. Theoretically, plasma exchanges using cryosupernatant or solvent–detergent prepared FFP may be more efficacious than using standard fresh frozen, although there are no clinical data to support this currently. Both cryosupernatant and solvent–detergent prepared FFP are deficient in highmolecular-weight VWF multimeric forms and thus may be less likely to stimulate further thrombosis. Daily plasma exchange should continue for a minimum of 2 days after complete remission. Platelet transfusions are contraindicted.

Concomitant therapy

Adjuvant corticosteroid therapy with pulsed methylprednisolone 1 g IV daily for 3 days can be considered. Low-dose aspirin (75 mg daily) should be commenced on platelet recovery (platelet counts >50×10^9/L). Red cell transfusion should be administered according to clinical need. Folate supplementation is required in all patients. Platelet transfusions are contraindicated in TTP unless there is life-threatening hemorrhage. Hepatitis vaccination is recommended [7].

Refractory disease

In the presence of refractory disease, intensification of plasma exchange should be considered. The use of

Ritoximab is emerging as a major advance in the management of acquired TTP. Having gained a place in salvaging patients not responding to plasma exchange, there is some evidence to suggest it induces faster remissions when it has been used early in the course of the disease [8].

In refractory TTP, advice should be sought from a specialist in this field. Vincristine 1 mg repeated every 3–4 days or intensive immunosuppression using either cyclosporin or cyclophosphamide has been used in severe refractory or recurrent TTP. Protein A column immunoabsorption may be considered. Urgent self-referral is advised if a patient develops symptoms suggestive of relapse. Splenectomy may reduce the risk of relapse.

Mortality

Prior to the advent of plasma exchange, mortality rates were in excess of 90%. With prompt plasma exchange, the mortality has fallen to 10–30%. Thirty-five percent do not have neurological involvement at presentation, but a reduced level of consciousness has been identified as a poor prognostic indicator with an overall survival of 54%. The average number of plasma exchange procedures required for remission was 15.8 (range 3–36) in one series.

HHUS

HUS is characterized by:
- microangiopathic hemolytic anemia,
- thrombocytopenia, and
- renal failure.

There may be associated multiorgan disease, including enterocolitis, neurological complications, liver, and pancreatic and cardiac dysfunction.

The epidemic form (D$^+$) is associated with:
- a prodromal illness,
- bloody diarrhea, and
- enterotoxin enterococcal (VTEC) infection.

Rare sporadic or atypical cases have:
- no prodrome, and
- may be associated with HIV, cytomegalovirus, or bacterial infection.

Secondary causes of HUS include:
- post–solid-organ or -bone marrow transplantation,
- drug exposure (pentostatin, cyclosporine, mitomycin C, heroin, and quinine),
- malignancy, and
- Systemic lupus erythematosus.

However, approximately 50% of HUS cases are associated with a mutation in one or more genes coding for proteins involved in regulation or activation of the alternative pathway of complement, such as factor H deficiency [9].

Laboratory investigations

Early stool culture is essential for the diagnosis of VTEC-associated HUS (*E. coli* 0157:H7) [10]. Other investigations are as for TTP.

Treatment of HUS

Management involves meticulous fluid and electrolyte balance and blood pressure control, with renal dialysis as required. Antimotility drugs and antibiotic treatment adversely affect the outcome and should be avoided. At present, there is no conclusive evidence that either FFP or plasma exchange improves outcome. Adjuvant treatment with antiplatelet agents, anticoagulation, antifibrinolytics, or IVIg is not recommended.

HELLP

HELLP is diagnosed by the presence of:
- hemolysis,
- elevated liver function tests, and
- thrombocytopenia

in the second and third trimesters of pregnant or postpartum woman.

It occurs in up to 10% of women with severe preeclampsia. Severe thrombocytopenia and abnormal liver function tests can occur in the absence of significant hypertension or proteinuria. Exacerbations may occur postpartum, and there is a recurrence risk of approximately 3% in subsequent pregnancies. HELLP occasionally presents postpartum, usually within 48 hours, but rarely as late as 6 days after delivery.

Common presenting symptoms include:
- nausea,
- malaise,
- epigastric or right upper quadrant abdominal pain,
- and edema.

Table 26.3 Differential diagnosis of pregnancy-associated thrombotic microangiopathy.

Diagnosis	Classic TTP	Postpartum HUS	HELLP	Preeclampsia
Time of onset	Usually <24 weeks	Postpartum	Usually >34 weeks	Usually >34 weeks
Histopathology of lesions	Widespread platelet thrombi	Thrombi in renal glomeruli only	Hepatocyte necrosis and fibrin deposition in periportal sinusoids	Glomerular endothelial hypertrophy and occlusion of placental vessels
Haemolysis	+++	++	++	+
Thrombocytopenia	+++	++	++	++
Coagulopathy	−	−	+/−	+/−
CNS symptoms	+++	+/−	+/−	+/−
Liver disease	+/−	++	+	+
Renal disease	+/−	+++	+	+
Hypertension	Rare	+/−	+/−	+++
Effect on fetus	Placental infarct can lead to IUGR and mortality	None, if maternal disease is controlled	Associated with placental ischemia and increased neonatal mortality	IUGR, occasional mortality
Effect on delivery	None	None	Recovery, but may worsen transiently	Recovery, but may worsen transiently
Management	Early plasma exchange	Supportive care +/− plasma exchange	Supportive, consider plasma exchange if persists	Supportive +/− plasma exchange

A neonatal mortality of 10–20% is attributed to placental ischemia. The maternal death rate is less than 1%. Delivery is the treatment of choice and is usually followed by complete recovery within 24–48 hours, although occasionally signs can persist for much longer.

Differential diagnosis

The differential diagnosis of pregnancy-associated thrombotic microangiopathy is shown in Table 26.3. Fever rarely occurs in HELLP and may be a useful distinguishing feature. Revision of a diagnosis of preeclampsia must be made when a thrombotic microangiopathy fails to resolve postpartum. There are no diagnostic assays. The differentiation of the thrombotic microangiopathies is based on history, physical examination, and routine laboratory studies [7,11].

Sepsis and the Systemic Inflammatory Response Syndrome (SIRS)

Sepsis constitutes the systemic inflammatory response to infection. It is the host response rather than the na-

ture of the pathogen that is the major determinant of patient outcome.

SIRS is manifested by two or more of the following:
- temperature >38°C or <36°C,
- heart rate >90 beats/minute,
- respiratory rate >20 breaths/minute or $PaCO_2$ <4.3 kPa, or
- white cell count >12 × 10^9/L, <4 × 10^9/L, or >10% immature forms.

Sepsis is defined as:
- SIRS resulting from documented infection.

Severe sepsis is associated with:
- organ dysfunction,
- hypoperfusion or hypotension, and
- a mortality rate of 30–50%.

Septic shock is defined as:
- severe sepsis with hypotension (systolic BP <90 mm Hg or a reduction of >40 mm Hg from baseline),
- in the absence of other causes for hypertension or inotropic or vasopressor treatment, and
- despite adequate fluid resuscitation.

Coagulation is activated in most patients with severe sepsis as evidenced by:

• elevated markers of thrombin turnover, such as thrombin–antithrombin complexes and prothrombin fragment $1 + 2$.

• Similarly, fibrinolysis is increased with elevated levels of D-dimer.

• Decreased protein C and antithrombin levels due to consumption are also common.

• Activation of coagulation may lead to depletion of circulating clotting factors and secondary DIC.

Treatment of SIRS

Recombinant human activated protein C (APC; Drotrecogin alfpha, activated) was licensed for adjunctive treatment of severe sepsis with multiorgan failure in 2001. It has anti-inflammatory, antithrombotic, and fibrinolytic properties. In the PROWESS trial [12], it was given as a continuous intravenous infusion and decreased absolute mortality of severely septic patients by 6.1%, resulting in a 19.4% relative reduction in mortality. The absolute reduction in mortality increases to 13% if the population treated is restricted to patients with an APACHE II (acute physiology and chronic ill health evaluation) score greater than 24.

The most frequent and serious side effect is bleeding. Severe bleeds increased from 2% in patients given placebo to 3.5% in patients receiving drotrecogin alpha. The risk of bleeding was only increased during the drug infusion time, and returned to placebo levels within 24 hours of stopping the infusion. Patients with a platelet count of $<30 \times 10^9$/L were excluded from the trials. Subsequent trials have been less favorable, and a recent study suggested the absence of a beneficial treatment effect, coupled with an increased incidence of serious bleeding suggest it should not be used in those with sepsis who are at low risk of death, such as those with single organ failure or an APACHE II score less than 25 [13].

Sequential Organ Failure Assessment (SOFA) score

SOFA is a scoring system to evaluate the severity of critically ill patients in the ICU. A severity score

Table 26.4 The SOFA score.

System	Description	Score
Respiratory system PaO_2/FiO_2 in mm Hg	$<400 \pm$ respiratory support	1
	$<300 \pm$ respiratory support	2
	<200 and respiratory support	3
	<100 and respiratory support	4
Cardiovascular system	MAP <70 mm Hg	1
Vasopressors in gamma/kg/ minute	Dopamine ≤ 5 or dobutamine	2
	Dopamine >5 or epi/norepinephrine ≤ 0.1	3
	Dopamine >15 or Epi/ Norepinephrine >0.1	4
Liver	20–32	1
Bilirubin µM/L	33–101	2
	102–204	3
	>204	4
Renal	100–170	1
Creatinine in µM/L or urine output in mL/day	171–299	2
	300–440 or <500 mL per day	3
	>440 or <200 mL/day	4
Coagulation	101–150	1
Platelets $\times 10^9$/L	51–100	2
	21–50	3
	<20	4
Glasgow coma score	13–14	1
	10–12	2
	6–9	3
	<6	4

is needed in clinical research studies to standardize reports, improve the understanding of the course of disease, and allow evaluation of new treatments. Estimates of morbidity serve as a reliable indicator of intensive care performance, allllowing comparison between medical centers, cost/benefit analyses, and evaluation of new therapeutic or management modalities.

The SOFA score has been designed to report morbidity and to objectively quantify the degree of dysfunction/failure of each organ daily in critically ill patients (see Table 26.4).

HIT

HIT is a transient drug-induced autoimmune pro-thrombotic disorder initiated by heparin. Heparin exposure can induce the formation of pathogenic IgG antibodies that cause platelet activation by recognizing complexes of platelet factor 4 (PF4) and heparin on platelet surfaces. Platelet activation results in thrombocytopenia and thrombin generation, with an increased risk of venous and arterial thrombosis [14].

HIT antibodies are directed against multiple neoepitope sites. Only a minority of PF4/heparin-reactive HIT sera activate platelets in vitro. Some HIT-IgG recognize PF4 bound to solid phase even in the absence of heparin. PF4 antibodies usually decline to undetectable levels within a few weeks or months of an episode of HIT, and there is no anamnestic response.
- The frequency of HIT varies widely depending on the type of heparin used and the patient group.
- Unfractionated heparin is associated with a higher incidence of HIT than fractionated heparin.
- Surgical patients have a higher frequency of HIT than either medical or obstetric patients with the same heparin exposure.
- Postoperative orthopedic patients receiving unfractionated heparin have the highest HIT frequency (up to 5%) and require more intense platelet count monitoring than pregnant women receiving LMWH, who have an almost negligible risk.

Laboratory diagnosis

HIT antibodies are detected using either:
- commercially available PF4-dependent antigen immunoassays, or
- functional assays of platelet activation and aggregation.

Clinically insignificant HIT antibodies are common in patents that have received heparin 5–100 days earlier. In the ICU setting, HIT is uncommon (0.3–0.5%), whereas thrombocytopenia from other causes is very common (30–50%).

For laboratory diagnosis of HIT antibodies, both antigen assays and functional (platelet activation) assays are available. Both tests are very sensitive (high negative predictive value) but specificity is poor, especially for the antigen assays, which will also detect nonpathogenic immunoglobulin M and immunoglob-ulin A class antibodies. Detection of immunoglobulin M or immunoglobulin A antibodies could potentially lead to adverse events, such as bleeding, if a false diagnosis of HIT prompts replacement of heparin by an alternative anticoagulant. Dosing regimens of the direct thrombin inhibitors are too high, especially in ICU patients. Assays of platelet activation are technically demanding, time consuming, and not available in some centers. Testing should be performed when HIT is clinically suspected.

Clinical diagnosis

The diagnosis of HIT should be based on:
- clinical abnormalities (thrombocytopenia with or without thrombosis), and
- a positive test for HIT antibodies, as outlined in Table 26.5.

Isolated HIT is the occurrence of thrombocytopenia without thrombosis. Retrospective cohort studies indicate that 25–50% of these patients develop clinically overt thrombosis after stopping heparin, usually within the first week. Subclinical thrombosis was found in 8 of 16 patients who underwent routine lower-limb duplex ultrasonography for isolated HIT. Early heparin cessation alone does not reduce the risk of thrombosis in patients with isolated HIT, so alternative anticoagulation is required.

About 25% of HIT patients receiving a heparin bolus develop signs or symptoms, such as fever, chills, respiratory distress, or hypertension. Transient global amnesia and cardiorespiratory arrest have also been reported. About 5–15% of HIT patients develop decompensated DIC.

Thombocytopenia does not usually develop until day 5–10 of heparin treatment and reaches a median nadir of 55×10^9/L. The platelet count falls below 150×10^9/L in around 90% of HIT cases. Hemorrhage and platelet counts below 10×10^9/L suggest an alternative cause, such as post-transfusion purpura. Patients who have received heparin within the last 100 days may have a fall in platelet count within one day of reexposure to heparin.

Treatment of HIT

Heparin should be stopped immediately, and not repeated, in those who develop thrombocytopenia or

Table 26.5 HIT diagnosis based on clinical and laboratory abnormalities.

Clinical	Laboratory
Thrombocytopenia (fall of >50%) with or without any of the following	A PAA using washed platelets Serotonin release assay Heparin-induced platelet activation test Microparticles by flow cytometry

A Venous thrombosis
  Coumarin-induced limb necrosis
  Deep vein thrombosis
  Pulmonary embolus
  Cerebral venous thrombosis
  Adrenal hemorrhagic infarction
	B PGA using citrated platelet-rich plasma

B Arterial thrombosis
  Lower limb thrombosis
  Cerebrovascular accident
  Myocardial infarction
  Other
	C Antigen assay
	  PF4/heparin-enzyme immunoassay (EIA)
	  PF4/polyvinyl sulphonate-EIA
	  PF4-dependent EIA detecting HIT IgG
	  Fluid phase EIA
	  Particle gel immunoassay

C Skin lesions
  Skin lesion at heparin injection site
  Skin necrosis
  Erythematous plaques	

D Acute systemic reaction to heparin	
E Hypofibrinogenemia secondary to DIC	

Abbreviations: PAA, platelet activation assay; PGA, platelet aggregation assay.

the original platelet count falls by 50%. Recent data indicate that, as HIT is strongly associated with thrombosis (odds ratio 12–40), an alternative anticoagulant should be commenced. For treatment of HIT, three alternative anticoagulants are approved: the direct thrombin inhibitors, lepirudin and argatroban, and the heparinoid, danaparoid (not approved in the United States). Prophylactic platelet transfusions are relatively contraindicated. Therapeutic doses of anticoagulants are recommended even in the absence of thrombosis.

Lepirudin (Refludan), a recombinant hirudin, is licensed for anticoagulation in HIT patients. The dose is adjusted according to the APTT and is 400 µg/kg initially by slow intravenous injection, followed by a continuous intravenous infusion of 150 µg/kg/hour (max. 16.5 mg/hour), adjusted to maintain the APTT between 1.5 and 2.5 times baseline. The APTT should be measured 4 hours after the start of treatment or after the infusion rate is altered, and then at least once daily. As lepirudin is renally excreted, the initial dose should be reduced by 50%, and subsequent doses by 50–85% in patients with mild renal impairment. Although the BNF (British National Formulary) advises that lepirudin should be avoided in severe renal failure, it has been used in severe renal failure or hemodialysis at a dose of 0.005–0.01 mg/kg/hour without initial bolus, with subsequent dose adjustment according to the APTT.

Argatroban is another alternative anticoagulant for use in HIT patients but is rarely used. It is a direct thrombin inhibitor, has hepatobiliary excretion, and increases the INR. The dose is 2 mg/kg/minute, without an initial bolus. An APTT target range of 1.5–3.0 times baseline is required. The dose must be reduced in liver failure. As argatroban increases the INR, a higher than ususal therapeutic target INR during warfarin co-therapy should be used.

Danaparoid sodium (Orgaran) is a heparinoid which may be used in HIT patients providing there is no evidence of cross-reactivity. Danaproid does not cross the placenta but is renally metabolized. It is given by intravenous injection at a dose of 2500 U (1250 U if body weight <55 kg, 3750 U if >90 kg), followed by an intravenous infusion of 400 U/hour for 2 hours, then 300 U per hour for 2 hours, then 200 U per hour for 5 days. Anti-Xa target range is between 0.5 and 0.8 anti-Xa U/mL and should be monitored in those with renal impairment or a body weight of over 90 kg. Danaproid given by subcutaneous injection has 100% bioavailability. The 24-hour intravenous dose can be divided into two or three daily injections.

Fondaparinux is a pentasaccharide that potentiates antithrombin and has anti-Xa activity. Despite being a synthetic heparin derivative, it does not generate HITT antibodies and has been used safely in those with suspected or confirmed HITT.

There is a 5–20% frequency of new thrombosis despite treatment of HIT patients with an alternative anticoagulant.

The current American College of Chest Physician guidelines [14] recommend that patients who are receiving heparin or have received heparin within the previous 2 weeks, they should be investigated for a diagnosis of HIT if the platelet count falls by ≥50%, and/or a thrombotic event occurs, between days 5 and 14 (inclusive) following initiation of heparin, even if the patient is no longer receiving heparin therapy when thrombosis or thrombocytopenia has occurred (Grade 1C). For patients with strongly suspected (or confirmed) HIT, whether or not complicated by thrombosis, we recommend use of an alternative, nonheparin anticoagulant [danaparoid (Grade 1B), lepirudin (Grade 1C), argatroban (Grade 1C), fondaparinux (Grade 2C), or bivalirudin (Grade 2C)] over the further use of unfractionated heparin (UFH) or low-molecular-weight heparin (LMWH) therapy or initiation/continuation of vitamin K antagonists (Grade 1B).

Management of thromboembolism in ICU

Massive pulmonary embolism

Venous thromboembolism (VTE) is an important cause of morbidity and mortality in ICU patients. Among patients who died in ICU, pulmonary emboli (PE) were reported in 7–27% of postmortem examinations. The mortality rate for PE is <8% when the condition is recognized and treated, but approximately 30% when untreated.

Massive PE has a mortality of 18–33% and may present with shock, dyspnea, and confusion. In patients with massive PE and hemodynamic instability, rapid risk assessment is paramount and bedside echocardiography has become the most popular tool. Multislice chest computed tomography (CT) is also useful for identifying patients who may benefit from thrombolysis or embolectomy. Cardiac biomarkers, including troponin and the natriuretic peptides, are sensitive markers of right ventricular function. Low levels of troponin, B-type natriuretic peptide (BNP), and NT-terminal proBNP are all highly sensitive assays for identifying patients with an uneventful clinical course. Multislice chest CT is not only useful to diagnose or exclude PE; it also is useful for risk assessment. A right-to-left ventricular dimension ratio >0.9 on the reconstructed CT four-chamber view identifies patients at increased risk of early death [15].

Treatment of PE

LMWH and fondaparinux are equal or superior in efficacy to UFH for the treatment of DVT and PE [16]. The benefit-to-risk ratio of thrombolysis in deep vein thrombosis (DVT) is dubious but is recommended for unstable patients with PE, although these patients represent <5% of all patients hospitalized for PE.

The streptokinase/urokinase PE thrombolysis trials showed that thrombolytic therapy successfully decreases pulmonary artery pressures acutely with improvements in the lung scan and arteriogram at 12 and 24 hours. There was no overall decrease in mortality in those receiving thrombolysis compared with those receiving heparin therapy. The use of thrombolytic treatment in patients with submassive PE remains controversial. Contraindications to thrombolysis include active internal bleeding, a stroke within 2 months, and an intracranial process such as neoplasm or abscess. Relative contraindications include surgery or organ biopsy within 10 days, uncontrolled hypertension, and pregnancy.

The dose of alteplase is 10 mg IV injection over 1–2 minutes followed by an IV infusion of 90 mg over 2 hours (max. 1.5 mg/kg in patients <65 kg). The dose of streptokinase is 250,000 U by IV infusion over 30 minutes, then 100,000 U every hour for up to 12–72 hours according to clinical condition, with monitoring of clotting parameters. A simplified algorithm for alteplase consisting of 0.6 mg/kg over 15 minutes has been used successfully in many centers, with equivalence to the standard regime demonstrated in two prospective randomized studies. Hemorrhagic complications are higher in patients with a recent invasive procedure, such as pulmonary angiogram or placement of an IVC filter. There is a reported incidence of intracranial hemorrhage of approximately 2%, with higher rates in the elderly and those with poorly controlled hypertension. The major hemorrhage rate ranges from 11% to 20%.

Two indications are widely recognized for inferior vena cava filters:
• The first is a permanent or temporary contraindication to anticoagulation, in patients with proximal DVT or PE.
• The second is the occurrence of PE or propagation of the thrombus in patients treated for DVT or recurrence in patients with PE [17].

The PREPIC study [18] demonstrated that, at 8 years, vena cava filters reduced the risk of PE but increased that of DVT and had no effect on survival. The authors concluded that, although their use may be beneficial in patients at high risk of PE, systematic use in the general population with VTE is not recommended. A Cochrane review concluded that further trials, especially with retrievable filters, are needed to assess vena caval filter safety and effectiveness [19].

Surgical intervention should be considered for patients whose condition worsens despite intensive medical treatment. A randomized study of embolectomy versus medical therapy is unavailable. Thrombolytic treatment fails in 15–20% of patients. The mortality after surgical embolectomy is around 30–40%, with a higher mortality in those with a longer duration of hemodynamic instability, a requirement for cardiopulmonary resuscitation and intubation, high doses of catecholamines, metabolic, and respiratory acidosis, and poor urine output. Early diagnosis and treatment leads to improved outcomes.

Thromboprophylaxis in the ICU

The critically ill are at substantially increased risk of VTE, which contributes significantly to their morbidity and mortality. PE is frequently seen at postmortem in these patients, the incidence being as high as 27%. The incidence of image-proven DVT in critically ill patients ranges from 10% to almost 100%, depending on the screening methods and diagnostic criteria used.

Most critically ill patients have multiple risk factors for VTE. Many risk factors predate ICU admission in particular recent surgery, immobilization, trauma, sepsis, malignancy, increased age, heart or respiratory failure, and previous VTE. These initial VTE risk factors are confounded by others, which are acquired on the ICU including immobilization, pharmacological paralysis, central venous catheterization, additional surgical procedures, sepsis, vasopressors, and hemodialysis.

Clinically undetected DVT may be present on admission to a critical care unit. Five studies using Doppler ultrasound, in a total of 990 patients reported a rate of 5.5% DVT on admission to ICU with rates up to 29% in patients not given thromboprophylaxis prior to ICU admission. Although the majority of DVTs are clinically silent and often confined to the calf veins, asymptomatic DVT can become symptomatic and lead to embolic complications. There is no way of predicting which at-risk patients will develop symptomatic VTE; it is, however, well recognized that massive PE frequently occurs without warning and is often fatal. PE is found in 15% of in-patients' deaths at postmortem.

Hospitalized patients recovering from major trauma have the highest risk of developing VTE. Without adequate thromboprophylaxis, patients with multisystem failure or major trauma have a DVT risk exceeding 50%, with PE being the third leading cause of mortality after the first day.

Despite extensive trials of thromboprophylaxis for medical and surgical patients, there are few for critical care patients. Extrapolating data relating to specific medical and surgical patients to the critically ill is not easy, for the risk–benefit ratio may be significantly different between these groups. There have been two systematic reviews of thromboprophylaxis [20,21].

With few exceptions, thromboprophylaxis should be used in all ICU patients. Decisions regarding the initiation and method of prophylaxis should be based on the balance of bleeding and thrombotic risk. Patients with a high risk of bleeding should be given mechanical prophylaxis with either graduated anti-embolic stockings alone or stockings combined with intermittent pneumatic compression devices until bleeding risk decreases and prophylaxis with heparin can be commenced.

Prophylaxis should be reviewed daily and altered as necessitated by the patient's clinical status. Prophylaxis should not be interrupted for procedures or surgery unless there is a particularly high bleeding risk. Procedures such as insertion or removal of epidural catheters should be planned to coincide with the nadir of anticoagulant effect. Table 26.6 outlines recommendations for prophylaxis in critically ill patients suggested by Geerts and coworkers [22].

Those that receive either suboptimal or no thromboprophylaxis should have Doppler ultrasound screening. Thromboprophylaxis should be continued until hospital discharge in those at high risk, and this period includes inpatient rehabilitation. The ACCP guidelines also recommend that thromboprophylaxis should be continued post discharge in those with continuing immobility.

Table 26.6 Suggested VTE prophylaxis in critically ill patients.

Bleeding risk	Thrombosis risk	Prophylaxis
Low	Moderate	Low-dose heparin (LDH) 5000 U sc bd or LMWH at prophylactic doses
Low	High	LMWH in thromboprophylactic doses
High	Moderate e.g medical or postoperative patients	Graduated compression stockings or intermittent pneumatic compression, and LMWH
High	High e.g major trauma, orthopedic surgery	Graduated compression stockings or intermittent pneumatic compression, and LMW

Table 26.7 Possible additional risk factors for VTE disease in renal transplant recipients.

Immunosuppressive agents
Cyclosporine
Corticosteroids
Muromonab-CD3 (OKT3)
Sirolimus
Mycophenolate Mofetil

Antiphospholipid antibodies
Elevated homocysteine levels
Nephrotic syndrome
Pretransplant continuous ambulatory peritoneal dialysis
Posttransplant erythrocytosis
Acute CMV infection

Special situations

Renal failure (thrombosis of vascular access, LMWH, uremia)

For continuous hemofiltration, UFH or LMWH is used commonly, although some units use prostacyclin or regional citrate. Regional citrate anticoagulation is gaining in popularity as studies have shown it is associated with prolonged filter survival, significantly decreased bleeding risk, and increased completion of scheduled filter life span when compared with heparin [23]. With the use of a heparin, an occasional need for antithrombin replacement is indicated in patients undergoing continuous hemofiltration, or other extracorporeal circulation procedures, if there are low plasma antithrombin levels.

Renal transplantation and thrombophilia

Some renal transplant recipients have an increased risk of thromboembolism. The hypercoagulability of these patients persists throughout life, but is most marked in the first 6 months after transplantation. In a large series published by the European Dialysis and Transplantation Association in 1983, 4.4% of deaths occurring in renal transplant recipients were secondary to pulmonary embolus [24,25].

The hypercoagulable state appears to be multifactorial, with proposed contributing factors, including:
• the procoagulant side effects of certain immunosuppressive agents,
• an increased prevalence of antiphospholipid antibodies,
• hyperhomocysteinemia,
• altered levels of hemostatic factors secondary to nephrotic syndrome,
• posttransplant erythrocytosis, and
• acute CMV infection.

The risk factors outlined in Table 26.7 should be sought in renal transplant patients. Prophylactic measures will be required in high-risk patients. Several immunosuppressive agents have been implicated in posttransplant venous thromboembolic disease.

Cyclosporine

Data concerning the thromboembolic complications associated with cyclosporine therapy are contradictory. Although cyclosporine has procoagulant effects in vivo, large clinical trials have failed to support a significant difference in thromboembolic events.

Steroids

The thrombotic effects of corticosteroids have been well described and include enhanced endothelial synthesis of VWF, impaired fibrinolysis due to suppression of tissue plasminogen activity and increased plasminogen activator inhibitor type 1 synthesis. Long-term steroid treatment results in a hypercoagulable hypofibrinolytic state.

Monoclonal antibodies

Muromonab-CD3 (OKT3) is an IgG2a murine monoclonal antibody that targets the CD3–T cell receptor complex. It has been used in the prophylaxis and treatment of acute graft rejection but has been largely replaced by newer antirejection drugs. Treatment with OK3 results in complement activation, cytokine release, coagulation activation, and an increased incidence of intragraft thrombosis, particularly when given in combination with steroids.

Sirolimus

This is an immunosuppressive agent and potent in vitro enhancer of platelet aggregation and secretion. In April 2002, the United States Food and Drug Administration warned of an increased incidence of hepatic artery thrombosis among liver transplant recipients treated with Sirolimus in combination with either cyclosporine or Tacrolimus. The situation has not been fully explored by clinical trials in renal transplant patients.

Mycophenolate

Mofetil is associated with in vivo platelet aggregation in normal subjects and uremic patients. However, this complication appears to be localized and related only to intravenous administration of MMF, with phlebitis and thrombosis in 4% of renal transplant recipients.

Antiphosphilipid antibodies

The prevalence of antiphospholipid antibodies in renal transplant recipients has been reported to be as high as 28%. The incidence of posttransplant thrombosis is significantly higher in antiphospholipid positive patients than in negative patients (26% and 8.5%, respectively). Renal artery thrombosis necessitating transplant nephrectomy has been reported, and was recurrent in a second renal transplant in two antiphospholipid antibody positive renal transplant recipients. These patients require adequate peritransplant anticoagulation.

Homocysteinemia

Stable renal transplant recipients have an excess prevalence of hyperhomocysteinemia, occurring in up to 70% of 207 patients in one series. The main determinant of serum homocysteine concentration was the level of renal function. Patients with hyperhomocysteinemia should be offered treatment dose folic acid.

Nephrotic syndrome

Nephrotic syndrome contributes to an increased thromboembolic risk by causing elevated levels of some coagulation factors (fibrinogen, factors V, VIII, and XIII) and decreased levels of some anticoagulant proteins (antithrombin and protein S), as well as being associated with thrombocytosis, platelet hypercoagulability, and hypofibrinolysis.

Peritoneal dialysis

A hypercoagulable state due to trans-peritoneal protein loss has been reported in patients undergoing continuous ambulatory peritoneal dialysis. These patients have higher levels of factors VII, IX, and X and fibrinogen. Transplanted peritoneal dialysis patients are more likely to suffer allograft thrombosis than patients treated with hemodialysis prior to transplantation.

Hematocrit

Erythrocytosis is defined as a hematocrit >52% in men and >49% in women. The incidence of posttransplant erythrocytosis in renal graft recipients is 8–22%. Long duration of dialysis, acquired cystic disease, polycystic kidney disease, graft artery stenosis, graft hydronephrosis, diabetes, smoking, and hypertension may contribute to its development. The incidence of thromboembolic complications is increased. Angiotensin converting enzyme inhibitors or angiotensin II receptor agonists may be used to reduce the hematocrit. Repeated phlebotomy is used in nonresponders.

Cytomegalovirus (CMV)

The CMV virus has a tropism for endothelial cells and can be found in venous or arterial walls. It has been suggested that CMV infection causes increased endothelial cell activation and thus a procoagulant state. In one series, 7 of 13 renal transplant recipients who presented with a thromboembolic event had a simultaneous CMV infection. All were nonhospitalized ambulatory patients.

Jehovah's Witnesses (JW)

Jehovah's witnesses (JW) do not accept transfusion of blood or its major components, based on the belief that to be transfused with blood is equivalent to eating it and therefore prohibited by scripture. Until 2000, any JW transfused with a prohibited blood product was expelled from the society and ostracised by other JWs. Since 2000, any JW who "wilfully and without regret" accepts blood transfusion is no longer expelled but instead "revokes his own membership by his own actions." Doctors should consider the possibility that individual JW patients have interpreted this change as allowing them to accept transfusion under certain circumstances. This will require clarification in a one-to-one consultation in absolute medical confidentiality [26].

The Association of Anaesthetists of Great Britain and Ireland (AAGBI) advise that, although it is unlawful to give blood to a patient who has refused it, "for unconscious patients, the doctor will be expected to perform to the best of his/her ability, and this may include giving blood" (AABI 1999). This would only apply when JW status is unclear and/or relatives/associates cannot produce an Advance Directive document.

Before dismissing the use of blood products, there must be a certainty that the patient is a committed JW, has independently and freely decided to refuse transfusion, and has thought this decision through to the point of death at the time of making an Advance Directive (living will) or additional consent to surgery.

A copy of the Advance Directive should be placed in the patient's notes and the contents respected. If life-threatening bleeding occurs and time allows, a doctor of Consultant status should discuss with the patient, or relative, the implications of withholding blood, and a clear, signed entry should be written in the patient's notes.

The 2000 Watch Tower directive stated that "primary components" of blood must be refused, but that "when it comes to fractions of the primary components, each Christian must conscientiously decide for himself."

Every JW should decide which products are acceptable to him/her during the consent process. All available blood products should be discussed, as interpretations of a "fraction of the primary component" may hypothetically include products such as leukocyte-depleted red cells and platelets, intravenous immunoglobulin, fibrinogen concentrates, and solvent–detergent treated FFP.

Most JW patients refuse autologous predonation because blood is separated from the body in storage. Normovolemic hemodilution and some forms of intraoperative cell salvage and hemodialysis may be acceptable because the extracorporeal blood remains in contact with the circulation. Hematological parameters should be optimized preoperatively. Meticulous surgical hemostasis, minimal access surgery, and systemic pre- and perioperative administration of antifibrinolytic agents (tranexamic acid or aprotinin) or desmopressin (DDAVP) should be considered. The use of topical hemostatic plasma fractionation products, such as fibrin glue, may be acceptable to some.

JW patients accept crystalloids and synthetic colloids, including dextran, hydroxyethylstarch, and gelatins (Haemaccel and Gelofusin) for circulatory support. Most requiring plasma exchange will refuse human albumin but may accept Hetastarch or protein A immunoabsorption as alternatives.

Recombinant blood products are acceptable to many JW. Epoetin beta (NeoRecormin) contains a trace of albumin, whereas Epoetin alpha does not contain albumin and so is more widely accepted. Epoetin alpha (Eprex) is licensed for the treatment of moderate anemia (hemoglobin concentration 10–13 g/100 mL) before elective orthopedic surgery in adults with expected moderate blood loss, to reduce exposure to allogeneic transfusion. It is given by subcutaneous injection (max. 1 mL per injection site), 600 U/kg every week for 3 weeks before surgery and on the day of surgery or 300 Units/kg daily for 15 days starting 10 days before surgery.

Supplementation with folic acid and oral iron, or intravenous folinic acid and iron, should be considered, particularly if the patient is maintained on erythropoietin. Frequency and amount of blood sampling should be minimized.

Granulocyte colony stimulating factor (G-CSF) is acceptable treatment for neutropenia. Recombinant activated factor VII (rFVIIa, NovoSeven) is licensed for the treatment of bleeding episodes in hemophiliacs with inhibitors, and has been used to treat bleeding in platelet disorders as well as those without a preexisting hemostatic disorder.

Recombinant factor VIII and XI, particularly second-generation products containing no albumin, facilitate therapy of hemophilia A and B in JW patients. DDAVP is a synthetic product suitable for use in mild hemophilia A and type 1 von Willebrand disease and uremia. Some patients with rare hemorrhagic disorders that currently require plasma-derived therapeutic products (e.g. type 2 or 3 vWD) will accept a purified fractionated product.

Some JW will regard their peripheral blood and bone marrow stem cell as a permissible fraction and consent to collection by leukapheresis or marrow aspiration. Specific treatment of the JW with other hematological disorders is beyond the scope of this chapter. There should be an open, full, and confidential discussion of all available options. JW exercise the right of any adult with capacity to refuse medical treatment and often carry advance directive cards indicating their incontrovertible refusal of blood.

Despite their belief regarding transfusion, JW do not have a higher mortality rate after traumatic injury or surgery. Transfusion requirements are often overestimated. Increased morbidity and mortality is rarely observed in patients with a hemoglobin concentration >7 g/dL, and the acute hemoglobin threshold for cardiovascular collapse may be as low as 3–5 g/dL. There are many modalities to treat the JW patient with acute blood loss. Treatment with recombinant human erythropoietin, albumin, and recombinant activated factor VIIa have all been used with success. Autologous autotransfusion and isovolemic hemodilution can also be used to treat patients who refuse transfusion. Hemoglobin-based oxygen carriers may play a future role as intravascular volume expanders in lieu of transfusion of red blood cell concentrates.

In conclusion, there are many treatment modalities available to assist in the care of JW patients, especially because their beliefs on the intricacies of the Blood Ban appear to be in flux.

References

1 Robinson S, Harrison C. Review: challenges in the management of thrombocytosis in young patients. *Clin Adv Hematol Oncol* 2008;6(2):137–8, 14

2 Guidelines for the use of platelet transfusions. *Br J Haematol* 2003;122:10–23.

3 Segal HC, Harrison P. Methods for counting platelets in severe thrombocytopenia. *Curr Hematol Rep* 2006;5(1):70–5.

4 Stasi R, Evangelista ML, Stipa E, Buccisano F, Venditti A, Amadori S. Idiopathic thrombocytopenic purpura: current concepts in pathophysiology and management. *Thromb Haemost* 2008;99(1):4–13.

5 Allen DL, Samol J, Benjamin S, Verjee S, Tusold A, Murphy MF. Survey of the use and clinical effectiveness of HPA-1a/5b-negative platelet concentrates in proven or suspected platelet alloimmunization. *Transfus Med* 2004;14(6):409–17.

6 Wahla A, Ruiz J, Nourredine N, Upadhya B, Sane D, Owen J. Myocardial infarction in thrombotic thrombocytopenic purpura. A single center experience and literature review. *Eur J Haematol* 2008;81:311–16.

7 Allford SL, Hunt BJ, Rose P, Machin SJ; Haemostasis and Thrombosis Task Force, British Committee for Standards in Haematology. Guidelines on the diagnosis and management of the thrombotic microangiopathic haemolytic anaemias. *Br J Haematol* 2003;120(4):556–73.

8 Scully M, Yarranton H, Liesner R, et al. Regional UK TTP Registry: correlation with laboratory ADAMTS 13 analysis and clinical features. *Br J Haematol* 2008;142:819–26.

9 Jokiranta TS, Zipfel PF, Fremeaux-Bacchi V, Taylor CM, Goodship TJ, Noris M. Where next with atypical hemolytic uremic syndrome? *Mol Immunol* 2007;44(16):3889–9.

10 Goldwater PN. Treatment and prevention of enterohemorrhagic Escherichia coli infection and hemolytic uremic syndrome. *Expert Rev Anti Infect Ther* 2007;5(4):653–63.

11 Hay JE. Liver disease in pregnancy. *Hepatology* 2008;47(3):1067–76.

12 Bernard GR, Vincent JL, Laterre PF, et al. Recombinant human protein C Worldwide Evaluation in Severe Sepsis (PROWESS) study group. Efficacy and safety of recombinant human activated protein C for severe sepsis. *N Engl J Med* 2001;344(10):699–709.

13 Abraham E, Laterre PF, Garg R, et al. Administration of Drotrecogin Alfa (Activated) in Early Stage Severe Sepsis (ADDRESS) Study Group. Drotrecogin alfa (activated) for adults with severe sepsis and a low risk of death. *N Engl J Med* 2005;353(13):1332–41.

14 Warkentin TE, Greinacher A, Koster A, Lincoff AM. Treatment and prevention of heparin-induced thrombocytopenia: American College of Chest Physicians Evidence-Based Clinical Practice Guidelines (8th Edition). *Chest* 2008;133(6 Suppl):340S–80S.

15 Kucher N, Goldhaber SZ. Risk stratification of acute pulmonary embolism. *Semin Thromb Hemost* 2006;32(8): 838–44.

16 Becattini C, Agnelli G, Emmerich J, Bura A, Weitz JI. Initial treatment of venous thromboembolism. *Thromb Haemost* 2006;96(3):242–50.

17 Emmerich J, Meyer G, Decousus H, Agnelli G. Role of fibrinolysis and interventional therapy for acute venous thromboembolism. *Thromb Haemost* 2006;96(3): 251–7.

18 PREPIC Study Group. Eight-year follow-up of patients with permanent vena cava filters in the prevention of pulmonary embolism: the PREPIC (Prevention du Risque d'Embolie Pulmonaire par Interruption Cave) randomized study. *Circulation* 2005;112(3): 416–22.

19 Young T, Tang H, Aukes J, Hughes R. Vena caval filters for the prevention of pulmonary embolism. *Cochrane Database Syst Rev* 2007;(4):CD006212.

20 Attia J, Ray JG, Cook DJ. Deep vein thrombosis and its prevention in critically ill adults. *Arch Intern Med* 2001;161:1268–79.

21 Geerts W, Cook D, Selby R, et al. Venous thromboembolism and its prevention in critical care. *J Crit Care* 2002;17:93–104.

22 Geerts WH, Bergqvist D, Pineo GF, et al. Prevention of venous thromboembolism: American College of Chest Physicians Evidence-Based Clinical Practice Guidelines (8th Edition). *Chest* 2008;133(6 Suppl):381S–453S.

23 Bagshaw SM, Laupland KB, Boiteau PJ, Godinez-Luna T. Is regional citrate superior to systemic heparin anticoagulation for continuous renal replacement therapy? A prospective observational study in an adult regional critical care system. *J Crit Care* 2005;20(2):155–61.

24 Kazory A, Ducloux D. Acquired hypercoagulable state in renal transplant recipients. *Thromb Haemost* 2004;91: 646–51.

25 Irish A. Hypercoagulability in renal transplant recipients. Identifying patients at risk of renal allograft thrombosis and evaluating strategies for prevention. *Am J Cardiovasc Drugs* 2004;4(3):139–49.

26 Hughes DB, Ullery BW, Barie PS. The contemporary approach to the care of Jehovah's witnesses. *J Trauma* 2008;65(1):237–47.

27 Transfusion

Adrian Copplestone

Introduction

The most common request to hematologists for help in the emergency management of patients in the hospital setting, relates to the control of hemorrhage and the use of blood products. Whereas most treatment involves the use of purified drugs, blood and blood products are derived from human blood donors. They are rarely pure; they are subject to biological variation and carry the risk of infection. This chapter discusses some of these issues and describes their use in specialized clinical settings.

Blood transfusion as a form of transplantation

Transfusion with red cells and other blood products is a form of tissue transplantation, which is made easier because the cells lack some or all of the HLA antigens. Because cells lack progenitor capacity, the benefit is temporary but allows time for the body's homeostatic processes to recover. However, the transfused cells contain surface proteins that are foreign to the host and give rise to an immune reaction. The common red cell blood grouping systems are listed in Table 27.1.

The ABO group

These most important antigens are as a result of the inheritance of enzymes causing alternative glycosylation of the red cell membrane.
• If individuals lack an A or B antigen, they make anti-A or anti-B, respectively, after exposure to these glycopeptides in food.

• Blood group O is due to the lack of A or B antigen and so these people develop anti-A and anti-B antibodies.
• Group AB people have both antigens and lack the anti-A and anti-B antibodies; see Table 27.2.

Individuals have naturally occurring circulating immunoglobulin M (IgM) antibodies to the A and B groups they lack. These antibodies are good at fixing complement, have the capacity to cause intravascular hemolysis, and can lead to disseminated intravascular coagulation (DIC). A useful scheme for remembering which ABO groups can be transfused to which patients is shown in Fig. 27.1. In allogeneic blood and marrow stem cell transplantation, the picture is more complex because patients take on the blood group of the donor, and hemolysis may occur during the period of changeover.

The Rhesus system

The next most important blood group system is the Rhesus (Rh), of which the D antigen is the most immunogenic. The use of Rh D-negative blood for Rh D-negative patients is partly to prevent immunization but also to prevent hemolytic disease of the newborn due to the transplacental passage of anti-D to Rh D-positive children of Rh-D negative mothers.

Red cell cross-matching

Just over 100 years ago, Landsteiner discovered blood groups. Transfusion from donor to patient became feasible when it was possible to determine blood groups and store the blood in an anticoagulated form. In

Table 27.1 Common red cell blood group systems.

Blood group	Gene location
ABO	9q34.1-q34.2
Rhesus	1p36.11
Lewis	19p13.3
Kell	7q33
Duffy	1q22-23
Kidd	18q11-q12
MN	4q28-31
Ss	4q28-31

Table 27.2 ABO antigen and antibodies.

Blood group	Antigen	Antibody
A	A	anti-B
B	B	anti-A
O	none	anti-A & B
AB	A & B	none

recent years, the speed of matching suitable blood for a patient has been enabled by:

• Monoclonal antibodies to achieve more consistent blood grouping results (phenotype).

• Knowledge of genetic basis of blood group to determine the genotype where relevant.

• Use of cell panels with wide representation of antigens to enable the exclusion of alloantibodies (antibody screening).

• Use of new technologies to enhance the antibody–antigen reaction (low ionic strength saline, gel tubes, microtiter plate capture).

Confidence in the blood group results and the detection of clinically relevant allo-antibodies has led to increasing acceptance of electronic cross-matching,

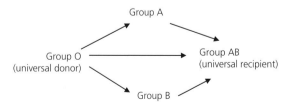

Figure 27.1 Choice of red cells by ABO group.

where the donor cells and patient serum are not actually tested against each other but a negative result is predicted.

These advances have dramatically reduced the time needed to supply suitable blood, enabling many operations to go ahead on a "blood grouped and screen basis." It also enables blood to be used in a more efficient manner and reduces waste because of expiry. However, the speed of the process may lead clinicians to forget that, when antibodies are present or develop, more steps are necessary to provide compatible blood and this takes longer.

Use of O-negative blood

In many emergencies where the blood group is not known, group O, Rh D-negative blood products may be required. If there is a shortage of group O blood, the Rh D-negative blood is reserved for children and women of child-bearing age. Men can be given group O Rh D-positive blood and only a proportion will make anti-D.

Risks of transfusion

Donor screening and testing have reduced the risks of transfusion, but it should always be remembered that this process can never be "100% safe." New infections emerge and sometimes the steps taken to improve blood safety adversely affect other blood products.

Infective risks

Infections can be transmitted by transfusion by a wide variety of organism. Examples are listed in Table 27.3.

Reducing risk

Donor screening is designed to select out potential donors who are at higher risk of infection because of lifestyle or travel. All donor blood is tested for:

• HBsAg,

• antibodies to HIV1 and HIV2,

• syphilis,

• hepatitis C virus,

Table 27.3 Examples of transfusion-transmitted infections.

Viruses	Hepatitis A
	Hepatitis B
	Hepatitis C
	HIV
	HTLV 1 & 2
	CMV
	EBV
	Parvovirus
	West Nile virus
Bacteria	Treponema pallidum (syphilis)
	Borrelia burgdorferi (Lyme disease)
	Staphylococcus spp.
	Diphtheroids
	Salmonella spp.
	Pseudomonas spp.
	Yersinia spp.
Protozoa	Plasmodium spp. (malaria)
	Toxoplasma gondii (toxoplasmosis)
	Trypanosoma cruzi (Chaga's disease)

Abbreviations: CMV, cytomegalovirus; EBV, Epstein–Barr virus; HTLV, human T cell leukaemia virus.

- human T cell leukaemia virus, and
- some donors for cytomegalovirus.

Despite these tests, there exist a small number of donors who are infected but lack antibody; this will be reduced further by nucleic acid testing using polymerase chain reaction technology to look for viral genome.

New agents (e.g. West Nile virus and SARS) continue to emerge as pathogens. Steps taken to reduce these risks include:

- donor lifestyle screening,
- antibody testing,
- leukodepletion, and
- DNA/RNA testing.

For plasma products, it is also possible to:

- heat treat,
- nanofilter, or
- disrupt lipid membranes with solvents, methylene blue, or psoralens with ultraviolet light.

Widespread leukodepletion was introduced in the UK in 1998 to reduce the risk of transmission of variant Creutzfeldt–Jakob Disease (vCJD). In addition,

there was a major shift of procurement of plasma for plasma products from areas without bovine spongiform encephalopathy (BSE), primarily the US. No test is currently available to detect the abnormal prion. BSE has been transmitted in sheep by transfusion, and in the UK, by 2008, there have been four cases of vCJD transmission by blood transfusion.

Transfusion reactions

Immediate hemolytic reactions

These are likely to be associated with shock, renal failure, and DIC. The most common cause is patients receiving the wrong blood, in 70% because of the labeling or checking errors at the bedside or in the laboratory. These errors are preventable by the adherence to clear transfusion protocols.

Delayed hemolytic reactions

These are usually caused by extravascular hemolysis and the boosting of allo-antibody levels.

Febrile transfusion reactions

Less common now that universal leukodepletion is in place, these are caused by the presence of cytokines and HLA antibodies. Urticarial and allergic reactions can still occur.

Transfusion-related acute lung injury

Transfusion-related acute lung injury (TRALI) is caused by donor leukocyte antibodies which cause adult respiratory distress syndrome. The patient becomes acutely short of breath and often requires artificial ventilation and circulatory support. TRALI needs to be distinguished from circulatory fluid overload, which can occur following the transfusion of large volumes, especially in older patients. In the UK, the number of cases of TRALI has fallen after the increased use of male plasma to make fresh frozen plasma (FFP), as males have less immunization by white cell antigens than females (related to pregnancy).

Immunization

Alloimmunization can affect the efficacy of transfusion, especially platelets. It may also affect the subsequent choice of donors for organ transplantation. Immunomodulation can follow transfusion with an

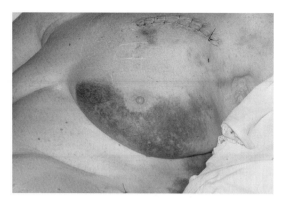

Figure 27.2 Post-transfusion purpura presenting with ecchymosis in a female patient with a platelet count of 10 × 10⁹/L, subsequently shown to be HPA-1a negative with anti-HPA-1a antibodies. Transfusion had been given preoperatively. Reprinted from Blood in Systemic Disease 1e, Greaves and Makris, 1997, with permission from Elsevier.

increase in infections and increase in relapse of carcinoma following surgery to patients who were transfused.

Post-transfusion purpura

Post-transfusion purpura (PTP; Fig. 27.2) is a rare complication where severe thrombocytopenia occurs approximately 1 week after transfusion. The recipient is usually HPA1a-negative and HLA DR3*1010 and has anti-HPA1a antibodies, although on rare occasions other platelet groups are implicated. Treatment is high-dose intravenous immunoglobulin (IVIg).

Blood products available

Red cells

Whole blood

Donor blood is anticoagulated in 10% citrate anticoagulant, and during storage, the labile coagulant factors V and VIII and platelets are lost within a few days. Little whole blood is used in the UK because transfusion practice has adopted a component approach.

Leukodepleted red cells in additive solution

These donor cells are collected in citrate anticoagulant, the white cells are removed by filtration, and the red cells are stored in saline, adenine, mannitol, and glucose (SAG-M). With storage at 4°C, the red cells have a 35-day shelf-life.

Washed red cells

For patients who have severe reactions to leukodepleted blood, or who have IgA deficiency, red cells washed in saline can remove plasma proteins that cause the reactions.

Frozen red cells

These are used for patients with rare blood groups. The red cells are frozen in glycerol as cryoprotectant and washed before use.

Platelets

Platelet concentrates are prepared from either:
• plateletpheresis of donors using a cell separator machine; or
• combining platelet-rich plasma from buffy coats and packed in four-donor pools.

At present, the shelf-life of platelet concentrates is only 5 days (with testing taking up the first 24–48 hours), but the use of additive solution may extend this to 7 days.

Platelets are used to correct bleeding resulting from thrombocytopenia or abnormal platelet function, with the exception of immune thromocytopenia purpura (ITP), thrombotic thrombocytopenia (TTP), and heparin-induced thrombocytopenia (HIT). The latter two conditions are associated with thrombosis, and platelet transfusions can exacerbate the disease.

Of the platelet concentrates made from blood donation or plateletpheresis, a significant quantity is given to patients with bone marrow failure. In recent years, the trigger level of platelet count at which platelet transfusion is given has been falling and is usually 10 × 10⁹/L. Counting platelets accurately at this level is difficult, even using modern automated blood counters. It is also not clear whether to give large doses of platelets or only treat if the patient has bleeding; several large trials are in progress. Patients may become refractory to repeated platelet transfusion and need more expensive HLA-matched platelets. Another area where large quantities of platelets are used is cardiac surgery. The combined problem is the use of antiplatelet drugs and cardiac–pulmonary bypass circuits. This is discussed in more detail in Chapter 19.

Fresh frozen plasma

FFP is used to correct coagulation deficiencies, and there has been considerable debate on the relative merits of different products.

In the ideal world, FFP would provide high concentrations of the relevant factor, be from a low number of screened regular donors, have a viral inactivation step in the production that does not adversely affect the coagulation factors, be procured in a country where BSE is not endemic, come from male donors (to reduce the risk of TRALI), and have appropriate ABO group.

The following are available:
• Single-donor FFP.
• Methylene blue-treated FFP for pediatric use is a single-donor product, procured in the US. In the UK, it is used primarily for children born after January 1, 1996 when the risk of vCJD from meat was minimized, but its use will extend to other age groups as it becomes more available.
• Solvent detergent FFP (Octaplas®) is a pooled product that is solvent treated to reduce the infective risks. It is used in large quantities in TTP because it is low in high-molecular-weight multimers of von Willebrand factor (VWF), but it has been associated with thrombosis because of protein S deficiency.

British Committee for Standards in Haematology (BCSH) guidelines suggest that:
• FFP should only be used to replace single inherited clotting factor deficiencies for which no virus-safe fractionated product is available. Currently, this applies mainly to factor V.
• FFP is indicated when there are demonstrable multifactor deficiencies associated with severe bleeding and/or DIC. However, FFP is not indicated in DIC with no evidence of bleeding.
• FFP should not be used to reverse warfarin effect in the absence of bleeding as it has an incomplete effect and is not an ideal product as large quantities are required. Vitamin K and prothrombin complex concentrate should be used when reversing coumarin anticoagulants in patients who are bleeding or at high risk of bleeding.
• Large quantities of FFP are used for correction of abnormal coagulation tests prior to invasive procedures, but the evidence base that this reduces bleeding is weak.

Cryoprecipitate and MB Cryo

Cryoprecipitate forms when FFP is thawed slowly, and the product, which is refrozen, is rich in fibrinogen and factors VIII and XIII. It is commonly used in the treatment of DIC to replace fibrinogen. Methylene blue-treated Cryo is available for children in the UK.

Cyrosupernatant and MB Cryosupernatant

The complementary product cryosupernatant has been used in conjunction with plasmapheresis in TTP as it lacks high-molecular-weight multimers of VWF; however, SDFFP is the recommended product in the UK.

Human albumin solution

The final product of the plasma fractionation process, human albumin solution (HAS), comes in two strengths: 4.5 g/dL and 20 g/dL (salt-poor albumin). It is an important colloid for maintaining the oncotic pressure in the intravascular compartment, and its main indication relates to replacing albumin in severe edematous states. Its use as plasma expander has largely been superseded by crystalloids and gelatin solutions.

Intravenous immunoglobulin

IVIg solutions are pooled normal human donor immunoglobulins. In the coagulation disorders, they are used as an immunomodulator for the treatment of ITP and PTP. Because supply cannot meet demand, most countries have adopted national clinical guidelines together with a demand management plan.

Coagulation factor concentrates

Concentrates are prepared from large pools of donor plasma. They all have steps to reduce viral contamination and most have steps to remove impure proteins. Increasing use of recombinant coagulation factors as these become available is being encouraged:
• Factor VIII for hemophilia A. Some of the intermediate purity products contain useful amounts of VWF as well.
• Factor IX for hemophilia B.
• VWF concentrates are now available for von Willebrand disease (VWD).
• Prothrombin complex concentrate (combined factors II, VII, IX, and X concentrate) is primarily used in

the correction of life-threatening hemorrhage in patients on oral anticoagulants.

• Individual concentrates for factors VII, X, and XIII and fibrinogen are available for patients with hereditary deficiencies.

Fibrin sealants

Mixing thrombin and fibrinogen forms "fibrin glue," which is applied to the site of bleeding and is a popular treatment in neurosurgery.

Autologous blood

In many situations, it is possible to use the patient's own blood and thereby avoid exposure to the risks of donor blood. However, there are still risks with using autologous blood, mainly related to bacterial infection and the blood being transfused to the wrong patient. A number of approaches are possible.

Predeposit donation

Blood is venesected prior to elective surgery and retained for up to 4 weeks. By retransfusing older blood during the collection process, up to 4 U of blood can be stored. Surgery must take place on the planned date or the blood may expire. In the UK, the use of predeposit donation has fallen as patients can be more anemic at the time of surgery, and if anemia can be corrected pre-admission, the patient can often withstand the loss of volume of blood that would have been transfused.

Cell salvage

Blood can be aspirated during an operation and washed red cells returned to the patient. This is useful in vascular surgery and is also finding a place in cardiac surgery, trauma, and obstetric patients.

Intraoperative hemodilution

Blood is venesected at the time of anesthesia, and crystalloid is used as fluid replacement. If bleeding occurs, less red cells are lost because of the lower hematocrit. At the end of the operation, the blood, which also contains coagulation factors and platelets, is retransfused.

Cell salvage from wound drains

Blood is drawn into a sterile container by suction and transfused. This application has been used extensively in orthopedic surgery and has reduced the need for blood in joint-replacement operations.

Drugs that reduce the need for transfusion

A number of drugs are used to either boost the hemostatic system or reduce fibrinolysis. Drugs that can increase the red cells mass are also important.

Desmopressin (DDAVP)

This analogue of antidiuretic hormone is used in mild hemophilia, VWD, and some platelet disorders. Endothelial stores of VWF are released. Repeated administration is subject to tachyphylaxis.

Tranexamic acid and other fibrinolytic inhibitors

These are useful in major surgery, but their use needs to be balanced against the risk of venous thromboembolism (VTE). They may also be used in patients with marrow failure who have mucosal bleeding from chronic thrombocytopenia in patients but are refractory to platelet transfusions.

Aprotinin (Trasylol®) is a bovine protease inhibitor that inactivates plasmin and kallikrein. It has been used in cardiac surgery in patients on cardiopulmonary bypass, with a reduction in the need for transfusion, reoperation for bleeding, and length of stay in ICU and hospital admission. In 2006, concerns of increased frequency of renal failure and multiorgan failure led to considerable discussion of its role. A suspension of marketing was agreed in November 2007.

Iron

There are many patients who have low iron stores or frank deficiency as a consequence of chronic hemorrhage, either through the disease process or the result of treatment (e.g. nonsteroidal anti-inflammatory drugs). Correction with small doses of iron to improve compliance can avoid the need for transfusion. Where anemia has developed slowly, patients can tolerate quite low hemoglobin levels. Treatment with iron and patience are much safer than "top-up transfusions."

Vitamins

Other vitamins (such as folic acid) may also be required in anemic patients with poor intake (elderly or malabsorption) or increased turnover (pregnancy).

Erythropoietin

Erythropoietin (rhEPO) can be useful to boost the erythron. Concomitant iron therapy may also be needed to achieve a rapid response. Its cost has restricted its use in clinical practice, but many patients with renal failure no longer require regular transfusion.

Recombinant activated factor VII

This recombinant protein (rFVIIa) was originally used in hemophiliacs with inhibitors, but it is now increasingly being used in patients with severe bleeding from multiple trauma or major bleeding in a critical care situation.

Use of blood products

How much to give?

The decision of when to transfuse and how much to give can be difficult [1–5]. In general, the rule should be to try to avoid transfusion if possible, but if it is necessary, to use sufficient quantities of the right product to achieve the desired effect (usually hemostasis).

Guidelines on the use of red cells have previously advised transfusion based on the reduction of red cell mass, but this can be difficult to estimate in clinical practice. As a result, "Hb triggers" have increasingly been used in the management of patients, particularly in the postoperative setting. In a landmark study [6], Hébert and coworkers showed that, in patients in a critical care unit, a restrictive transfusion policy (Hb trigger 7.0 g/dL, aim Hb 7–9 g/dL) had a lower mortality than a more liberal policy (Hb trigger 10 g/dL, aim Hb 10–12 g/dL), with the possible exception of patients with acute myocardial infarction and unstable angina.

Although Hb trigger levels are easy for clinical teams to use, other factors also affect the Hb level, and the Hb trigger level may need to be adjusted for individual patients based on comorbidities. Other measures may usefully aid the decision as to whether to transfuse, such as the rate of postoperative bleeding. Where this has been measured for a cohort of patients (e.g. postcardiac bypass surgery), deviations from the usual course can be spotted more rapidly and appropriate action taken. Similarly, if more attention was paid to improving anemia preoperatively, there would be less need for transfusion.

Assessment of hemorrhage

In situations where patients are bleeding, the first question is to determine whether this is surgically correctable. Simultaneously, blood should be sent for blood count and coagulation studies. The prothrombin time (PT) and activated partial thromboplastin time (APPT), combined with supplementary tests (fibrinogen level, thrombin time, equal volume mix with normal plasma) usually give an indication as to the type of hemostatic defect. Confirmation with specific factor levels can follow if necessary.

Blood sampling is important as these patients often have multiple cannulae, and it is important that the sample is not taken through a line contaminated with heparin. The drug chart should be examined especially for anticoagulants, antifibrinolytics, and antiplatelet drugs. Caution must be taken with blood count samples, as patients may be inappropriately transfused if taken from lines running intravenous fluids.

Near patient testing

Because coagulation tests take at least 20 minutes to complete (and usually longer, taking sample transport into account), there has been a move to use near patient testing (NPT) with a number of different devices.
- Whole blood clotting time: ACT; this is used in cardiac surgery to monitor heparin effect.
- PT and APTT devices (e.g. Coaguchek®): these are designed mainly for testing patients on oral anticoagulants.
- Thromboelastogram: the TEG® is described in more detail in Chapter 19, and is used in liver and cardiac units. It gives information relating to platelet function, clot strength, and fibrinolysis within approximately 15 minutes.
- Platelet function analyses (PFA-100®): an in vitro bleeding time test whose current role is determining mild VWD and platelet defects.

Although many hematologists dislike NPT equipment as being "uncontrolled" and lacking some of the strict supervision of laboratory procedures, the immediacy of results will lead to their increased use, and both laboratory and clinical teams should work together to define their role in decision making.

Importance of good communication

When dealing with complex patients, there needs to be good communication between the clinical team and the transfusion, hematology, and coagulation laboratories. The hematologist is ideally suited to advise on suitable blood products, facilitate testing to minimize delays, ensure that blood products are dispatched rapidly, and anticipate future requirements, especially if the source of supply is off-site.

Special situations

Disseminated intravascular coagulation

DIC often requires transfusion of coagulation factors and platelets (see Chapter 12). Consumption of products may be dramatic, and regular coagulation tests are required to guide therapy, although treatment is based on the degree of bleeding and organ failure rather than abnormalities in the tests. To reverse the process, the underlying cause must be treated.

Massive transfusion

The replacement of the blood volume with stored blood lacking platelets and factors VIII and V leads to mucosal bleeding and generalized ooze at operative sites. Recognition of the condition and correction with platelet and FFP transfusion, based on laboratory clotting studies, is usually all that is required. Antifibrinolytic drugs can help but their use can increase the risk of VTE. The military use of "shock packs" (red cells, thawed frozen plasma and platetets) early in the management of patients with multiple injury is being increasingly used in civilian practice, in an attempt to prevent the generalized bleeding syndrome that occurs in these patients.

Cardiac surgery

Cardiac surgery uses approximately 10% of the blood supply and is a major user of FFP, second only to critical care units (FFP) and oncology (platelets). This is discussed in detail in Chapter 19.

Obstetrics

Major hemorrhage in obstetrics is an emergency. It can occur for a number of reasons (Table 27.4). It can

Table 27.4 Causes of major hemorrhage in obstetrics.

Ectopic gestation
Abortion
Placental abruption
Placenta previa
Postpartum: atonic uterus, trauma due to childbirth, coagulation disorders

be dramatic, and in rare cases of maternal mortality, the severity of the situation has often not been recognized. It requires immediate resuscitation, using the group O Rhesus D-negative emergency blood if necessary, and ABO-matched blood, FFP, and platelets dispatched without delay. Further hematological support will depend on coagulation studies. DIC may be present.

Every obstetric unit should have a major hemorrhage protocol, agreed with the hematology laboratory. Good communication with the clinical team, laboratory, and hematologist is essential.

Pediatrics

Neonates and young children have a number of considerations with respect to hemostasis and transfusion:
• Their size means that much smaller volumes are used.
• Donor exposure should be kept to a minimum.
• Their relatively immature immune systems mean that they may not make some antibodies (e.g. anti-A and anti-B), so blood grouping will be different to adults (i.e. no reverse grouping available).
• Often group O red cells are used, but the plasma should not contain high-titer anti-A or anti-B antibodies. Similarly, note should be taken when using large volumes of FFP or platelets as red cell hemolysis resulting from ABO incompatibility has been reported.
• Their blood may contain maternal IgG antibodies (e.g. hemolytic disease of the newborn).
• Neonates who have received transfusion in utero, and children with immunodeficiency, require irradiated blood products (to reduce the risk of transfusion-associated graft-versus-host disease).
• Severe coagulation disorders may present in the neonatal period. Coagulation studies can be difficult

to perform and repeated tests will lead to institutional anemia.

• Neonatal thrombocytopenia may have an infective or immune basis. Treatment depends on the cause.

Jehovah's Witnesses

Jehovah's Witnesses belong to the Watch Tower Bible and Tract Society. They believe that transfusing blood is equivalent to eating it, and this is prohibited by scripture. Although they refuse transfusion, they accept modern medical care and technology. As mentally competent adults, they have a right to refuse treatment. The situation is more complex in unconscious adults and children. Exactly which blood product is refused is an individual decision, although often guided by church elders (Table 27.5).

Surgery should be planned to minimize blood loss, with good consultation between patient, surgeon, anesthetist, and hematologist. The patient should sign an Advance Directive.

Table 27.5 Acceptance of blood products by Jehovah's Witnesses.

Refused	Accepted	Variable
Red cells	Crystalloids	Albumin
White cells	Synthetic colloids	Immunoglobulin
Platelets	EPO	Vaccines
Plasma	GCSF	Coagulation factors
	rFVIIa	Cell salvage
	Organ transplant	

Abbreviations: EPO, erythropoietin; GCSF, granulocyte colony-stimulating factor; rFVIIa, recombinant factor VIIa.

Hemovigilance and regulation of transfusion

A decade ago, recognition that sometimes transfusion can harm patients resulted in the setting up of Serious Hazards of Transfusion (SHOT) scheme in the UK.

Cumulative data 1996–2006

Numbers of cases reviewed (n=3770)
* Formerly DTR

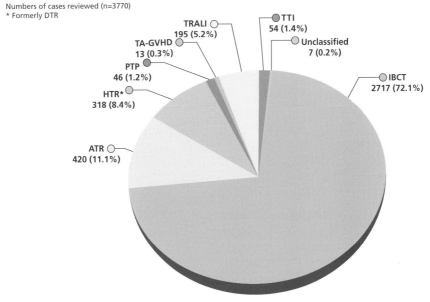

TRALI 195 (5.2%)
TTI 54 (1.4%)
TA-GVHD 13 (0.3%)
Unclassified 7 (0.2%)
PTP 46 (1.2%)
IBCT 2717 (72.1%)
HTR* 318 (8.4%)
ATR 420 (11.1%)

Comparison of report types 1996–2006

Figure 27.3 Reports of adverse events to Serious Hazards of Transfusion scheme. ATR, acute transfusion reactions; DTR, delayed transfusion reaction; HTR, hemolytic transfusion reactions; IBCT, Incorrect blood component transfused; PTP, post-transfusion purpura; TA-GVHD, transfusion associated graft versus host disease; TRALI, transfusion related acute lung injury; TTI, transfusion transmitted infection.

This is a voluntary confidential reporting scheme that has been copied in many other countries. Analysis of adverse events has been invaluable in improving the safety of transfusion. The type of errors is shown in Fig. 27.3. In the 3770 cases reported, there were 109 deaths and 315 cases of major morbidity. The annual reports give details and recommendations to improve transfusion practice.

In Europe, Blood Safety Directives have been incorporated into national legislation (Blood Safety and Quality Regulations in the UK). Reporting of adverse events is mandatory. There needs to be full traceability from donor to patient with records retained for 30 years (in view of vCJD risks). Transfusion laboratories have to maintain a quality management system and are subject to inspection.

In the US, transfusion laboratories are regulated by the Food and Drug Agency. All deaths relating to transfusion need to be reported. Hospitals can apply for accedition from the Joint Commission for Accreditation for Healthcare Organisations, the College of American Pathologists, and American Association of Blood Banks.

Conclusions

Good transfusion practice [7,8] in treating coagulation disorders is a combination of thinking ahead to reduce the need for transfusion and using the appropriate product in the right quantity. Clear documentation of the reasons for transfusion and good institutional protocols also help.

References

1 British Committee for Standards in Hematology (BCSH). Guidelines for the use of platelet transfusions. *Br J Haematol* 2003;122:10–23.
2 BCSH. Clinical use of red cell transfusion. *Br J Haematol* 2001;113:24–31.
3 BCSH. Guidelines for the administration of blood and blood components and the management of transfused patients. *Transfus Med* 1999;9:227–39.
4 BCSH. Guidelines for the use of fresh frozen plasma, cryoprecipitate and cryosupernatant. *Br J Haematol* 2004; 126:11–28. Amendment: http://www.bcshguidelines.com/pdf/FFPAmendment_2_17_Oct_2007.pdf.
5 BCSH. Guidelines on the management of massive blood loss. *Br J Haematol* 2006;135:634–41.
6 Hébert PC, Wells G, Blajchman MA, et al. A multicenter, randomized, controlled clinical trial of transfusion requirements in critical care. *N Engl J Med* 1999;340: 409–17.
7 McClelland DBL. Handbook of Transfusion Medicine, 4th edition, 2007. Available from: http://www.transfusionguidelines.org.uk/docs/pdfs/htm_edition-4_all-pages.pdf.
8 Murphy MF, Pamphilon DH. *Practical Transfusion Medicine* (3rd edition). Oxford: Blackwell Science, 2008.

Web sites of interest

BCSH guidelines: http://www.bcshguidelines.com.
Blood transfusion toolkit: http://www.transfusionguidelines.org.uk.
Serious Hazards of Transfusion: http://www.shotuk.org.

Appendix 1 Reference ranges

Steven Kitchen and Michael Makris

Background

Interpretation of any laboratory result requires its comparison with a reference range or reference interval. There are detailed guidelines making recommendations about establishment of reference intervals in general [1]; and the importance of the reference interval is confirmed by its presence in the US Clinical and Laboratory Imporvement Ammendments (CLIA) legislation, which requires that laboratories verify that any manufacturer's stated reference intervals are appropriate for the laboratories patient population [2]. This is particularly true for tests of hemostasis, where it is also the case that relatively subtle local differences in relation to sample collection, processing, and testing may have an impact on the results obtained locally. This means that reference ranges for use in hemostasis must be established or at the very least validated locally. The reference range is influenced not just by the biological variability between subjects in health, but also includes the variability associated with the analytical process; so even if the population is the same for two centers, the local validation is still required to take account of the analytical variability in that particular center so that it fully reflects the local conditions.

There are essentially two types of reference interval, the most common of which is health-associated. This is based on the results obtained for a particular test when performed in healthy normal individuals. The second type of reference interval can be described as decision-based [3] and describes the specific limits used for making a clinical decision used to diagnose or manage particular patient groups. In the latter case, the intervals are defined using groups other than healthy normal subjects. This chapter will deal mainly with health-associated reference intervals.

The reference interval derived from healthy normal subjects is more commonly referred to as the normal range. The selection of individuals for testing and method of data handling used for construction of reference ranges is important. Health is not well defined, and results of some coagulation tests are influenced by age, sex, hormone replacement therapy, some oral contraceptive pills, blood group, and other variables, which means that, in some instances, a reference range established by analysis of a carefully matched control group might be required.

Selection of subjects

The reference range should be established by analyzing a representative subset of subjects drawn from the same population as the test samples. This process is not straightforward because of the many factors that influence levels of hemostatic factors and therefore the results of laboratory tests in this area. The most appropriate group of subjects to use for establishment of a reference range is one which has been matched for age, sex, diet, lifestyle, etc. to the patient population. In practice, however, a more pragmatic approach can be successfully taken provided that the selection criteria are taken into account when making use of the data. A useful practical approach is to select normal subjects and adopt inclusion/exclusion criteria before analysis. A simple questionnaire can be used to identify subjects taking medications, which may influence results who can then be excluded. Because there is the possibility to identify unexpected abnormalities during testing, apparently normal subjects may have lifestyle or health insurance implications as a result of taking part. The authors recommend the use of written informed consent so that subjects can choose in advance of recruitment whether they wish to be informed of any such findings. Once this is in place, subjects can be recruited from the general population, from blood donors, or from hospital staff. It is normally unacceptable to use hospital patients even if they are carefully selected because, by definition, they are unlikely to meet the "normal" criteria.

The demographics of the normal subjects used to establish a reference interval need to be considered because, for example, concentrations of factors VII, VIII:C, and IX and fibrinogen increase with age. In the case of FVIII:C and von Willebrand factor (VWF), there are highly significant differences according to the blood group of the subject [4], with levels approximately 25% lower in group O individuals compared with non-O blood groups. However, many centers do not take this latter effect into account when screening for von Willebrand disease (VWD) because the clinical management will normally depend on the actual levels of FVIII and VWF in relation to the clinical needs of the patient irrespective of blood group.

For some tests of hemostasis, sex needs to be taken into account. The lower limits of protein S activity in women compared with men are probably sufficiently great (approximately 20% different at age under 45 years) that a sex-specific reference range is warranted, and where this is not done, the sex of the patient should be taken into account when interpreting results obtained by some methods. This is also the case for homocysteine determinations (approximately 25% lower in females).

Recently the ISTH SSC subcommittee on Womens Health Issues published guidelines on the preanalytical conditions related to the patients physiological state and other exogenous factors which need to taken into account when performing laboratory tests of hemostasis in women [5]. This includes a review of the evidence for the effects of physical stress (up to 10-hour persistence of a 2.5-fold increase in FVIII/VWF, for example), mental stress (increase in FVII and VWF after acute mental stress), hormone effects [6], circadian variations, and the effects of posture and diet. Some general recommendations were made that were not restricted to investigation of female patients. These were as follows:
• Abstain from intense physical exercise for 24 hours prior to venipuncture.
• Use an envoirement where physical and mental stress are lessened.
• Abstain from fatty foods and smoking on the morning of venipuncture.
• Obtain samples early in the morning (7–9 am) after sitting in a relaxed position for 20–30 minutes.

As discussed elsewhere in this chapter, such conditions should only be used for blood collection from normal subjects for establishment of reference intervals if the conditions are also used for patient blood sample collection.

Reference intervals may be required for patient groups other than healthy normal subjects to take account of particular physiological or pathological states. Because of considerable variations in the concentration of clotting factors during pregnancy and development, specific normal ranges for neonatal, pediatric, and pregnant subjects should be available. This is a particular problem where, because of ethical and practical reasons, it is virtually impossible for each laboratory to establish their own neonatal normal ranges, so many laboratories use the same published ranges in newborns. Data on the expected results of clotting tests in older children have also been published. For these studies, it is important to note that ranges for screening tests are only appropriate for the particular technique used in the study, whereas the results of clotting factor assays are normally influenced much less by the method employed and may therefore be a useful guide to centers employing other techniques.

In some cases, the effects of drugs on coagulation tests should be taken into account. For example, if attempting to diagnose protein C (PC) or protein S (PS) deficiency during oral anticoagulant therapy, a reference range constructed from subjects receiving oral anticoagulant prophylaxis is necessary to take account of the reductions in PC and PS induced by the therapy.

In general, establishing these types of group-specific reference ranges may not always be practical, and for many hemostatic parameters, it may be of debatable clinical value.

Number of subjects required

The number of normal subjects required for analysis and construction of a normal range depends on a number of issues. From a statistical validity aspect, the International Federation of Clinical Chemistry and International Committee for Standardisation in Haematology have indicated that the number of subjects required is at least 40 but that this should preferably be 120 to obtain reliable estimates [7]. However, for many tests of hemostasis, the effect of increasing numbers of subjects from 25–30 up to much larger numbers leads to entirely minor and clinically irrelevant differences in the calculated ranges, and in these cases, 25–30 is probably adequate. A CLSI guideline [8] addressing the PT and APTT considered that the full 120 normal values should be tested by manufacturers when they first develop new methods, but for practical purposes, individual laboratories can obtain a close approximation by testing a minimum of 20 individuals that encompass the age range that patient testing will include. The same guideline reminds the reader that the reference intervals are only a guide to be used in conjunction with the patients clinical picture. The World Federation of Haemophilia laboratory manual considers that 30 is an adequate number of normal subjects for construction of reference ranges for hemostasis tests used in the investigation of bleeding disorders [9].

Processing of samples

When constructing normal ranges, the samples from normal subjects should be collected, processed, and analyzed locally using identical techniques to those used for the analysis of the patient samples. If the normal practice is for samples to be stored deep frozen for batch analysis, then this should also be done for normal samples. If patient samples are processed after a delay during which samples are transported to the laboratory over several hours, then a similar delay should

be used between collection of samples and testing for the samples from normal subjects used to derive reference intervals. The literature and reagent manufacturer's information should only be used as a guide. Adopting a manufacturer's range without local validation can lead to misdiagnosis; and in one study of 23 genetically confirmed protein S-deficient subjects, all 23 were sucessfully identified as abnormal using a locally detemined reference range (even though only 20 normal subjetcs were analysed to derive this), whereas 4 deficient subjects would have been misclassifed as normal based on the manufacturer's stated reference range for one particular technique [10].

Change in reagent lot numbers

In the case of some APTT reagents, there is sufficient variation between different production lots or batches of the reagent to affect the results obtained. It is particularly important to check that any change in APTT reagent lot number does not affect results for patients receiving unfractionated heaprin, because there are reports that, for some reagents at least, there can be clinically important differences in the therapeutic range for different lots of the same type of reagent [11]. In this case, it is necessary to reassess the therapeutic range before introducing a new lot number. A method to assess whether a small difference between different lots is sufficient to require a full establishment of a new theapeutic range has been described [8]. A change in reagent lot number could also affect the reference range for other screening tests including the PT as well as global test of hemostasis, such as thrombin generation tests, thrombelastograghy/thomboelastometry, and tests that screen the protein C pathway, including activated protein C resistance tests.

Data analysis

The reference or normal range is usually constructed from individual results in such a way that it contains 95% of the reference distribution. When the results are normally distributed, the normal range is conventionally calculated to be the mean ± 2 standard deviations, which includes 95% of the population. If the results are not normally distributed, other statistical tests, such as log transformation, should be used first to obtain a normally distributed population. In some cases, non-parametric methods may be used to identify the central 95% of values.

Results of normal subjects can be inspected graphically to identify skewedness or particularly to identify outliers amongst the group. Any outliers (i.e. any result that lies unexpectedly far from the majority of others) should then be excluded from calculations. This can be done statistically using a discordancy test, which identifies extreme outliers amongst the set of results using the deviation from the sample mean and taking account of the estimated variance as described by Barnett and Lewis [12], but visual inspection of the data in the form of a bar chart showing the number of observations (vertical axis) against the relevant test result interval (x-axis) is often sufficient [8]. For some tests, the exclusion of outliers can have an important impact on the calculated reference range [13], but it may be useful to calculate the reference range with and without the inclusion of potential outliers, because in many areas of hemostasis testing, this frequently shows that the calculated range is largely unaffected either way, provided a large enough group of subjects have been tested. Because of some of these issues, it is important that those who make interpretations of patient results against reference ranges keep in mind that the reference range should only be a guide to use alongside all other available clinical information.

Examples of locally determined reference ranges

As discussed above, it is important that a full reference range is established when a newly developed method is introduced or if there has been a significant modification, which may require analysis of up to 120 subjects for fully valid data to be obtained. As mentioned above, the CLSI guideline [1] recognizes that an abbreviated version using a minimum of 20 subjects may be used for validating the transfer of reference values among comparable analytical platforms. Furthermore, there are a number of laboratory tests in hemostasis where agreement between ranges derived in different centers by different techniques/reagents can be expected to be in good agreement. This should be the case, for example, in relation to many clotting factor assays, where data from external quality assessment programs throughout the world demonstrate that different reagents/methods are associated with the same laboratory results on average. For this reason, we have included some examples of locally determined reference ranges below from our own center in Sheffield, UK at the time of publication of this book (table 1).

Table 1 Normal ranges in the Authors' Laboratory in 2009.

Test	Method	Range	No. of subjects
Bleeding disorders			
FVIII:C	One stage assay	58–209 IU/dL	25–30
VWF:Ag	ELISA	46–146 IU/dL	25–30
VWF:RCo	Visual Agglutination	50–172 IU/dL	25–30
FIX	APTT based	62–144 IU/dL	25–30
FII	PT-based	84–132 IU/dL	25–30
FV	PT-based	66–126 U/dl	25–30
FVII	PT-based	61–157 IU/dL	25–30
FX	PT-based	74–149 IU/dL	25–30
FXI	APTT-based	60–150 U/dL	25–30
FXII	APTT-based	50–180 U/dL	25–30
FXIII	Pentapharm assay	59–163 U/dL	20
α_2-Antiplasmin	Chromogenic	67–103 U/dL	20
Thrombotic disorders			
Antithrombin activity	Chromogenic	85–131 IU/dL	80
Antithrombin antigen	ELISA	83–124 IU/dL	30
Protein C activity	Chromogenic	79–142 IU/dL	80
Protein C antigen	ELISA	75–131 IU/dL	25–30
Protein S total	ELISA	71–136 IU/dL	80
Protein S free	Latex	Males 74–143 IU/dL	40
		Females 67–125 IU/dL	40

Pregnancy normal ranges

Few laboratories have specific normal ranges for pregnant subjects. It is rarely necessary to have a precise range, but it is important for clinicians to be aware of the range and type of changes that occur during this period. Table 2 from a published study indicates some of the hemostatic variables that change during pregnancy. Shown are the mean values and the calculated normal ranges from the mean ±2 standard deviations [14].

Table 2 Normal ranges in pregnancy (adapted from reference 14).

Variable (Non pregnant normal range)		Pregnancy (Weeks Gestation)				Post partum	
		10–15	23–25	32–34	38–40	1	8
Classic APCR (>2.3)	mean	2.89	2.74	2.64	2.66	2.87	3.16
	normal range	2.33–3.45	2.18–3.30	2.16–3.12	2.02–3.30	2.09–3.65	2.34–4.00
Modified APCR (V depleted) (>2.0)	mean	2.63	2.59	2.57	2.62	2.68	2.71
	normal range	2.39–2.87	2.35–2.83	2.35–2.79	2.36–2.88	2.40–2.96	2.43–2.99
FVIII:C u/ml (0.50–2.0)	mean	1.41	1.69	2.06	2.31	2.24	1.25
	normal range	0.51–2.31	0.81–2.49	1.02–3.10	1.43–3.19	0.86–3.62	0.49–2.01
Fibrinogen g/dl (2.0–4.0)	mean	3.3	3.5	4.1	4.5	4.6	2.6
	normal range	2.1–4.5	2.3–4.7	2.9–5.3	3.5–5.5	3.2–6.0	1.8–3.4
Protein C u/ml (0.70–1.25)	mean	0.95	1.04	1.02	1.00	1.16	1.02
	normal range	0.65–1.25	0.68–1.40	0.64–1.40	0.62–1.38	0.76–1.56	0.68–1.36
Free Protein S u/ml (0.63–1.12)	mean	0.62	0.53	0.51	0.51	0.59	0.74
	normal range	0.36–0.88	0.35–0.71	0.33–0.69	0.31–0.71	0.27–0.91	0.52–0.96
DDimer ng/ml (<120)	mean	35	81	130	193	251	11
	normal range	0–93	0–175	0–286	0–417	0–867	0–22

Neonatal normal ranges

Adult reference intervals should not be used to interpret results obtained in neonates because there are important differences in the results obtained [15–17].

Reference values for coagulation tests in the healthy full-term infant during the first 6 months of life are shown in table 3. Values shown are mean with the normal range based on mean ±2 standard deviations [16].

Table 3 Normal ranges for neonates and children (adapted from reference 16).

Tests	Day 1	Day 5	Day 30	Day 90	Day 180	Adult
PT (sec)	13.0 (10.1–15.9)*	12.4 (10.0–15.3)*	11.8 (10.0–14.2)*	11.9 (10.0–14.2)*	12.3 (10.7–13.9)*	12.4 (10.8–13.9)
INR	1.00 (0.53–1.62)	0.89 (0.53–1.48)	0.79 (0.53–1.26)	0.81 (0.53–1.26)	0.88 (0.61–1.17)	0.89 (0.64–1.17)
APTT (sec)	42.9 (31.3–54.5)	42.6 (25.4–59.8)	40.4 (32.0–55.2)	37.1 (29.0–50.1)*	35.5 (28.1–42.9)*	33.5 (26.6–40.3)
TCT (sec)	23.5 (19.0–28.3)*	23.1 (18.0–29.2)	24.3 (19.4–29.2)*	25.1 (20.5–29.7)*	25.5 (19.8–31.2)*	25.0 (19.7–30.3)
Fibrinogen (g/l)	2.83 (1.67–3.99)*	3.12 (1.62–4.62)*	2.70 (1.62–3.78)*	2.43 (1.50–3.79)*	2.51 (1.50–3.87)*	2.78 (1.56–4.00)
F II (u/ml)	0.48 (0.26–0.70)	0.63 (0.33–0.93)	0.68 (0.34–1.02)	0.75 (0.45–1.05)	0.88 (0.60–1.16)	1.08 (0.70–1.46)
F V (u/ml)	0.72 (0.34–1.08)	0.95 (0.45–1.45)	0.98 (0.62–1.34)	0.90 (0.48–1.32)	0.91 (0.55–1.27)	1.06 (0.62–1.50)
F VII (u/ml)	0.66 (0.28–1.04)	0.89 (0.35–1.43)	0.90 (0.42–1.38)	0.91 (0.39–1.43)	0.87 (0.47–1.27)	1.05 (0.67–1.43)
F VIII (u/ml)	1.00 (0.50–1.78)*	0.88 (0.50–1.54)*	0.91 (0.50–1.57)*	0.79 (0.50–1.25)*	0.73 (0.50–1.09)	0.99 (0.50–1.49)
VWF (u/ml)	1.53 (0.50–2.87)	1.40 (0.50 (2.54)	1.28 (0.50–2.46)	1.18 (0.50–2.06)	1.07 (0.50–1.97)	0.92 (0.50–1.58)
F IX (u/ml)	0.53 (0.15–0.91)	0.53 (0.15–0.91)	0.51 (0.21–0.81)	0.67 (0.21–1.13)	0.86 (0.36–1.36)	1.09 (0.55–1.63)
F X (u/ml)	0.40 (0.21–0.68)	0.49 (0.19–0.79)	0.59 (0.31–0.87)	0.71 (0.35–1.07)	0.78 (0.38–1.18)	1.06 (0.70–1.52)
FXI (u/ml)	0.38 (0.10–0.66)	0.55 (0.23–0.87)	0.53 (0.27–0.79)	0.69 (0.41–0.97)	0.86 (0.49–1.34)	0.97 (0.67–1.27)
F XII (u/ml)	0.53 (0.13–0.93)	0.47 (0.11–0.83)	0.49 (0.17–0.81)	0.67 (0.25–1.09)	0.77 (0.39–1.15)	1.08 (0.52–1.64)
Antithrombin (u/ml)	0.63 (0.39–0.87)	0.67 (0.41–0.93)	0.78 (0.48–1.08)	0.97 (0.73–1.21)*	1.04 (0.84–1.24)*	1.05 (0.79–1.31)
Protein C (u/ml)	0.35 (0.17–0.53)	0.42 (0.20–0.64)	0.43 (0.21–0.65)	0.54 (0.28–0.80)	0.59 (0.37–0.81)	0.96 (0.64–1.28)
Protein S (u/ml)	0.36 (0.12–0.60)	0.50 (0.22–0.78)	0.63 (0.33–0.93)	0.86 (0.54–1.18)*	0.87 (0.55–1.19)*	0.92 (0.60–1.24)

*Values are indistinguishable from those of the adult.

Conclusion

In general, the normal range should be used only as a guide and an aid to clinical interpretation in conjunction with all other available relevant clinical information. The most appropriate normal reference range is one that has been established locally using the same system as for patient samples. It is important to use a technique for which such a local range is in broad agreement with the published literature.

References

1 CLSI. How to Define and Determine Reference Intervals in the Clinical Laboratory: Approved Guideline (2nd Edition). Wayne, PA: Clinical and Laboratory Standards Institute, 2000:Document C28-A2.

2 Clinical Laboratory Improvement Amendments of 1988 (CLIA) 42 CFR section 493.1253, part (b) (1) (ii) (2003).

3 Freidberg RC, Souers R, Wagar EA, Stankovic AK, Valenstein PN. The origin of reference intervals: a college of American Pathologists Q-probes study of "Normal ranges" used in 163 clinical laboratories. *Arch Pathol Lab Med* 2007;131:348–57.

4 Gill JC, Endres-Brooks J, Bauer PJ, Marks WJ, Montgomery RR. The effect of ABO blood group on the diagnosis of von Willebrand's disease. *Blood* 1987;69:1691–5.

5 Blomback M, Konkle BA, Manco-Johnson MJ, Bremme K, Hellgren M, Kaaja R, on behalf of the ISTH SSC on Womens Health Issues. *J Thromb Haemost* 2007;5:855–8.

6 Lowe GDO, Rumley A, Woodward M, et al. Epidemiology of coagulation factors, inhibitors and activation markers: the third Glasgow MONICA survey I. Illustrative reference ranges by age, sex and hormone use. *Br J Haematol* 1997;97:775–84.

7 Solberg HE on behalf of International Federation of Clinical Chemistry (IFCC) and International Committee for Standardization in Hematology (ICSH), IFCC Expert panel on Reference values. Approved recommendation on the theory of reference values. Part 5 Statistical treatment of Collected Reference values. Determination of reference limits. *J Clin Chem Clin Biochem* 1987;25:645–56.

8 CLSI. One Stage Prothrombin Time (PT) Test and Activate Partial Thromboplastin Time (APTT) Test: Approved Guideline (2nd Edition). Wayne, PA: Clinical and Laboratory Standards Institute, 2008:Document H47-A2.

9 Kitchen S, McCraw (2000). Diagnosis of haemophilia and other bleeding disorders: a laboratory manual. Available from: http://www.wfh.org/publications.

10 Jennings I, Kitchen S, Cooper P, Makris M, Preston FE. Sensitivity of functional protein S assays to protein S deficiency: a comparative study of 3 commercial kits. *J Thromb Haemost* 2003;1:1112–17.

11 Shojania AM, Tetreault J, Turnbull G. The variations between heparin sensitivity of different lots of APTT reagents produced by the same manufacturer. *Am J Clin Pathol* 1988;89:19–23.

12 Barnett V, Lewis T. *Outliers in Statistical Data*. Chicester: John Wiley, 1978:91–3.

13 Horn PS, Feng L, Yanmei L, Pesce AJ. Effect of outliers and non-healthy individuals on reference interval estimation. *Clin Chem* 2001;47:2137–45.

14 Kjellberg U, Ansdersson NE, Rosen S, Tengborn L, Hellgren M. APC resistance and other haemostatic variables during pregnancy and puerperium. *Thromb Haemost* 1999;81:527–31.

15 Andrew M, Paes B, Milner R, et al. Development of the human coagulation system in the full-term infant. *Blood* 1987;70:165–72.

16 Andrew M, Paes B, Johnston M. Development of the hemostatic system in the neonate and young infant. *Am J Pediatr Hematol Oncol* 1990;12:95–104.

17 Andrew M, Vegh P, Johnston, Bowker J, Ofosu F, Mitchell L. Maturation of the hemostastic system during childhood. *Blood* 1992;80:1998–2005.

Index